Consent, Benefit, and Risk in Anaesthetic Practice

D1378421

Consent, Benefit, and Risk in Anaesthetic Practice

Jonathan G Hardman
Associate professor and reader and Honorary Consultant
Anaesthetist, University of Nottingham,
Queen's Medical Centre Campus,
Nottingham University Hospitals NHS Trust,
Nottingham, United Kingdom

Iain K Moppett
Associate professor and Honorary Consultant Anaesthetist,
University of Nottingham, Queen's Medical Centre Campus,
Nottingham University Hospitals NHS Trust,
Nottingham, United Kingdom

Alan R Aitkenhead
Professor and Honorary Consultant Anaesthetist,
University of Nottingham,
Queen's Medical Centre Campus,
Nottingham University Hospitals NHS Trust,
Nottingham, United Kingdom

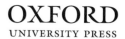

OXFORD
UNIVERSITY PRESS

OXFORD
UNIVERSITY PRESS

Great Clarendon Street, Oxford OX2 6DP

Oxford University Press is a department of the University of Oxford.
It furthers the University's objective of excellence in research, scholarship,
and education by publishing worldwide in

Oxford New York

Auckland Cape Town Dar es Salaam Hong Kong Karachi
Kuala Lumpur Madrid Melbourne Mexico City Nairobi
New Delhi Shanghai Taipei Toronto

With offices in

Argentina Austria Brazil Chile Czech Republic France Greece
Guatemala Hungary Italy Japan Poland Portugal Singapore
South Korea Switzerland Thailand Turkey Ukraine Vietnam

Oxford is a registered trade mark of Oxford University Press
in the UK and in certain other countries

Published in the United States
by Oxford University Press Inc., New York

© Oxford University Press, 2009

The moral rights of the author have been asserted
Database right Oxford University Press (maker)

First published by Oxford University Press 2009

All rights reserved. No part of this publication may be reproduced,
stored in a retrieval system, or transmitted, in any form or by any means,
without the prior permission in writing of Oxford University Press,
or as expressly permitted by law, or under terms agreed with the appropriate
reprographics rights organization. Enquiries concerning reproduction
outside the scope of the above should be sent to the Rights Department,
Oxford University Press, at the address above

You must not circulate this book in any other binding or cover
and you must impose the same condition on any acquirer

British Library Cataloguing in Publication Data

Data available

Library of Congress Cataloging in Publication Data

Data available

Typeset in Minion by Cepha Imaging Private Ltd., Bangalore, India
Printed in Great Britain
on acid-free paper by
the MPG Books Group

ISBN 978–0–19–929–6873

10 9 8 7 6 5 4 3 2 1

Oxford University Press makes no representation, express or implied, that the drug
dosages in this book are correct. Readers must therefore always check the product
information and clinical procedures with the most up-to-date published product
information and data sheets provided by the manufacturers and the most recent codes of
conduct and safety regulations. The authors and the publishers do not accept responsibility
or legal liability for any errors in the text or for the misuse or misapplication of material in
this work. Except where otherwise stated, drug dosages and recommendations are for the
non-pregnant adult who is not breast-feeding.

Contents

Section 4 **Personal perspectives**

Contributors

Alan R Aitkenhead
Professor and Honorary Consultant
Anaesthetist, University of Nottingham,
Queen's Medical Centre Campus,
Nottingham University Hospitals NHS
Trust, Nottingham, United Kingdom

Oliver R Dearlove
Consultant Anaesthetist, Royal
Manchester Children's Hospital, Central
Manchester and Manchester Children's
University Hospitals NHS Trust

Elizabeth A Flockton
Specialist Registrar, University of
Liverpool, Critical Care Research Unit,
School of Clinical Sciences, The Duncan
Building, Daulby Street, Liverpool,
United Kingdom

Ronnie J Glavin
Scottish Clinical Simulation Centre,
Stirling Royal Infirmary, Stirling,
United Kingdom

Jonathan G Hardman
Reader and Honorary Consultant
Anaesthetist, University of Nottingham,
Queen's Medical Centre Campus,
Nottingham University Hospitals NHS
Trust, Nottingham, United Kingdom

Simon P Holbrook
Clinical Lecturer in Anaesthesia,
University of Leeds, St James' University
Hospital, Leeds Teaching Hospitals NHS
Trust, Leeds, United Kingdom

Philip M Hopkins
Professor of Anaesthesia and Honorary
Consultant Anaesthetist, University of
Leeds, St James' University Hospital,
Leeds Teaching Hospitals NHS Trust,
Leeds, United Kingdom

Simon J Howell
Senior Lecturer and Honorary
Consultant Anaesthetist, University of
Leeds, Leeds General Infirmary, Leeds
Teaching Hospitals NHS Trust, Leeds,
United Kingdom

Jennifer M Hunter
Professor of Anaesthesia, University of
Liverpool, Critical Care Research Unit,
School of Clinical Sciences, The Duncan
Building, Daulby Street, Liverpool,
United Kingdom

Bertie Leigh
Senior Partner, Hempsons Solicitors,
London, United Kingdom

Adam C March
Specialist Registrar in anaesthesia &
intensive care, Queen's Medical Centre
Campus, Nottingham University
Hospitals NHS Trust, Nottingham,
United Kingdom

Robert A McCahon
Consultant Anaesthetist, Queen's
Medical Centre Campus, Nottingham
University Hospitals NHS Trust,
Nottingham, United Kingdom

Iain K Moppett
Associate Professor and Honorary
Consultant Anaesthetist, University of
Nottingham, Queen's Medical Centre
Campus, Nottingham University
Hospitals NHS Trust, Nottingham,
United Kingdom

Michael H Nathanson
Associate Professor and Honorary
Consultant Anaesthetist, University of
Nottingham, Queen's Medical Centre
Campus, Nottingham University
Hospitals NHS Trust, Nottingham,
United Kingdom

Ozzie Newell
Secretary and Treasurer of the
Nottingham Stroke Research Consumer
Group, Nottingham, United Kingdom

Felicity S Plaat
Consultant Anaesthetist, Hammersmith
Hospital, Imperial NHS Trust, London,
United Kingdom

Bernard Riley
Consultant in anaesthesia and intensive
care, Queen's Medical Centre Campus,
Nottingham University Hospitals NHS
Trust, Nottingham, United Kingdom

Wendy E Scott
Consultant Anaesthetist, Derby City
General Hospital, Derby Hospitals NHS
Foundation Trust, Derby,
United Kingdom

Henry J Skinner
Consultant Anaesthetist, City Hospital
Campus, Nottingham University
Hospitals NHS Trust, Nottingham,
United Kingdom

Scott Wallace
Consultant Anaesthetist, Charing Cross
Hospital, Imperial College Healthcare
NHS Trust, London, United Kingdom

Stuart M White
Consultant Anaesthetist, Brighton and
Sussex University Hospitals NHS Trust,
United Kingdom

Robert J Winter
Consultant in anaesthesia and intensive
care, Queen's Medical Centre Campus,
Nottingham University Hospitals NHS
Trust, Nottingham, United Kingdom

Foreword

Dr William Harrop-Griffiths MA MBBS FRCA

Consultant Anaesthetist, Imperial College Healthcare NHS Trust, London, UK

"Informed consent is a process, not a piece of paper".

Recently, I was involved in a difficult case that threw light on our current concepts of informed consent and the difficulties that can arise through the strict interpretation of written guidelines. A woman was scheduled to undergo a therapeutic surgical procedure for a painful medical condition. She had seen the same surgeon on three occasions in the outpatient clinic and had agreed with him that she would undergo the procedure. He had carefully and patiently explained the risks and benefits of undergoing surgery in a way that she understood. He had documented this discussion and the risks that he had described in the patient's notes. On admission to the hospital for surgery, she had made clear to the nurse admitting her that she had a good understanding of the nature of her surgery and of its intended benefits. The surgeon who had seen her in the outpatient clinic and who was scheduled to perform the operation saw her on the day of surgery and talked her through the procedure again. The anaesthetist visited her before surgery and he got the impression that she had been well prepared and fully informed about what was to happen to her that day. She walked to the operating theatre, lay on the operating table and offered her arm to the anaesthetist for venous cannulation and induction of anaesthesia. After induction of anaesthesia and while she was being prepared for surgery, the scrub nurse asked to see the consent form. It could not be found. Although almost all of the stages of the consent process for this patient had been completed, one step had been inadvertently omitted – the signing of the consent form by the patient. A vigorous debate ensued in which the surgeon insisted that the process of consent was adequate and that surgery should continue while the scrub nurse argued that because written hospital guidelines demanded that a signed consent form be available before surgery could commence, the procedure should be abandoned. The anaesthetist insisted that all should act in the best interests of the patient but there was no general agreement as to what exactly this was. Managers were involved; they supported the scrub nurse's views and the patient was woken up by a reluctant anaesthetist. On emergence to full consciousness, the patient was very angry that she had not undergone surgery and demanded that she be allowed to sign the consent form so that she could be anaesthetised again and surgery could proceed. She had made complex social and childcare arrangements to allow her to undergo surgery on that day and was becoming increasingly distressed by the medical complaint that first brought her to the surgeon. The clinician responsible for clinical ethics in the hospital was consulted, and he took the view that the patient did not have capacity to provide written consent to surgery at that stage as she had just had a general anaesthetic. The patient did not undergo surgery that day.

As in so many complex ethical situations in contemporary clinical practice, there are no easy answers. In the scenario I describe above, the views of each of the protagonists are supportable, and yet the ultimate outcome was arguably not in the patient's best interests. Consent to undergo treatment is usually a straightforward matter that is the stuff of routine and everyday practice. However, it is also the subject of an expanding amount of increasingly complex legislation throughout the developing and developed world. The bodies responsible for medical practice in many countries produce lengthy guidance documents on informed consent. As the focus of medical practice rightly swings towards the choices and rights of patients and away from the simple will of the doctors, consent is becoming an increasingly important matter about which no sensible doctor would fail to be knowledgeable. However, anaesthesia is a medical intervention for which there is no universal agreement for the need for express, written consent. This fact underlines the need for anaesthetists to be aware of the concepts related to the consent process and to have a firm grasp of the risks and benefits of the different approaches and techniques that they can offer to their patients. This publication is therefore very timely.

The editors of this book have brought together leading experts not only on the legal aspects and ethics of consent, but also on anaesthetic management in a number of subspecialty areas. After an introductory section that sets the overall scene, there follows detailed discussion of the areas of clinical practice in which difficulties with consent are most likely to be encountered, followed by a section in which the risks and benefits of various aspects of anaesthetic practice are described, assessed and interpreted. Finally, a lawyer and a patient provide fascinating personal views of consent. All in all, this is a compelling, challenging and critical area of anaesthetic practice. No other publication brings together all the threads that will enable and equip the anaesthetist to provide his or her patient with a full and fair description of the risk and benefits of anaesthesia while providing the anaesthetist with a detailed knowledge base of the key facts relating to consent in contemporary anaesthetic practice.

The editors and authors are to be congratulated for the production of such a comprehensive and comprehensible treatment of a potentially complex topic. I think that it will rapidly become an accepted and authoritative reference text and I would encourage all anaesthetists to read it.

London, January 2009

Section 1

Consent

Chapter 1

Generic aspects of consent

Alan R Aitkenhead

Public expectations of health care have changed dramatically over the last 10–20 years, particularly in relation to the involvement of patients in determining treatment options and the selection of the most appropriate treatment plan. Paternalistic actions of doctors, which involved telling the patient what treatment they were going to receive, without discussing the risks and benefits of various options, is no longer acceptable. This has been reflected in decisions reached by the courts in cases in which patients have entered litigation on the basis that inadequate information was given to them before treatment, and that they were unaware of risks of complications that subsequently materialized. Although most claims of this nature are brought against surgeons, similar claims are likely in relation to anaesthetic procedures. Complaints about lack of information or inadequate consent can also result in a doctor being reported to regulatory authorities. It is therefore necessary for anaesthetists to be aware of current issues surrounding provision of information and obtaining consent for anaesthesia in various categories of patient.

Introduction

This chapter refers predominantly to the legal situation in England and Wales. Broadly similar principles apply in other jurisdictions in the developed world, but details may differ, and each jurisdiction has its own case law.

The competent adult patient has a fundamental right under common law to give, or to withhold, consent to examination, investigation, or treatment. This is a basic principle of health care. Any treatment, investigation, or physical contact with the patient undertaken without consent may amount to battery[§]. It is highly unlikely that a healthcare professional would be charged with criminal assault for treating a patient without consent; a criminal charge would be appropriate only if harm was intended or was an obviously foreseeable risk. Battery by medical practitioners is regarded by the General Medical Council (GMC) as an offence that may constitute serious professional misconduct and may also result in employers invoking disciplinary procedures.

Patients consent to treatment after receiving information about the treatment and about material risks, which may be associated with the treatment. A material risk is

[§] A battery is an unauthorized physical contact. In an assault, the victim is caused to fear that a battery is about to occur. In most medical cases in which unauthorized physical contact occurs, there is no assault.

one to which a reasonable person in the patient's position would be likely to attach significance. If a foreseeable complication materializes from a risk that was not mentioned, the patient may argue that consent for the procedure would not have been given if the risk of that complication had been explained. This has two potential consequences in law.

The patient may argue that the consent was invalid, and that performance of the procedure amounted to battery as a result of failure to obtain 'informed consent'. Outside the United States of America, this found little favour with the Courts, although recent decisions suggest that this position may have changed (see Chapter 2).

Alternatively, the patient may argue that, by refusing to undergo the procedure, if appropriate warnings had been given, the complication would have been avoided. If this argument is successful, then the patient is entitled to compensation for the consequences of the injury, even if the injury occurred despite all reasonable care in undertaking the procedure. Thus, in contrast to claims for negligent treatment, it is not necessary for the patient to show that the standard of care in performance of the procedure was inadequate; it is necessary only to demonstrate that the warnings that were given did not conform to an acceptable standard and, if the warning had been given, the patient would not have consented to undergo the procedure.

In theory, the test in law is based on a comparison between the risks that were explained and the risks that a reasonable doctor would have mentioned[1]. In clinical negligence claims, which centre on the standard of clinical care, often involving very complex issues, judges rely on expert evidence to determine the standard of care, which would have been regarded as appropriate, by a reasonable and responsible body of medical opinion at the time; judges have no experience in medical practice, and must base their judgements on the opinions of doctors who have experience in the relevant field. However, judges are actual or potential patients, and are able to form their own view as to the adequacy of information provided to a patient, irrespective of evidence about the risks, which a reasonable doctor would have mentioned. Consequently, it cannot be assumed that judges will accept an argument that most doctors would not have explained a potential risk before the patient consented to undergo the procedure if, in the opinion of the judge, that risk should have been explained.

The GMC[2] believes that successful relationships between doctors and patients depend on trust. To establish that trust, doctors must respect the autonomy of patients, including their right to decide whether or not to undergo any medical intervention even where a refusal may result in harm to themselves or in their own death. Patients must be given sufficient information, in a way that they can understand, to enable them to exercise their right to make informed decisions about their care. The Department of Health[3] has stated that doctors are expected to be aware of the legal principles set by relevant case law in this area. Doctors must take appropriate steps to find out what patients want to know and ought to know about their condition and its treatment.

Anaesthesia is a non-therapeutic intervention, with no benefit to the patient other than the benefit of allowing surgery or a complex diagnostic test to take place. The public perception is that it is simple and safe. The fact is that it is fairly safe (and not simple) but is associated with a number of complications, which may lead to injury. However, because it is perceived to be safe and is non-therapeutic, patients who suffer complications, which lead to injury, often allege that inadequate information was provided by the anaesthetist (e.g. in relation to regional blocks).

Consent in adults

Consent can be given voluntarily by an appropriately informed person who is competent to consent to the intervention in question.

Voluntariness of consent

Consent must be given voluntarily and freely, without pressure or undue influence either to accept or refuse treatment. Such pressure can come from partners or family members or from other carers. Doctors should be alert to this possibility and, if necessary, should arrange to see the patient alone. The views of healthcare professionals on the perceived benefits of a treatment must not lead to coercion to accept the treatment.

While competent adults have an absolute right to refuse treatment in its entirety, doctors are not obliged to treat the patient who refuses specific components of treatment if these components are important in determining the success of the treatment. If a patient refuses consent for a component of a procedure when refusal is regarded by the doctor as resulting in increased risk to the patient, then it may be necessary to refuse to treat the patient. Doctors have a responsibility to provide what is, in their judgement, treatment that has the most favourable predicted outcome for the patient. For example, if a patient scheduled to undergo elective oesophago-gastrectomy refused consent for insertion of a central venous catheter and arterial catheter after being told of the risks of these procedures, it would be wrong for the anaesthetist to coerce the patient into agreeing to the same; however, if no reasonable body of opinion would support undertaking the operation without a central venous catheter and arterial catheter, then proceeding with the operation without the information that these catheters would provide would be regarded as professional misconduct. Consequently, while there must be no coercion, anaesthetists must be prepared to refuse elective treatment if the patient's decision compromises the anaesthetist's ability to provide a safe level of care.

Consent may be implied by the conduct of the patient for many of the physical contacts between healthcare workers and patients—for example, co-operation during physical examination for preoperative assessment or for attachment of monitoring apparatus. Consent may be implied if a conscious patient co-operates during venepuncture, or during performance of a local or regional anaesthetic block. Although consent implied in this manner would make it difficult for a patient to succeed in a claim for trespass, it cannot be taken as an indication that material risks have been explained and understood. Express consent should be obtained for any procedure that carries a material risk.

Provision of appropriate information

To be properly informed, a patient needs to understand, in broad terms, the nature and purpose of the procedure, and relevant potential complications or side-effects. Consent is agreement to the proposal of another. However, before agreeing to medical examination, investigation, or treatment, patients should be provided with sufficient information to allow them to decide whether or not to proceed. Until the last few years, it was standard practice to offer almost no information to patients unless they asked direct questions about risks and benefits; a paternalistic approach was adopted, with the expectation that patients would agree to whatever their doctor recommended. For a variety of reasons, including a number of recent legal cases, changes in society, and access to almost unlimited information through the internet, that approach has become unacceptable.

In the case of Sidaway[1], a patient who underwent surgery to the cervical spine was paralysed as a result of damage to the spinal cord. Mrs Sidaway's claim was based on the failure to warn her of the risk of damage to the cord (estimated to be a risk of less than 1%) or to warn her of a combined risk of damage to a nerve root and/or spinal cord (estimated at 2%). It was found that the surgeon had told her of the possibility of disturbing a nerve root, but had not mentioned the risk of spinal cord damage. It was also found that a responsible body of neurosurgeons would not have discussed death or paralysis because this would have frightened the patient. The case was eventually considered in the House of Lords, and the Law Lords, who found in favour of the hospital on a majority decision, made a number of observations.

> The doctor cannot set out to educate the patient to his own standard of medical knowledge of all the relevant factors involved. He may take the view, certainly with some patients, that the very fact of his volunteering, without being asked, information of some remote risk involved in the treatment proposed, even though he describes it as remote, may lead to that risk assuming an undue significance in the patient's calculations.
>
> It is a matter of clinical judgement to determine what degree of disclosure of risks is best suited to assist a particular patient to make a rational choice as to whether or not to undergo a particular treatment.
>
> Whether or not failure to disclose a risk or cluster of risks in a particular case constitutes a breach of the doctor's duty is a matter to be decided principally on the basis of expert medical evidence. Having heard the evidence it is for the judge to decide whether a responsible body of medical opinion would have approved of non-disclosure in the circumstances of the case.

This is the *Bolam* test[4]; a doctor is not guilty of negligence if his practice conformed to that of a responsible body of medical opinion held by practitioners skilled in the field in question. However, the Law Lords left it open for a judge to override expert medical opinion.

> A judge may come to the conclusion that, even in the absence of expert witnesses, disclosure of a particular risk was so obviously necessary to an informed choice on the part of the patient that no reasonably prudent medical man would fail to make it.

In December 1987, a female patient underwent marsupialization of a Bartholin's cyst. The operation was performed under general anaesthesia, but a caudal block was undertaken after she was unconscious, in order to provide intra-operative and post-operative analgesia. Postoperatively, she was unable to move her legs and had no control over her bladder. There was considerable improvement over the next 48 h, but a neurological abnormality persisted, affecting predominantly her left foot. It was accepted that caudal block had not been discussed with her before anaesthesia, and it was alleged that performance of the caudal block was therefore a trespass. The court accepted that, in 1987, a responsible body of anaesthetists would not have told a patient specifically that a caudal block would be performed after induction of general anaesthesia. Judgement was in favour of the Defendants[5]. The judge rejected the suggestion made by the patient that she should have been informed of each component of her anaesthetic, saying that this sectionalized approach would encourage the 'deplorable' prospect of actions being brought in trespass rather than negligence.

> If one is to treat the administration of an injection for analgesic purposes while the patient is generally anaesthetized (e.g. the caudal block) as something requiring separate consent, why should separate consent not also be sought for an injection of, for example, morphine to provide analgesia when the patient begins to come around from the general anaesthetic.
>
> In my judgement, there is no realistic distinction between omitting to tell a patient that while she is under a general anaesthetic a tube will be put in her trachea and omitting to tell her that while she is under a general anaesthetic a needle will be put into her caudal region to provide postoperative analgesia.

In view of the recommendations of the Association of Anaesthetists of Great Britain and Ireland (AAGBI)[6], that patients should be informed if a local anaesthetic block is to be used (see following paragraphs), this precedent might not help an anaesthetist charged in similar circumstances now.

Since Sidaway, judgements in a number of negligence cases (relating both to the provision of information and to the standard of treatment given) have shown that courts are willing to be critical of a 'responsible body' of medical opinion, particularly if that opinion does not withstand logical analysis. It is now clear that the courts will be the final arbiter of what constitutes responsible practice, particularly with regard to consent, although the practice of responsible practitioners remains influential.

In 1992, the High Court of Australia affirmed the determination of the Supreme Court of New South Wales that a doctor has a duty to warn a patient of any material risk involved in a proposed treatment[7]. In this case, Ms Whitaker became essentially blind after an unsuccessful operation on her right eye caused sympathetic ophthalmia in her left eye. Although there was no question that the surgery had been performed with the requisite skill and care, Ms Whitaker sued because her ophthalmologist, Dr Rogers, had failed to warn her of the possibility (approximately 1 in 14 000) that sympathetic ophthalmia could develop. The Court considered that a risk was material if a reasonable person in similar circumstances would attach significance to the risk, or if the doctor is, or should be, cognizant that the particular patient would express concern about the risk. Ms Whitaker had enquired about possible complications and had expressed specific concern that her 'good eye' should not be harmed, but Dr Rogers did not inform her of the potential risks associated with the surgery, and reassured her. It was determined that it was for the court to adjudicate on what was an appropriate standard of care; the *Bolam* principle was rejected.

A more recent English Court of Appeal judgement[8] stated that it will normally be the responsibility of a doctor to inform a patient of 'a significant risk'.

> If there is a significant risk which would affect the judgement of a reasonable patient, then in the normal course it is the responsibility of the doctor to inform the patient of that significant risk, if the information is needed so that the patient can determine for him or herself as to what course he or she should adopt.

The GMC[2] advises that doctors should do their best to find out about patients' individual needs and priorities when providing information. If the patient asks specific questions about the procedure and associated risks, these should be answered truthfully. If the doctor believes that to follow these guidelines in full would have a deleterious effect on the patient's health, this view, and the reasons for it, should be recorded in the patient's notes. The mere fact that the patient might become upset by hearing the information, or might refuse treatment, is not sufficient to justify withholding the information.

The Professional Conduct Committee of the GMC paid no heed to the Bolam principle when considering allegations of assault against an anaesthetist who inserted an analgesic suppository during general anaesthesia without seeking the patient's consent. The events took place in a dental surgery, and the patient was fully clothed. The Committee was told that it was not standard practice to seek specific consent for insertion of an analgesic suppository, but reached the conclusion that the patient had been assaulted[9]. Standard practice changed almost overnight.

In all but the most recent cases outside the United States of America, a patient would obtain damages if it could be demonstrated not only that there had been insufficient disclosure of information, but also the failure to disclose information altered outcome; the patient had to demonstrate that, if appropriate information had been given, then treatment would have been declined.

Once again, it was the High Court of Australia, which led the way in eroding this principle[10]. The facts and outcome were essentially the same as those in the more recent English case of *Chester v Afshar*, the outcome of which was ultimately determined in a majority decision in the House of Lords[11]. This case, and its implications, is discussed in detail in Chapter 22. Ms Chester suffered from lumbar disc protrusion resulting in severe low-back pain, resistant to treatment by epidural injections. Latterly, she could hardly walk, and had reduced control of her bladder. She was referred to Mr Afshar, a neurosurgeon, who advised surgery, but was found not to have warned her of the 1–2% risk of cauda equina syndrome associated with surgery. She underwent the surgery three days later, and the risk materialized, causing a severe neurological deficit in her left leg. Ms Chester said that, if she had been warned of that risk, she would have cancelled the operation and sought a second opinion. Had she done so, the second (or, if she so chose, a third) opinion would have confirmed that surgery was indicated, and was associated with a 1–2% risk of cauda equina syndrome. The Lords of Appeal found that, in all probability, she would then have agreed to surgery.

The judgement was in favour of Ms Chester. Even though she was already suffering neurological impairment and would have continued to do so, probably progressively, without surgery, and even though she would have agreed to surgery after taking a second (or third) opinion, thereby accepting the risk of cauda equina syndrome, which was no greater in Mr Afshar's hands than any other surgeon's, it was determined that she was entitled to compensation for infringement of the *right* to be warned of 'a significant risk of the surgery', 'special disadvantages and dangers', or 'possible serious risks'.

This judgement has immense implications, yet their extent is not clear. The Lords of Appeal seem to have accepted the American concept of 'informed consent' (that patients should be warned of all potential risks before agreeing to treatment), a concept, which hitherto had been regarded outside the United States of America as unhelpful to patients; if presented with several pages listing all potential complications, how could the patient make a balanced decision about the risks and benefits of agreeing to treatment? The judgement in *Chester v Afshar* appears to uphold a policy of autonomy; the patient is entitled to receive information, and failure to provide the information should be compensated financially even if the provision of the information ultimately would not have caused the patient to refuse treatment, and therefore, would have not have altered the risk that the complication materialized.

What the Lords of Appeal failed to address was the definition of a 'serious risk'. Were they referring to *any* risk of a serious consequence, or a common occurrence (the term used by the Royal College of Anaesthetists to describe complications with an incidence of around 1%) of a risk of a serious consequence, or a common occurrence of *any* risk? The safe view would be that patients should be warned of any risks that have consequences that are more than transient[12]. It is probably for this reason that the AAGBI has now recommended[6] that patients should be provided with information booklets, which describe virtually every complication that can occur in association with anaesthesia, including rare complications such as death.

With specific regard to anaesthesia, the AAGBI has recommended[6] that the following factors should be considered. These recommendations were made after the *Chester v Afshar* judgement in the House of Lords was known.

- The process of consent should begin before the anaesthetist and patient meet. The patient should be provided with an information leaflet relevant to the anaesthetic technique envisaged. Many hospitals have devised their own information leaflets, with varying degrees of success[13]. There are also commercially available leaflets, and leaflets published by the Royal College of Anaesthetists[14], which set out clearly a wide range of potential complications, with a guide to the frequencies of their occurrence. Written information should be available in a range of languages. Braille and large-print versions should be available where there is impaired vision, and translators or readers should be available for patients who are unable to read the written information provided.

- Patients must be given sufficient time to come to a considered view after they have been provided with relevant information. It is neither desirable nor practical for all information to be provided to patients at the preoperative visit, and unacceptable for new information to be provided in the anaesthetic room, other than in exceptional circumstances.

- The amount and nature of information disclosed to the patient should as far as possible be determined by the question: 'What would *this* patient regard as relevant when coming to a decision about which of the available options to accept?'[1,7]

- In broad terms, patients must understand what they are consenting to, and anaesthetists should tell the patient what procedures they intend to undertake, why these procedures are to be used, what the significant, foreseeable risks of these procedures are, and what the significant, foreseeable consequences of these risks might be.

- Information should be provided about what may be expected as part of the proposed anaesthetic technique, e.g. fasting, the administration and effects of premedication, transfer from the ward to the anaesthetic room, insertion of an intravenous cannula, application of monitoring equipment, induction of general or local anaesthesia, monitoring throughout surgery by the anaesthetist, transfer to the recovery room, and return to the ward. Intra-operative and postoperative analgesia, fluids and anti-emetic therapy should also be described.

- Where appropriate, information should be given about postoperative recovery in a critical care environment.

- Information should be provided about alternative anaesthetic techniques, where appropriate. Patients do not have to agree to the anaesthetist's preferred anaesthetic technique; however, the anaesthetist does not have to agree to use a technique of the patient's choice if it is clearly inappropriate.

- Commonly occurring side-effects such as nausea and vomiting, numbness after local anaesthetic techniques, suxamethonium pains, and post-dural puncture headache should be discussed if relevant.

- Rare but serious complications such as awareness, nerve injury, disability (stroke, deafness, and blindness), and death should be provided in written information, with an estimate of the incidence of the risk. Anaesthetists must be prepared to discuss these risks at the preoperative visit if the patient asks about them.

- Specific risks or complications that may be of special significance to the patient should be discussed, e.g. the risk of vocal cord damage if the patient is a professional singer.

- Any increased risk from anaesthesia and surgery relating to the patient's medical history, the nature of the surgery, and the urgency of the procedure should be discussed.

- If local or regional anaesthetic techniques are proposed, the risks and benefits in comparison to other analgesic techniques should be discussed.

- In patients in whom only a local or regional anaesthetic technique is to be used, the risk of intra-operative pain and the risks and benefits of using sedatives or converting to general anaesthesia should be discussed.

- Where appropriate, the benefits and risks of associated procedures such as central venous catheterization should be discussed.

- Day-stay patients must be supplied with clear and comprehensive pre- and postoperative instructions and told that, when they leave the premises, they must be accompanied by a responsible adult, instructed not to drive for at least 24 h but to check with their own insurance company in case longer prohibition applies.

- All patients should be given the opportunity to ask questions, and honest answers should be provided.
- Many questions relate to the operation itself. The anaesthetist should not provide information about the surgical procedure beyond his or her capability, but should ensure that an appropriate person discusses the surgical procedure and answers the patient's questions before anaesthesia is induced.
- The amount and the nature of information that should be disclosed to the patient should, as far as possible, be determined by assessing what he or she regards as relevant when coming to a decision about which, if any, of the available options should be accepted. Detailed information should not be forced upon patients who have indicated clearly that they do not want to hear it, but written information should be left in case they decide later they would like to know it.

More detailed consideration of the manner in which information should be provided is described in Chapter 2 and a patient's perspective is presented in Chapter 23

Clear information is particularly important when students or trainees carry out procedures to further their own education. If the procedure will further the patient's care (e.g. inserting an intravenous cannula, which will be used for administration of drugs or fluids) then, assuming the student is appropriately trained in the procedure, the fact that it is carried out by a student does not alter the nature and purpose of the procedure. It is therefore not a legal requirement to tell the patient that the clinician is a student, although it is good practice to do so. In contrast, where a student proposes to conduct a physical examination, which is not part of the patient's care, then it is essential to explain that the purpose of the examination is to further the student's training and to seek consent for that to take place. This is particularly important if the examination is to take place during general anaesthesia.

Competence to give consent

A competent adult is a person who has reached 18 years of age, and who has the capacity to make decisions on his or her own behalf regarding treatment. That capacity is present if the patient can comprehend and retain information provided about treatment, including the consequences of having or not having the treatment; believes that information; and weighs that information in the balance to arrive at a choice[15]. No other person can consent to treatment on behalf of a competent adult. Patients may be competent to consent to some interventions but not to others. Adults are presumed to be competent to provide consent, but where any doubt exists, the capacity of the patient to give consent should be assessed. This assessment and the conclusions drawn from it should be recorded in the patient's notes.

A patient's capacity to comprehend and believe information, and to make a balanced choice, may be affected by factors such as confusion, panic, shock, fatigue, pain, or medication. However, the existence of such factors should not be assumed automatically to render the patient incapable of providing consent. An apparently unreasonable decision by the patient does not imply necessarily that the patient lacks competence. The competent adult patient is entitled to make a decision, which is based on their own belief or value system, even if it is perceived by others to be irrational, as long as the patient understands the consequences of that decision.

Additional procedures

During an operation, it may become evident that the patient would benefit from an additional procedure that was not within the scope of the original consent. If it would be unreasonable to delay the procedure until the patient regains consciousness, it may be justified to perform the procedure on the grounds that it is in the patient's best interests. For example, this could apply to insertion of invasive monitoring catheters in a patient who bled unexpectedly, or insertion of an epidural catheter for postoperative pain control if the nature of the operation changed. However, the procedure should not be performed merely because it is convenient. In addition, if a patient has refused specific procedures before anaesthesia, then this refusal must be respected.

Consent to video recordings and clinical photography

Photographs and video recordings of treatment may be used both as a medical record and as a tool for teaching, audit, or research. The Department of Health does not regard it as necessary to obtain consent for images which will be used solely as part of the medical record. However, if the images are to be used for teaching, audit, research, or publication, patients must be made aware that they can refuse without their care being compromised. It is now standard practice to obtain written consent for images to be taken for any purpose other than to form part of the medical record.

Form of consent

The AAGBI does not believe[6] that a formal signed consent form is necessary for anaesthesia and anaesthesia-related procedures, because it is the process of consent itself which is important, and a signed form does not increase the validity of consent. However, the anaesthetist should make a record of the anaesthetic techniques (e.g. general anaesthesia, regional anaesthesia, local anaesthesia, or a combination) that have been discussed with and agreed by the patient, and list the material risks that have been explained.

Duration of consent

In general, consent remains valid for an indefinite duration unless it is withdrawn by the patient. However, the GMC recommends that a doctor should inform the patient if new information has become available about the proposed intervention after consent was sought but before the intervention is undertaken, and that consent is reconfirmed. If the patient's condition has changed significantly in the intervening time, it may be necessary to seek consent again, on the basis that the likely benefits or risks of the intervention may also have changed.

Refusal of consent

Competent adult patients have a right to refuse treatment with or without good reason. If a competent adult makes a voluntary and informed decision to refuse treatment, this decision must be respected, except in circumstances defined by the Mental Health Act (1983). This is the case even where refusal of consent may result in the death of the patient and/or the death of an unborn child, whatever the stage of the pregnancy.

If a patient refuses to consent to the anaesthetic technique which the anaesthetist believes to be the most appropriate, then reasonable attempts can be made to persuade the patient that the proposed technique or procedure carries the least risk of adverse sequelae. The advantages and disadvantages of the proposed procedure in relation to alternatives, and the reasons for the advice, should be explained clearly. However, it is not acceptable to coerce patients into accepting a specific form of treatment.

Occasionally, a refusal of treatment appears so bizarre or irrational that it raises the possibility of mental disorder. If this is considered to be a possibility, then a psychiatric opinion should be sought.

Withdrawal of consent

A competent patient is entitled to withdraw consent at any time, including during the performance of a procedure. In anaesthetic practice, this may occur immediately before induction of anaesthesia, during the performance of a local or regional block, or during operations performed under local or regional anaesthesia. If a patient does object during treatment, the procedure should be stopped if this is possible. The reasons for the patient's concerns should be established, and the consequences of not completing the procedure explained. If stopping the procedure would put the life of the patient at risk, it is probably best to continue until this risk no longer applies.

Self-harm

Patients who have deliberately harmed themselves present special difficulties to health-care professionals if they refuse treatment. If the patient is able to communicate, an assessment of mental capacity should be made as soon as possible. A patient who is judged not to be competent may be treated on the basis of temporary incapacity (see following paragraphs). Patients who have attempted suicide and are unconscious should be given emergency treatment if any doubt exists about either their intentions or their capacity when they took the decision to attempt suicide.

However, competent patients have the right to refuse treatment. The Department of Health recommends that a psychiatric assessment should be obtained if a competent patient who has harmed himself or herself refuses treatment. If the use of the Mental Health Act (1983) is not appropriate, then the refusal must be respected. If practitioners have good reason to believe that a patient genuinely intended to end his or her life and was competent when that decision was taken, and are satisfied that the Mental Health Act is not applicable, then treatment should not be forced on the patient although attempts should be made to encourage him or her to accept help.

Adults without capacity

The Mental Capacity Act 2005[16] provides a statutory framework to empower and protect vulnerable people who may not be able to make their own decisions. It clarifies who can take decisions in specific situations, and enables people to plan ahead for a time when they may lose capacity.

The Act applies to individuals who are 16 years of age or older and who are in England or Wales, and came into effect in full in October 2007. Scotland has its own legislation, the Adults with Incapacity Act 2000, which contains similar principles. Northern Ireland currently has no similar legislation, and common law applies. The Mental Capacity Act relates to the management of property and financial affairs, and healthcare and personal welfare matters. In relation to health care, there are a number of situations in which the Act may influence management of patients by surgeons and anaesthetists.

The Act is underpinned by five key principles:

- Every adult has the right to make his or her own decisions and must be assumed to have the capacity to do so unless proved otherwise.
- An individual must be given all appropriate help in understanding what is proposed, before it is concluded that he§cannot make a competent decision.
- Individuals must retain the right to make what may be seen to be eccentric or unwise decisions.
- Any decision made on behalf of individuals without capacity must be in their best interests.
- Anything done for an individual without capacity should be the least restrictive of his basic rights and freedoms.

Assessing lack of capacity

An individual lacks capacity in relation to a matter, if, at the time, he is unable to make a decision for himself because of an impairment of, or a disturbance in, the functioning of the mind or brain, making him unable:

(a) to understand the information relevant to the decision;

(b) to retain that information;

(c) to use or weigh that information as part of the process of making the decision; or

(d) to communicate the decision, whether by talking, by using sign language or by any other means.

An individual should not be regarded as unable to understand information if he is able to understand an explanation of the matter in a way that is appropriate to the circumstances, using, if necessary, simple language, visual aids, or any other means. The fact that an individual is able to retain information for only a short period of time does not prevent him from being regarded as able to make a decision. A lack of capacity cannot be presumed merely by reference to an individual's age, appearance, the presence of a specific disease or diagnosis, or any aspect of behaviour, which might lead others to make unjustified assumptions about capacity.

Best interests

If an individual lacks capacity, the person who determines what is in his best interests must take into account a number of factors.

---

§ The individual may, of course, be female. The term 'he' is used only for the purpose of brevity.

- How likely is it that the individual will at some future time have capacity, and if so, when is that likely to be?
- If possible, the individual should participate in decision-making as far as he is able.
- Consideration must be given, as far as is reasonably ascertainable, to the individual's past and present wishes and feelings (and in particular any relevant written statement made when he had capacity), the beliefs and values that would be likely to influence his decision if he had capacity, and other factors that he would be likely to consider if he was able to do so.
- If it is practicable and appropriate to consult them, views should be obtained from anyone named by the individual as someone to be consulted, anyone engaged in caring for the individual or interested in his welfare, anyone with lasting power of attorney (see following paragraphs), and any deputy appointed for the person by the Court of Protection.
- If the decision relates to life-sustaining treatment, the person must not, in considering whether the treatment is in the best interests of the individual, be motivated by a desire to bring about his death.

Acts in connection with care or treatment

Provided that a person reasonably believes that an individual lacks capacity and it will be in the individual's best interests for a particular decision to be made, the person does not incur any liability, which he would not have incurred if the individual had the capacity to consent and had consented. This does not alter civil or criminal liability for negligence and does not apply if an advance directive exists and is relevant.

Lasting Powers of Attorney (LPA)

An LPA is a legal document in which an individual (the donor), who must be at least 18 years of age and have capacity, confers on another person, the donee (who must also be at least 18 years of age), authority to make decisions in circumstances in which the individual no longer has capacity. An individual can appoint more than one donee and may appoint them to act jointly or to act in respect of some matters only (e.g. one donee might be appointed to look after financial matters and another to deal with healthcare decisions).

An LPA does not authorize the donee to perform any act which is intended to restrain the donor, unless the donee reasonably believes that the donor lacks capacity, or that it is necessary to restrain the donor in order to perform the act as a means of preventing harm, and that the act is a proportionate response to the likelihood of the donor suffering harm and proportionate to the seriousness of the harm. The authority does not extend to making decisions if the donor regains capacity, is overruled by relevant advance directives but does extend to giving or refusing consent to the carrying out or continuation of treatment by a healthcare worker. However, the LPA does not authorize the giving or refusing of consent to the carrying out or continuation of life-sustaining treatment unless there is express provision to that effect in the document.

The court of protection and deputies

The Court of Protection is a new, specialist court, which has jurisdiction to deal with decision-making for adults who lack capacity. It may sit on any day and any time, and at any place in England or Wales. In relation to its jurisdiction, it has the same powers, rights, privileges, and authority as the High Court. Applications to determine whether a proposed action is lawful (e.g. withdrawal of nutrition and hydration of patients in a permanent vegetative state) will now be dealt with by the Court of Protection. Other cases may be referred there if there are ethical dilemmas in untested areas or conflicts between healthcare professionals and family members.

The Court of Protection may appoint a deputy if no LPA exists. The deputy has the powers of a donee under an LPA, except that the deputy cannot refuse consent to the carrying out or continuation of life-sustaining treatment, and can authorize restraint only if authorized to do so by the Court (in addition to the restrictions placed on donees).

Advance decisions

An advance decision is a decision made by a person of 18 years of age or more, who has the capacity to do so, that if at a later time, in circumstances which can be specified, he lacks capacity to consent to the carrying out or continuation of treatment, the treatment is not to be carried out or continued. An advance decision does not affect the liability of a person for carrying out or continuing treatment unless the decision is, at the material time, valid and applicable to the treatment. An advance decision is not valid if the individual has withdrawn the decision at a time when he had capacity to do so, or, under an LPA, has conferred authority on a donee to give or refuse consent to the treatment to which the advance decision relates, or if, at the material time, the individual has capacity to give or refuse consent.

An advance decision is not applicable to the treatment in question if that treatment is not that specified in the advance decision, or if there are reasonable grounds for believing that circumstances exist, which the individual did not anticipate at the time of the advance decision and which would have affected his decision if he had anticipated them. It is not applicable to life-sustaining treatment unless the decision is verified by a statement to the effect that it is to apply to treatment even if life is at risk, which must be signed and witnessed. However, with these *caveats*, an advance decision that is valid and which relates to the treatment in question must be respected.

Research

Research involving an individual who lacks capacity may be lawfully carried out if a Research Ethics Committee agrees that the research is safe, relates to the person's condition, and cannot be done as effectively using people who have mental capacity. The research must produce a benefit to the individual that outweighs any risk, or, if it is to derive new scientific knowledge, it must be of minimal risk to the individual and be carried out with minimal intrusion or interference with their rights. Carers or nominated third parties must be consulted and must agree that the individual would want to join an approved research project. If the individual shows any signs of resistance or indicates in any way that he does not wish to take part, he must be withdrawn from the project immediately.

Additional provisions

The Act includes two additional provisions to protect vulnerable individuals.

An independent mental capacity advocate (IMCA) is a person appointed to support an individual who lacks capacity but has nobody to speak for him. The IMCA makes representations about the individual's wishes, feelings, beliefs, and values and brings to the attention of the decision-maker all factors that are relevant to the decision. The IMCA can challenge the decision-maker on behalf of the individual lacking capacity if necessary. NHS Trusts are required to make provision for appointment of an IMCA for an incapacitated patient who has no family members, carers, or close friends.

The Act introduces a new criminal offence of ill-treatment or neglect of an individual who lacks capacity. A person found guilty of such an offence may be liable to imprisonment for up to five years.

Implications for anaesthetists

In a dire emergency, it is still reasonable, in a patient who, after careful consideration, is considered to lack capacity to consent to or refuse treatment, to provide life-saving treatment which is considered to be in the patient's best interests. In patients who require management in an intensive care unit (see Chapter 5), or those who are considered to lack capacity to consent to elective or semi-elective surgery, steps must be taken to involve the patient's carers, and to establish whether a valid LPA or advance directive exists, or whether a deputy has been appointed by the Court; if not, then it is necessary to involve an IMCA before proceeding with treatment. Only life-saving emergency treatment may be given without IMCA representation unless a valid LPA or advance directive exists.

Temporary incapacity

An adult who usually has capacity may become temporarily incapable, e.g. whilst under a general anaesthetic or sedation, or, for example, as a result of confusion, panic, shock, fatigue, pain, or medication after a road traffic accident. Unless a valid advance refusal of treatment is applicable to the circumstances, the law permits interventions that are necessary to be made and no more than is reasonably required in the patient's best interests pending the recovery of capacity. If a medical intervention is thought to be in the patient's best interests but can be delayed until the patient recovers capacity and can consent to (or refuse) the intervention, it must be delayed until that time.

Referral to the court of protection

The courts have identified certain circumstances when referral should be made to them, for a ruling on lawfulness, before a procedure is undertaken. Circumstances relevant to anaesthesia are sterilization for contraceptive purposes and withdrawal of nutrition and hydration from a patient in a persistent vegetative state.

In Re F[17], the House of Lords considered the power of a court to authorize sterilization of an adult woman who did not have the capacity to give consent; she was 36 years old but had the mental capacity of a child of 4 years. She had become involved in a relationship but medical staff felt that a pregnancy would be 'disastrous from a psychiatric point of view'. The House of Lords concluded that, in these circumstances, sterilization was permissible and lawful because it was in the patient's 'best interests'. 'Best interests' was to be taken in a wide sense so as to include public interest but, in the area of non-therapeutic sterilization, was not to include the convenience of those responsible for the patient's care.

> The overriding consideration is that [doctors] should act in the best interests of the person who suffers from the misfortune of being prevented by incapacity from deciding for himself what should be done to his own body, in his own best interests.

Females who become pregnant incur risks associated with pregnancy and delivery, and these risks are avoided if sterilization is performed. An application was made by the mother of a young male adult with Down's syndrome to authorize his sterilisation because there was a possibility that he might have sexual intercourse and cause a pregnancy[18]. It was unlikely that he would be able to tolerate vasectomy under local anaesthesia, and therefore he would be subjected to the finite, although very small, risks associated with general anaesthesia. The Court decided that it was not in the patient's best interests to be sterilized, and public interest or the interest of females whom he might impregnate was irrelevant. The application was rejected.

Children and young people

In England and Wales, the legal position concerning consent and refusal of treatment by those under the age of 18 is different from the position for adults, in particular where treatment is being refused.

Young people aged 16–17 years

People aged 16 or 17 years can give consent for any surgical, medical, or dental treatment. As for adults, consent is valid only if it is given voluntarily by an appropriately informed patient capable (using the same criteria as for adults) of consenting to the particular intervention. However, unlike adults, the refusal of a competent person aged 16–17 years may, in certain circumstances, be over-ridden by either a person with parental responsibility (Table 1.1) or a court, if the child is likely to suffer harm as a result of their refusal.

It is not legally necessary to obtain consent from a parent in addition to that of the young person. However, it is good practice to involve the family in the decision-making process, unless the young person specifically wishes to exclude them.

If a young person of 16 or 17 years of age is not competent to give consent, then the consent of a parent should be sought, unless immediate treatment is required to prevent death or permanent injury.

Children under 16 years of age

This subject is dealt with in Chapter 7.

Mental Health Act (1983)

Treatment for mental disorder may proceed without obtaining the patient's consent if the patient is liable to be detained under the Mental Health Act. The Mental Health Act does not contain provisions to enable treatment of physical disorders without

Table 1.1 People who may have parental responsibility

The child's parents if married to each other at the time of conception or birth

The child's mother, but not father, if they were not married, unless the father has acquired parental responsibility via a court order or a parental responsibility agreement, or the couple subsequently marry

The child's legally appointed guardian is one of the following :

 ♦ Courts may appoint a guardian for a child who has no parent with parental responsibility

 ♦ Parents with parental responsibility may also appoint a guardian in the event of their own death

A person in whose favour the court has made a residence order concerning the child

A Local Authority designated in a care order in respect of the child

A Local Authority or other authorized person who holds an emergency protection order in respect of the child

An individual acting on behalf of a person with parental responsibility and with their express permission, in loco parentis, (e.g. a childminder, or staff at a boarding school)

consent, either for detained patients, or for people who may be suffering from mental disorder but who are not detained under the Mental Health Act, unless the physical disorder arises from the mental disorder, or is judged to be contributing to the mental disorder.

Neither the existence of mental disorder nor the fact of detention under the Mental Health Act should give rise to an assumption of incapacity. The patient's capacity must be assessed in every case in relation to the particular decision being made. The capacity of a person with mental disorder may fluctuate.

References

1. *Sidaway v. Board of Governors of Bethlem Royal Hospital and the Maudsley Hospital* (1985) AC 871.
2. General Medical Council. Seeking patients' consent: the ethical considerations (1998) London.
3. Department of Health.Good practice in consent implementation guide: consent to examination or treatment (2001) London
4. *Bolam v Friern Hospital Management Committee* (1957) 1 WLR 582.
5. *Davis v Barking, Havering and Brentwood HA* (1994) 4 Med LR 85.
6. Consent for Anaesthesia. Association of Anaesthetists of Great Britain and Ireland (2006) London.
7. *Rogers v Whitaker* (1992) 4 Med LR 79.
8. *Pearce v United Bristol Healthcare NHS Trust* (1999) 48 BMLR 118.
9. Mitchell J. (1995). A fundamental problem of consent. *British Medical Journal*, **310**, 43–8.
10. *Chappell v Hart* (1998) 72 ALJR 1344.
11. [2004] UKHL 41. http://www.parliament.the-stationery-office.co.uk/pa/ld200304/ ldjudgmt/jd041014/cheste-1.htm (last accessed 19th December 2008).

12. Wheat K. (2005). Progress of the prudent patient: consent after *Chester v Afshar*. *Anaesthesia*, **60**, 215–9.

13. White L and Turner J. (2003). Learning from existing practice: a process of evaluation. In *Raising the Standard: Information for patients*, pp. 33–69. Royal College of Anaesthetists and Association of Anaesthetists of Great Britain and Ireland, London.

14. Royal College of Anaesthetists, London. http://www.rcoa.ac.uk/index.asp?PageID=69 (last accessed 19th December 2008).

15. Re MB (*an adult: medical treatment*) (1997) 2 FLR 426 (CA).

16. Department for Constitutional Affairs. *The Mental Capacity Act 2005*. http://www.opsi.gov.uk/acts/acts2005/ukpga_20050009_en_1 (last accessed 1st December 2008).

17. *Re F* (1989) 2 WLR 1025 (1989) 2 All ER 545.

18. *Re A (Male Sterilisation)* (2000) 1 FLR 549, 557.

Chapter 2

Conveying risks and benefits

Iain K Moppett

In order for consent to be valid, patients must be given information in a form that they can understand. There has been much research to investigate information provision, both in the setting of normal clinical practice and clinical trials. Relatively little research has been related directly to anaesthesia, so extrapolation from investigations involving surgical or research consent is necessary.

Several related factors have to be considered when delivering information to patients. These are:

- Who can obtain consent and when should this be done?
- What information does the patient wish to know?
- Does the patient understand the information?
- Will the patient remember the information at a later date?
- Will the information provided be of benefit to the patient?
- Will the information provided be of harm to the patient?
- Will the information provided be considered sufficient by the regulatory authorities or courts of law should a problem arise?

Who can obtain consent and when should this be done?

The General Medical Council (GMC) guidelines on consent state:

> If you are the doctor providing treatment or undertaking an investigation, it is your responsibility to discuss it with the patient and obtain consent, as you will have a comprehensive understanding of the procedure or treatment, how it is carried out, and the risks attached to it. Where this is not practicable, you may delegate these tasks provided you ensure that the person to whom you delegate:
>
> - Is suitably trained and qualified;
> - Has sufficient knowledge of the proposed investigation or treatment, and understands the risks involved;
> - Acts in accordance with the guidance [from the GMC].
>
> You will remain responsible for ensuring that, before you start any treatment, the patient has been given sufficient time and information to make an informed decision, and has given consent to the procedure or investigation.

For some patients this is relatively straightforward, if the anaesthetist who will anaesthetize sees the patient preoperatively. For others it may be more difficult. Patients may be seen by colleagues who will not be administering anaesthesia, either as part of a formal preoperative assessment process or due to changes in theatre lists. Provided the information given to the patient is of an appropriate standard and is germane to what the actual anaesthetic procedures will involve, then this should not matter. Clearly, where a different approach is to be taken (e.g. general rather than spinal anaesthesia), the attending anaesthetist will need to be satisfied that the patient has been given adequate information and time to consent to the changed technique.

With increasing 'day of surgery' admissions, the timing of information provision is becoming more important. Although some healthcare organisations have systems in place whereby every patient is seen by an anaesthetist in a preoperative assessment clinic, many do not. Therefore, the patient may not meet an anaesthetist until shortly before surgery. Most guidance requires adequate time for patients to take in information. UK GMC Guidance[1] is that:

> [You should] allow patients sufficient time to reflect, before and after making a decision, especially where the information is complex or the severity of the risks is great.

Similarly, the Association of Anaesthetists of Great Britain and Ireland (AAGBI) guidance states:

> it is neither practical nor desirable for all information to be provided to patients at the preoperative meeting with the anaesthetist.

These statements necessitate that some information is given to patients a reasonable time before their operation. Such information will not necessarily be provided by an anaesthetist. Specially trained nurses are capable of taking consent for surgical procedures, and there is no reason why the same cannot apply to anaesthesia, provided the guidance regarding delegation is followed. Written information is likely to be the mainstay of information provision, although this cannot replace good verbal communication between the anaesthetist and patient. If general anaesthesia or sedation is required for dental treatment, the General Dental Council holds the dentist responsible for ensuring that the patient (or, in the case of children, a parent) has all the necessary information about the benefits and risks of anaesthesia at the time that the decision is taken to recommend the treatment[2]. If an anaesthetist is involved at the time of treatment, then it is his or her responsibility to ensure that the risks and benefits are understood by the patient, and to obtain consent for anaesthesia.

What information does the patient wish to know?

The answer to this question seems simple. Ask the patient. Various studies have shown that most patients or their carers wish to know more about the procedures they are to undergo than physicians think they do[3–8]. One study found that over 80% of obstetric patients wanted to know about common, less-severe side-effects of regional anaesthesia, and over 70% wanted to know about rarer but more severe complications such as permanent neurological deficit, high spinal block, and meningitis[9]. However, the majority of studies have found that most patients are content with the amount of information they receive[7,10]. When asked, around 50% of patients state they want written information, although 20% do not read the written information[11].

However, the information that patients or their carers say they want may depend upon the amount they are given. Garden and colleagues' study of 45 cardiac surgical patients found that around two-thirds of patients thought that any one of three anaesthesia information leaflets (minimal, standard, or full disclosure), if given on its own, was 'just right'. However, if all three leaflets were given together, two-thirds felt that too much information was withheld from the 'minimal' leaflet[6]. Various small surveys have found that a minority of patients want 'minimal' anaesthetic information, and approximately equal numbers wish for 'standard' or 'full disclosure'[10,12]. Conversely, Moores and colleagues[13], in a study of over 400 Scottish patients, found that at the point when 'consent' had been obtained, two-thirds had no further questions about their anaesthetic. The questions asked by the investigating anaesthetist up to that point were gathering information for the anaesthetist; no information was given. Of the one-third of patients who asked further questions, two-thirds of the questions were about anaesthesia, covering the expected range of topics: awareness, postoperative nausea, safety, etc.

The amount of information that patients and their carers want may be affected by various factors. Women appear to want to know more than men[14,15]. This extends to what they wish to know when their child is to be anaesthetized. A U.S. study found that mothers were more likely to want to hear all possible risks, whereas fathers were more likely to want to know only about those that are likely to occur[16]. Patients under 50 years of age generally want to know more than their elders[15,17]. Parents want to know more about risks for their children than for themselves[8,18]. There may be cross-cultural differences: Australian patients in the 1990s wanted to know more about risks than Scottish or Canadian ones[17], whereas Jamaicans[14] and Japanese[18] appeared to desire less information. Anxious patients do not appear to wish to know less, even though they may fear the information that is presented to them[5].

Does the patient understand the information?

Given that patients generally want information and are satisfied with what they receive, do they understand it? Most studies in this area have investigated understanding of surgery or research methods. Usually, patients say they understand[19], but, if tested directly, frequently do not. Providing written information may increase the ability of patients to recall information[20] but there is little evidence to suggest that it actually increases understanding. There may be several reasons for this.

+ First, physicians have invested much time and intellectual effort into understanding their field of expertise. Patients cannot be expected to match this after reading a short summary leaflet and having a few minutes of discussion with the physician.

+ Second, the mode of information presentation may not be appropriate. A few studies have assessed the readability of written information for consent for research studies. A New Zealand study found that subject information leaflets for medical research had Flesch reading ease indices of around 53 compared to 67 for magazine articles and 48 for newspaper editorials[21]. A Scottish study of ENT patient information found that around of a quarter of patients had reading abilities less than those which would be required to read the standard surgical consent form. Some of the information leaflets at that time required graduate-level reading ability[22]. For comparison, the current patient information leaflets from the UK Royal College of Anaesthetists[23] have a Flesch reading ease of around 60. The patient information page from the Canadian Anaesthetists' Society has a Flesch reading ease of just under 40[24], and the Australian Information leaflet index is around 45[25]. Readability scores should not be used as the sole means of assessing whether patients will understand a specific leaflet as they do not necessarily correlate[26], and they can be relatively easily manipulated by creating documents with very short sentences, regardless of whether they actually make sense. Similar issues apply to the provision of verbal information. Approximately, 50% of verbal information in physician–patient interactions is misunderstood. This appears to be because of the same issues as with written information: jargon, poor structure, and a mismatch between the imparted information and the ability of patients to understand. More information provision does not necessarily translate into better understanding. There may be an inverse 'U'-shaped relationship between information given and information understood[27]. Unfortunately, there is no realistic way of assessing the optimum amount of information for any individual patient.

- Third, appropriately presented information, which should be understandable by the patient, may still be misunderstood due to cognitive factors. Every person interprets the information they are given in the light of their own experience. Information that is in disagreement with this 'personal schema' may be misinterpreted: so-called cognitive dissonance[28–30]. This may be more of a problem with the elderly due to a greater life experience, although most anaesthetists will have encountered patients who place more reliance on anecdotal or family experience of adverse events than on published medical evidence[29].

Documents written purely by healthcare professionals may not be as well understood as those that have significant involvement of representative patients. This is probably for several reasons: lay people tend to remove the unnecessary jargon; the language level is appropriate to the intended readership; the information that patients want to read is included[31].

Patients who have a first language different to the healthcare professional may present a specific challenge. The use of family as interpreters, although convenient, is fraught with problems. Patients may not wish to discuss sensitive issues via a family member. The information coming from the physician may be paraphrased by the family member. Most anaesthetists will have experienced consultations where long questions seem to be translated into much shorter questions to the patient, or long answers from the patient end up as 'No.' Because many patients who receive information in their own language misunderstand that information, it is hardly surprising that non-professionals translating technical information make mistakes. For these reasons, professional interpreters should be used wherever possible. Even then, there is no guarantee of accuracy, especially when technical information is involved[32].

Where written information is concerned, it should be borne in mind that translations may not be perfect. Furthermore, many non-native language speakers may not be able to read their preferred language, so providing written information may not solve all problems.

The presentation of statements concerning risk has received some attention in published literature. Notwithstanding the fact that physicians and health purchasers[33,34] make different choices about the effectiveness of treatments dependent upon the way results are reported, patients' understanding of risk may not reflect what physicians think they have presented. In qualitative terms, people are generally more accepting of self-inflicted risk than that which is imposed[35], even when the absolute risk of harm weighs heavily towards self-inflicted risk. As an example, consider smokers who are concerned primarily about the risk of epidural abscess. Furthermore, timing affects the perceived severity of risk: immediate and long-lasting injuries are given greater importance than distant or short-duration problems. Adams and Smith argue that these factors explain some of the reasons why patients think anaesthesia is so risky, despite its relative safety[36]. Patients lose complete control for the duration of anaesthesia, and the complications, although rare, may have immediate and long-term consequences (e.g. paraplegia, hypoxic brain damage). Humans struggle to comprehend the wide range of risks, tending to overestimate rare risks and underestimate common ones.

Risks tend to be interpreted in a 'self-serving' fashion. 'Good risks' such as survival tend to be overestimated when referring to one's self, and 'bad risks' such as death tend to be underestimated[37]. Conversely, when the same risks are applied to others, the opposite tends to occur—bad things happen to other people. Compounding this problem is the issue of invulnerability. Patients may agree with the reported risks but believe that these risks do not apply directly to them. The number of anaesthetists who smoke is testament to the strength of this effect.

Regardless of the inaccuracy with which people interpret risk information, the presentation of the data affects what is understood in important ways. People prefer to give risk information in qualitative, verbal terms, but prefer to receive risk information in numeric terms[37]. Various publications have urged the use of words rather than numbers because very few patients (or doctors) truly understand probabilities and these are the media of communication in normal life. However, although some words have well-defined meanings (certain, never), the phrases used to describe intermediate risk are interpreted differently among subjects and are dependent upon to whom the probability refers[37]. As with numeric risks, verbal likelihood terms are interpreted in self-optimistic fashion when compared to the same terms referring to other 'random' individuals[37].

Despite this uncertainty, verbal likelihood scales are common in anaesthetic practice. United Kingdom drug information leaflets use the Calman verbal scale[38], the UK Royal College of Anaesthetists information documents[23] use a modified, and numerically defined, version of the scale, and the Canadian on-line and Australian published information use an undefined set of phrases[24,25] (Table 2.1). Although the data on which to estimate risk may be flawed and imprecise, patients prefer to be given numerical estimates of risk. In reality, these tend to be no more precise than verbal

Table 2.1 Comparison of risk scales

Level of risk	Calman Scale[38]	RCoA leaflets[23]	Population comparison[39] (One person in)
1 in 1 to 1 in 9		Very common	A family
1 in 10 to 1 in 99	High	Common	
1 in 100 to 1 in 999	Moderate	Uncommon	A street
1 in 1000 to 1 in 9999	Low	Rare	A village
1 in 10 000 to 1 in 1 000 000	Minimal	Very rare	A small town
1 in 1 000 000 to 1 in 9 999 999	Negligible		A city
1 in 10 000 000 to 1 in 99 999 999			A province or country
1 in 100 000 000 to 1 in 999 999 999			A large country

descriptions, because many risks are expressed as 'between 1 in 100 and 1 in 1000'. Referencing these numbers to the patient's world may provide the best way forward to create comprehensible risks, which have some scientific validity. One method proposed to achieve this is the population scale. Risks are compared to the proportion of individuals in a segment of a population such as family, village, or town (Table 2.1)[39].

A further issue, which has to be acknowledged, is the effect of the context of a risk statement, known as positive or negative framing. Patients are more likely to accept treatments described as having a 90% success rate than those with a 10% failure rate, despite both statements referring to the same risk[40]. Clearly, this means that the same information given to a patient in different forms may lead to the patient coming to different decisions. Relative and absolute risks are particularly problematical in this regard. This is most clearly demonstrated with information regarding obstetric anaesthetic risk. It is generally quoted that general anaesthesia is 'riskier' than regional anaesthesia, and the relative risk may be higher. However, the absolute risk of either technique is low. Quoting relative risks is likely to persuade patients to opt for regional anaesthesia. Absolute risks probably make the situation much less clear.

Will the patient remember the information at a later date?

Recall of information given, regardless of the medium, is generally poor[41,42]. Clearly, this has important implications for the doctor–patient relationship and for legal proceedings, should adverse events occur. Because of this poor recall, some have questioned the validity of informed consent. Others argue that whether or not patients remember what they were told is irrelevant to their ability to make a decision on the basis of that information at that time[43]. One study investigating anaesthesia specifically found that around two-thirds of patients stated that they had no or very little recall of a preoperative information document[11]. Similar findings hold for surgical consent[44,45]. Providing written information in addition to verbal information may improve recall if evidence from the wider medical literature can be extrapolated to anaesthesia[19,28,46–50], although some studies have found that the mode of information provision has little effect on recall[51,52]. The enhancing effect of written information may be larger for serious risks (e.g. death, nerve injury)[20,41].

Some groups of patients appear less likely to recall information, regardless of the mode of presentation. These include the elderly, those with fewer years of formal education, and those who believe that their health is not under their own control[53]. Information that is contradictory to previously held beliefs is less likely to be recalled[54,55], whereas information that is 'welcome' is more likely to be retained than 'unwelcome' news. The emotional state of the patient also influences subsequent recall. As with most learning, there is a degree of state dependency, such that information is best recalled when the subject is in a similar emotional state as when they were given the information[29]. Moderate anxiety when information is given enhances recall, whereas excessive or no anxiety tend to impair subsequent recall[29]. As expected from educational research, variety of presentation and repetition of information seem to enhance recall of medical information[56].

There is limited published evidence regarding use of online materials as part of the consent process, but the information which is available suggests that, if prepared appropriately, on-line resources can be as good as paper materials[57].

Will the information be of benefit or harm to the patient?

When information for consent first became an important issue, there was much concern in the medical community about the detrimental effects that too much information could have on the patient[13], and this attitude is still expressed[58,59]. This concern was stated explicitly in a commentary by a solicitor on a UK case in which an anaesthetist was found guilty of serious professional misconduct for administering a suppository to an anaesthetized dental patient without her consent.

> It is not clear from the [GMC] committee's decision how far it took account of the fact that—perhaps uniquely in the context of anaesthetics—the reason for not frightening a patient before a medical procedure is not merely humane. It is also scientific, as it is more difficult and dangerous to anaesthetize an apprehensive patient who has raised catecholamine concentrations. It is not the apprehensive patient who exercises the right to walk out who is the problem for the anaesthetist, it is the apprehensive patient who stays behind and submits to operation. It was pointed out that the problem of frightened patients is particularly relevant in the case of day patients who do not receive any premedication[60].

Most anaesthetists would probably find this statement somewhat extreme and the AAGBI guidelines on consent state:

> Good clinical practice has moved in advance of the law with respect to paternalism and the withholding of information on grounds of 'therapeutic privilege'. Information must not be withheld because the anaesthetist feels it may deter a patient from undergoing a beneficial procedure[61].

Despite this, and the fact that patients want the information, most anaesthetists are reluctant to tell patients directly about serious but rare events such as death, largely for fear of deterring patients from having beneficial operations. There is little if any evidence to support this practice. Although there may be valid ethical debate about the relative importance of autonomy (patient choice) versus beneficence (doing good for the patient), most Western societies currently place far more moral and legal emphasis on autonomy than beneficence. The published evidence also suggests that informing patients of risks of surgery[7,62,63] or anaesthesia[38,20] does not increase anxiety overall, although clearly this may not be true for an individual patient. One Swiss study found that a small number (7%) of women were more anxious after receiving a standardized operation-specific leaflet[64]. Even those patients who think that information will make them anxious want to know the information[5]. Interestingly, it does not seem to make much difference to what patients decide to do[65]. Unfortunately, despite this, current UK case law deems it negligent for a doctor to fail to warn of a 'significant' risk even if the patient would still have proceeded with the same course of action had they been warned (i.e. patients have a right to be informed of any 'significant' risk). Given that there is very little hard evidence to recommend any one form of anaesthesia or analgesia over another in terms of overall risk for most patients, it may be difficult in today's moral and legal climate to justify withholding risk information in order to prevent patients choosing the 'wrong' course. However, it is unclear from current case law whether a 'significant' risk refers to any clinically significant risk, irrespective of frequency, or to a clinically significant risk with a relatively high incidence (around 1 in 100).

Key points

- Patients generally want more information than is provided; if more information is provided then they want more
- Patients do not understand most of what they are told
  - Mismatch of professional and patient knowledge
  - Information too complicated
  - Discordance between what patients believe and what they are told
- Patients do not recall much of what they are told
  - Failure to understand
  - Possibly improved by the use of written information
  - Possibly improved by improved structure of information
  - Recall influenced by emotional state, age, education, and health beliefs
- Anxiety is not increased by more information
- Patient satisfaction improves with better consent procedures
  - Not linked to understanding or recall of information provided
  - No evidence of improved outcomes in relation to anaesthesia

Record keeping

Historically, anaesthetists have been poor at recording information regarding consent. However, the changing medicolegal climate has encouraged change. The AAGBI guidance[61] is that:

> ... it is essential for health professionals to document clearly both a patient's agreement to the intervention and the discussions which led up to that agreement.

There is no requirement for a separate signed consent for anaesthesia in the United Kingdom, although the surgical consent form stipulates the type of anaesthesia discussed. From a medicolegal standpoint, documenting a discussion of risks and benefits provides some evidence that such a discussion took place. More importantly, one cannot document such a discussion if it has not taken place. The anaesthetic record of the 'consent process' therefore provides a prompt for the anaesthetist to ensure that the patient is aware of the risks and benefits of the intended anaesthetic procedures.

Best practice

There is no single template for best practice in providing information for patients, but broad principles do exist.

- Patients generally want more information than is currently given, and they are not made unduly anxious when it is provided. Significant information about anaesthesia should therefore be included by default in information given to patients.
- Written information should be in a form and style appropriate to the patient group.
- Automated software can help in guiding the appropriate reading level, although having the document read by representatives of the patient group is more important.
- There is no perfect method of describing risk, although patients prefer numerical values. A combination of techniques may be beneficial.
- Repetition of information encourages understanding and probably recall.
- Translation by family members is to be avoided if possible, although even professional interpreters make mistakes.
- Written information is a complement to, not a replacement for, verbal communication with an appropriate healthcare professional.
- A written record of the information concerning risks and intended benefits of anaesthetic techniques should be made.

Key points

- Factors affecting perception of risk
  - Patients prefer numerical risks over verbal ones
  - Numerical risks are not necessarily any more precise than verbal ratings
  - Numerical risks, provided that they have some scientific basis, are likely to be easier to defend at a later date

Key points *(continued)*

- ◆ Patients tend to misinterpret risk due to:
  - • Variable translation of verbal to numerical risks
  - • Self-optimistic interpretation
  - • Perceived invulnerability
  - • Positive or negative framing
- ◆ Doctors as well as patients misinterpret risk

References

1. General Medical Council. (1998). *Seeking patients' consent: The ethical considerations.* General Medical Council, London.

2. General Dental Council.(1998). *Maintaining Standards: Guidance to Dentists on Professional and Personal Conduct.* General Dental Council, London.

3. Bellew, M., Atkinson, K.R., Dixon, G., and Yates, A. (2002). The introduction of a paediatric anaesthesia information leaflet: an audit of its impact on parental anxiety and satisfaction. *Paediatric Anaesthesia,* **12,** 124–30.

4. Burns, P., Keogh, I., and Timon, C. (2005). Informed consent: a patients' perspective. *Journal of Laryngology and Otology,* **119,** 19–22.

5. Dawes, P.J. (1994). Informed consent: what do patients want to know? *Journal of Royal Society of Medicine,* **87,** 149–52.

6. Garden, A.L., Merry, A.F., Holland, R.L., and Petrie, K. J. (1996). Anaesthesia information–what patients want to know. *Anaesthesia and Intensive Care,* **24,** 594–8.

7. Ivarsson, B., Larsson, S., Luhrs, C., and Sjoberg, T. (2005). Extended written preoperative information about possible complications at cardiac surgery–do the patients want to know? *European Journal of Cardio-thoracic Surgery,* **28,** 407–14.

8. Kain, Z.N., Wang, S.M., Caramico, L.A., Hofstadter, M., and Mayes, L.C. (1997). Parental desire for perioperative information and informed consent: a two-phase study. *Anesthesia and Analgesia,* **84,** 299-306.

9. Kelly, G.D., Blunt, C., Moore, P.A., *et al.* (2004). Consent for regional anaesthesia in the United Kingdom: what is material risk? *International Journal of Obstetric Anesthesia,* **13,** 71–4.

10. Chapman, M.V. and Wolff, A.H. (2002). Consent for anaesthesia. *Anaesthesia,* **57,** 710.

11. Rosique, I., Perez-Carceles, M.D., Romero-Martin, M., Osuna, E., and Luna, A. (2006). The use and usefulness of information for patients undergoing anaesthesia. *Medicine and Law,* **25,** 715–27.

12. El-Sayeh, S. and Lavies, N.G. (2003). Preoperative information about anaesthesia–is more better? *Anaesthesia,* **58,** 1119–20.

13. Moores, A. and Pace, N.A. (2003). The information requested by patients prior to giving consent to anaesthesia. *Anaesthesia,* **58,** 703–6.

14. Crawford-Sykes, A.M. and Hambleton, I.R. (2001). Patients' desire for peri-operative information: Jamaican attitudes. *West Indian Medical Journal,* **50,** 159–63.

15. Lonsdale, M. and Hutchison, G.L. (1991). Patients' desire for information about anaesthesia. Scottish and Canadian attitudes. *Anaesthesia*, **46**, 410–2.

16. Litman, R.S., Perkins, F.M., and Dawson, S.C. (1993). Parental knowledge and attitudes toward discussing the risk of death from anesthesia. *Anesthesia and Analgesia*, **77**, 256–60.

17. Farnill, D. and Inglis, S. (1994). Patients' desire for information about anaesthesia: Australian attitudes. *Anaesthesia*, **49**, 162–4.

18. Yoneyama, E., Kamitani, K., Nagakawa, T., *et al*. [The evaluation of the preoperative interviews using information sheets]. *Masui*, **47**, 1002–6.

19. Chan, T., Eckert, K., Venesoen, P., Leslie, K., and Chin-Yee, I. (2005). Consenting to blood: what do patients remember? *Transfusion Medicine*, **15**, 461–6.

20. Inglis, S. and Farnill, D. (1993). The effects of providing preoperative statistical anaesthetic-risk information. *Anaesthesia and Intensive Care*, **21**, 799–805

21. Murphy, J., Gamble, G., and Sharpe, N. (1994). Readability of subject information leaflets for medical research. *New Zealand Medical Journal*, **7**, 509–10.

22. Kubba, H. (2000). Reading skills of otolaryngology outpatients: implications for information provision. *Journal of Laryngology and Otology*, **114**, 694–6.

23. Royal College of Anaesthetists. (2003). *You and your anaesthetic*, 2nd edition. Royal College of Anaesthetists, London

24. Canadian Anesthesiologists' Society. (2007). *Anesthesia & You*. http://www.cas.ca/public/anesthesia_and_you/ (last accessed 10th December 2008).

25. Australian Society of Anaesthetists.(2004). *Anaesthesia & You*. Australian Society of Anaesthetists, Edgecliff. http://www.asa.org.au/pageBANK/documents/Anaesthesia%20You%20brochure%2023%20March%2007.pdf (last accessed 10th December 2008).

26. Taub, H.A., Baker, M.T., and Sturr, J.F. (1986). Informed consent for research. Effects of readability, patient age, and education. *Journal of American Geriatric Society*, **34**, 601–6.

27. Lynoe, N. and Hoeyer, K. (2005). Quantitative aspects of informed consent: considering the dose response curve when estimating quantity of information. *Journal of Medical Ethics*, **31**, 736–8.

28. Dillon, M.F., Carr, C.J., Feeley, T.M., and Tierney, S. (2005). Impact of the informed consent process on patients' understanding of varicose veins and their treatment. *Irish Journal of Medical Science*, **174**, 23–7.

29. Kessels, R.P. (2003). Patients' memory for medical information. *Journal of the Royal Society of Medicine*, **96**, 219–22.

30. Kiss, C.G., Richter-Mueksch, S., Stifter, E., Diendorfer-Radner, G., Velikay-Parel, M., and Radner, W. (2004). Informed consent and decision making by cataract patients. *Archives of Ophthalmology*, **122**, 94–8.

31. Kusec, S., Oreskovi, S., Skegro, M., Korolija, D., Busi, Z., Horzi, M. (2006). Improving comprehension of informed consent. *Patient Education and Conuseling*, **60**, 294–300.

32. Simon, C.M., Zyzanski, S.J., Durand, E., Jimenez, X., and Kodish, E.D. (2006). Interpreter accuracy and informed consent among Spanish-speaking families with cancer. *Journal of Health Communication*, **11**, 509–22.

33. Bucher, H.C., Weinbacher, M., and Gyr, K. (1994). Influence of method of reporting study results on decision of physicians to prescribe drugs to lower cholesterol concentration. *British Medical Journal*, 761–4.

34. Fahey, T., Griffiths, S., and Peters, T.J. (1995). Evidence based purchasing: understanding results of clinical trials and systematic reviews. *British Medical Journal*, 1056–9.

35. Keeney, R.L. (1995). Understanding life-threatening risks. *Risk Analysis*, **15**, 627–37.

36. Adams, A.M. and Smith, A.F. (2001). Risk perception and communication: recent developments and implications for anaesthesia. *Anaesthesia*, **56**, 745–55.

37. Smits, T. and Hoorens, V. (2005). How probable is probably? It depends on whom you're talking about. *Journal of Behavioral Decision Making*, **18**, 83–96.

38. Calman, K.C. (1996). Cancer: science and society and the communication of risk. *British Medical Journal*, **313**, 799–802.

39. Calman, K.C. and Royston, G.H. (1997). Risk language and dialects. *British Medical Journal*, **315**, 939–42.

40. Malenka, D.J., Baron, J.A., Johansen, S., Wahrenberger, J.W., and Ross, J.M. (1993). The framing effect of relative and absolute risk. *Journal of General Internal Medicine*, **8**, 543–8.

41. Brown, T.F., Massoud, E., and Bance, M. (2003). Informed consent in otologic surgery: prospective study of risk recall by patients and impact of written summaries of risk. *Journal of Otolaryngology*, **32**, 368–72.

42. Kriwanek, S., Armbruste, C., Beckerhinn, P., Blauensteier, W., and Gschwantler, M. (1998). Patients' assessment and recall of surgical information after laparoscopic cholecystectomy. *Digestive Surgery*, **15**, 669–73.

43. Leigh, B. (2006). Consent--an event or a memory? A judicial view. *Journal of Bone and Joint Surgery. British Volume*, **88**, 16–8.

44. Shurnas, P.S. and Coughlin, M.J. (2003). Recall of the risks of forefoot surgery after informed consent. *Foot and Ankle International*, **24**, 904–8.

45. Vallance, J.H., Ahmed, M., and Dhillon, B. (2004). Cataract surgery and consent; recall, anxiety, and attitude toward trainee surgeons preoperatively and postoperatively. *Journal of Cataract and Refractive Surgery*, **30**, 1479–85.

46. Ashraff, S., Malawa, G., Dolan, T., and Khanduja, V. (2006). Prospective randomised controlled trial on the role of patient information leaflets in obtaining informed consent. *Australian and New Zealand Journal of Surgery*, **76**, 139–41.

47. Chan, Y., Irish, J.C., Wood, S.J., *et al.* (2002). Patient education and informed consent in head and neck surgery. *Archives of Otolaryngology- Head and Neck Surgery*, **128**, 1269–74.

48. Langdon, I.J., Hardin, R., and Learmonth, I.D. (2002). Informed consent for total hip arthroplasty: does a written information sheet improve recall by patients? *Annals of Royal College of Surgeons of England*, **84**, 404–8.

49. Layton, S. and Korsen, J. (1994). Informed consent in oral and maxillofacial surgery: a study of the value of written warnings. *British Journal of Oral and Maxillofacial Surgery*, **32**, 34–6.

50. Pesudovs, K., Luscombe, C.K., and Coster, D.J. Recall from informed consent counselling for cataract surgery. (2006). *Journal of Law and Medicine*, **13**, 496–504

51. Graham, P. (2003). Type of consent does not influence patient recall of serious potential radiation toxicity of adjuvant breast radiotherapy. *Australasian Radiology*, **47**, 416–21.

52. Turner, P. and Williams, C. Informed consent: patients listen and read, but what information do they retain? *New Zealand Medical Journal*, **115**, U218.

53. Lavelle-Jones, C., Byrne, D.J., Rice, P., and Cuschieri, A. (1993). Factors affecting quality of informed consent. *British Medical Journal*, **306**, 885–90.

54. Okun, M.A. and Rice, G.E. (2001). The effects of personal relevance of topic and information type on older adults' accurate recall of written medical passages about osteoarthritis. *Journal of Aging and Health*, **13**, 410–29.

55. Rice, G.E. and Okun, M.A. (1994). Older readers' processing of medical information that contradicts their beliefs. *Journal of Gerontology*, **49**, 119–28.

56. Moseley, T.H., Wiggins, M.N., and O'Sullivan, P. (2006). Effects of presentation method on the understanding of informed consent. *British Journal of Ophthalmology*, **90**, 990–3.

57. Varnhagen, C.K., Gushta, M., Daniels, J., *et al.* (2005). How informed is online informed consent? *Ethics and Behavior*, **15**, 37–48.

58. Mishra, P.K. (2005). Detailed preoperative information-cruelty or improving quality of informed consent. *European Journal of Cardiothoracic Surgery*, **28**, 910–1, author reply 911.

59. Tobias, J.S. and Souhami, R.L. (1993). Fully informed consent can be needlessly cruel. *British Medical Journal*, **307**, 1199–201.

60. Mitchell, J. (1995). A fundamental problem of consent. *British Medical Journal*, **310**, 43–6.

61. Association of Anaesthetists of Great Britain & Ireland. (2005). *Consent for Anaesthesia*, 2nd edition. Association of Anaesthetists of Great Britain & Ireland, London.

62. Kerrigan, D.D., Thevasagayam, R.S., Woods, T.O., *et al.* (1993). Who's afraid of informed consent? *British Medical Journal*, **306**, 298–300.

63. Stanley, B.M., Walters, D.J., and Maddern, G.J. (1998). Informed consent: how much information is enough? *Australian and New Zealand Journal of Surgery*, **68**, 788–91.

64. Ghulam, A.T., Kessler, M., Bachmann, L.M., Haller, U., and Kessler, T.M. (2006). Patients' satisfaction with the preoperative informed consent procedure: a multicenter questionnaire survey in Switzerland. *Mayo Clinic Proceedings*, **81**, 307–12.

65. Paci, E., Barneschi, M.G., Miccinesi, G., Falchi, S., Metrangolo, L., and Novelli, G.P. (1999). Informed consent and patient participation in the medical encounter: a list of questions for an informed choice about the type of anaesthesia. *European Journal of Anaesthesiology*, **16**, 160–5.

Section 2

Clinical contexts for consent

Chapter 3

Obstetrics

Wendy E Scott

Pregnancy is a physiological process. In some instances, it may, however, become a pathological state. Women may choose to conceive, carry the child to term, and deliver the child. Accidental or forced conception, a wanted embryo that develops with an abnormality, or a woman's change of mind, may result in a termination of that pregnancy. Women have opportunities from conception onwards, to exercise their right to continue with the pregnancy, or to have it terminated—within the legal restriction of the Abortion Act[1] and the Human Fertilization and Embryology Act 1990[2].

Women themselves, by way of pressure groups and support groups such as the National Childbirth Trust and the Birthday Trust, or women's magazines and other media channels, are very much in the forefront of educating other women as regards opportunities and 'rights' around issues of pregnancy, labour, and delivery. This form of education has the inherent problem that it may be biased and incomplete. There is a significant swing away from hospital deliveries to home deliveries, the incidence of which is thought to be anything between 4% and 10%. Accurate information is not easily obtainable[3]. The UK government publication in 1993 entitled 'Changing Childbirth'[4] proposed greater choice for women in many aspects of their care, including the place to give birth. Obstetricians do not have professional responsibility for women who wish to have a home confinement or who wish to be delivered in a midwifery-led unit, unless subsequently referred to them. General practitioners have become less involved in maternity care. Many women never access their general practitioner during pregnancy. The midwife is the lead health professional responsible for that woman. A woman with an uncomplicated pregnancy and straightforward delivery may go through the entire pregnancy and labour without seeing an obstetrician.

Over the last few years, there has arisen, mainly from outside the medical profession, but also some within the profession, the expectation that doctors are, and should be, surplus to requirement as regards normal pregnancy, which is seen as an entirely physiological process. There has been a trend to move from a medical model to a social model of pregnancy.

When complications arise, or a woman is 'high risk' because of her own previous medical problems, she will either be under the shared care of a midwife and obstetrician or completely under the care of the obstetrician, seeing her midwife only for routine checks during the pregnancy.

Identification of women who are high-risk and the recognition of a developing complication during the pregnancy are areas that are potentially problematic. Many midwives (soon to be the majority) practising in acute maternity units, are 'direct entry', i.e. are not nurses and may have only minimal training in recognizing and looking after sick patients.

Anaesthetists are service providers for the obstetric population, providing, when requested, analgesia and anaesthesia. It can happen that the anaesthetist is presented with a woman who has not been examined by a doctor for potential medical problems. Recognition of previous medical problems, the diagnosis of developing medical problems, and the recognition of future risk are often left to midwives who may be relatively junior and totally untrained in anything except 'normality.'

3.1

An anaesthetist was requested to go to Room 9 on Labour Ward to perform an epidural on a primiparous woman. On questioning regarding allergies, it transpired the woman had a true allergy to lignocaine. Recently, she had been in an accident and her jaw was wired. The midwife had not thought it was necessary to inform the anaesthetists prior to her arriving in labour. Fortunately for everyone, the woman went on to have a normal spontaneous vaginal delivery.

This is an example of the importance of early antenatal referral of high-risk women[5]. In order that these women are referred, the problem needs to be recognized and an appropriate referral made.

An anaesthetist may be involved in the care of a pregnant woman at each and every stage from conception onwards. Indeed, the involvement may even be prior to conception, if working in areas of fertility where women are being investigated under anaesthesia for infertility problems, e.g. laparoscopy and dye, or in egg harvesting. Until conception is confirmed, the issue of consent is as for any other procedure for which the anaesthetist would be asked to give an anaesthetic.

In some hospitals, anaesthetists are asked to obtain written consent for anaesthetic procedures. Other hospitals rely on a 'tick box' protocol listing the side-effects and complications of a procedure, which the anaesthetist must mention and discuss with a woman prior to starting the procedure. Anaesthetists are obliged to follow the consent process employed by their trust or institution. The process of gaining consent should have been 'risk assessed' and deemed to be legally robust and appropriate by the organization.

Very early in their anaesthetic career, anaesthetists are required to provide anaesthesia for women who have experienced early fetal loss, i.e. who are having an evacuation of retained products of conception.

In this situation, consent for the surgery is gained by the obstetrician so unless the anaesthetist intends to use suppositories for postoperative pain relief, for which explicit permission, usually verbal, is required, the anaesthetist relies on the consent obtained by the surgeon. The anaesthetist does see and assess the woman for fitness for anaesthesia and explains the anaesthetic procedure.

However, if anaesthesia is for termination of pregnancy, issues around consent become more complicated. An anaesthetist in England and Wales has the right to refuse to give any anaesthetic care directly related to the termination procedure. The Abortion Act allows an anaesthetist to decline to anaesthetize a woman for termination of pregnancy for reasons of conscience. However, if that woman subsequently bleeds heavily as a result of the procedure, it is the duty of any anaesthetist, if asked to do so, to resuscitate and provide anaesthetic care for the woman. If a woman undergoing a late termination for fetal abnormality requests pain relief in the form of an epidural, she should receive it. In this situation, an anaesthetist can almost always be found who is prepared to provide an epidural block.

An anaesthetist who agrees to perform anaesthesia for the procedure of termination of pregnancy must ensure that all the necessary legal documents are signed by the requisite clinicians, prior to the procedure; otherwise he or she is involved in what could be construed by some as an illegal abortion.

3.2

A consultant anaesthetist was asked by a consultant obstetrician to anaesthetize a 15-year-old girl for a termination of pregnancy. The only person with her was her 15-year-old partner. The obstetrician had counselled the patient and suggested it would be a good idea for the girl to tell her parents. She refused. The obstetrician felt that the girl displayed the necessary degree of what is known as 'Gillick Competence'[6]. The consultant anaesthetist, knowing that he must not act as a technician but that he has a duty as a doctor, also saw and talked to the girl with and without her partner. He also agreed that she was mature enough to understand the issues and they respected her wishes that her parents were not informed.

The following issues need to be considered in the aforementioned situation:

- The age and level of understanding of the girl must be assessed to ascertain whether consent is truly valid. In 1985, there was a judgement by The House of Lords against Victoria Gillick. The ruling allowed a girl under the recognized age at which a person is usually considered competent, which in England and Wales is 16 years[7], to give valid consent for treatment, if the healthcare professional assessed her as being able to understand the consequences of the treatment. In this case, it allowed the girl to exercise her own choice over matters of birth control without consent or the knowledge of her mother.

- It is important to ensure that discharge is to a safe and caring environment and also to ensure that counselling and birth control are provided to try to prevent future unwanted conceptions. Matters of sexual health can also be addressed.

- If the obstetrician and anaesthetist are concerned about any aspect of the case (e.g. possible child abuse, prostitution, or whether Gillick competence is applicable), they must involve Social Services and the Trust Solicitors.
- Awareness of child protection issues is important.

Anaesthesia for incidental pathology during pregnancy, e.g. appendicitis, carries a small but increased risk to the woman. There is also an increased risk of fetal loss[8]. The physiological changes that a woman undergoes between conception and delivery increase the risks of anaesthesia. The point of maximum risk is not necessarily term but depends on the gestation of the pregnancy in relation to any underlying pathology. For example, in women with valvular heart disease, one point of potential decompensation is at 28–32 weeks' gestation due to the increase in cardiac output, which occurs at that time. For an elective procedure, that cannot or will not be postponed until after delivery, the safest time from the point of view of fetal loss is the middle trimester.

3.3

An ENT surgeon listed a woman, who was 12 weeks pregnant, for nasal surgery. She was experiencing what is one of the known 'complications' of pregnancy, namely, congested nasal passages, increasing her inability to breathe through her nose. She was snoring at night. Her partner was complaining. The anaesthetist explained to her that, although the safest time to give her an anaesthetic was during the second trimester, there was a small but recognizable risk of her losing the baby and she was suffering from a self-limiting condition, which would be likely to resolve when she was no longer pregnant.

The ENT surgeon complained to the anaesthetist that he was unnecessarily scaring the patient, that the anaesthetist was giving advice beyond his expertise, and it was the prerogative of the ENT surgeon to perform surgery when he had a gap on his operating list. The woman underwent a nasal polypectomy in the middle trimester without any problems to her or the baby.

There are a number of issues to consider in this situation.

- It is the duty of every doctor involved in the care of a pregnant woman to give all the necessary information in order that she can exercise her choice in full knowledge and understanding of all the facts. Ideally, specialists should confine themselves to a discussion about risks specific to their specialty, but if appropriate information has been omitted by the surgeon, and an anaesthetist is to be involved in the procedure, the anaesthetist has a duty to provide the missing information if competent to do so.
- If the anaesthetist feels that the patient does not have all the necessary information but that he or she is unable to advise on the risks of surgery, then the anaesthetist should make arrangements for the surgeon to do so; a meeting between the surgeon, anaesthetist, and patient may be the best way of resolving the problem.

- All risks, benefits, and alternative options should be discussed with the woman and documentation of the discussion written in the notes. Mention should be made of the risk to the fetus. The consent form, if she agrees to proceed, should also mention what was discussed.
- A decision to proceed rests entirely with the patient. It is often appropriate to discuss matters with her partner, but the partner has no right to contradict her decision.
- The woman's midwife or obstetrician should be informed of the proposed operation (if it is an emergency procedure, the duty obstetrician should be informed) and advice sought with regards to pregnancy issues. A midwife should listen for the fetal heart pre- and postoperatively, and it may be appropriate to arrange a scan after the procedure to ensure the ongoing viability of the fetus.
- The anaesthetist should give the safest anaesthetic, avoiding drugs that are contraindicated in pregnancy, and being aware that there are potentially two patients to consider.

The anaesthetist who is asked to provide epidural analgesia during labour, whether for a woman under midwifery-led care or under the care of an obstetrician, is often placed in a difficult situation, because this may be the first time that the woman has met an anaesthetist. Ideally, during her antenatal care, the woman will have received information about all methods of pain relief that will be available to her when she is in labour so that she has time to consider the information and make a choice based on written information sheets or discussions with an unbiased professional, through an interpreter if necessary.

How can the anaesthetist ensure that the necessary written information is given, that it is in an intelligible form, and that it is read and understood by the woman? The obstetric anaesthetists in an anaesthetic department must take ownership of the written information, should ensure that written information is in language appropriate to the reader, and should take steps to ensure that, if the woman cannot read it, the information is explained to her. They should also ensure that information divulged by other staff, for example, by midwives, is accurate and unbiased.

Information about epidural block must be provided at some time during the antenatal period. Written information is often handed out by a midwife in leaflet form some time after 20 weeks' gestation. Women are deluged with information, and often the leaflet on pain relief in labour is overlooked or lost. Antenatal classes are frequently not offered, but if they are, women do not always attend. In many places, and for a variety of reasons, anaesthetists no longer have the opportunity to be involved in the antenatal education of women. This means that the reality is that an anaesthetist is often faced with trying to explain serious and potentially life-threatening complications of a procedure that is non-therapeutic and non-diagnostic (when used only for analgesia in labour) to a woman writhing in pain who may well be under the influence of pethidine or another opioid analgesic. It is a situation that is less than ideal.

Midwives, in their desire to encourage birth to be a normal physiological process, may not always explain the pros and cons of epidurals in an unbiased manner. Instead of giving women increased choice, midwives may effectively be denying women what is the most effective form of pain relief.

To gain legal consent for a procedure, the law states that a person needs to have capacity. There is a potential anomaly in pregnancy. It is usually the case that, to gain consent from a non-pregnant individual, the patient must not be under the influence of opioid analgesics, or in distress, when information is given and consent taken. Women giving consent in labour have often been given an opioid analgesic, and may be in pain and distress. It can be difficult, especially where there are language difficulties, to gauge the knowledge and understanding of the woman. Under a ruling by the then Lady Butler-Sloss, a woman in labour is deemed competent not only to give consent to the major operation of Caesarean section but is also considered competent to refuse to have a Caesarean section even if her life and that of the baby are at risk[9]. There was no concession with regard to the woman having been given opioid analgesics. It could constitute civil or criminal assault if an anaesthetist and obstetrician were to force a woman to have a procedure for which she had not given consent.

The Court of Appeal in Re MB (1997) 2 FLR 426 stated as follows:

> A person lacks capacity if some impairment or disturbance of mental functioning renders the person unable to make a decision whether to consent to or refuse treatment. That will occur when:
>
> (a) The patient is unable to comprehend and retain information which is material to the decision, especially as to the likely consequences of having or not having the treatment in question
>
> (b) The patient is unable to use the information and weigh it in the balance as part of the process of arriving at the decision

While a competent woman has an absolute right to refuse any intervention irrespective of the potential outcome, a pregnant woman may be considered to lack capacity if she has a proven mental disorder in which capacity is lacking, but not just because she suffers from a mental disorder *per se*. The 1997 ruling also declares that if someone is in great pain, their judgement may be impaired to such an extent that capacity is lacking. The extent of pain required for this to be considered in an obstetric context has yet to be determined. Clearly, if a patient is unconscious or heavily sedated, capacity is at least temporarily lost. The procedure can be carried out in the patient's 'best interest' ideally with the agreement of a multidisciplinary team including the Trust legal advisers.

A woman can refuse to have an intravenous cannula inserted. To force her would be an assault; to leave her could result in her own death and/or the death of her baby. A woman who is mentally competent and who refuses to take advice must take ownership of her decisions. To make these decisions, she must be in possession of all the facts. The key things to remember, should such a situation arise, are that an attempt should be made to obtain a unanimous consensus of all heath professionals involved in her care and there should be careful documentation of the difficulties that are being encountered. Ideally, the woman should countersign the notes. The Trust's legal advisers should be contacted for advice, and kept abreast of the developing situation. It is also advisable to seek legal advice where there is time over a woman with presumed lack of capacity when a Caesarean is about to be performed where no valid consent can be obtained.

3.4

A primiparous woman presented in labour with her birth plan. It clearly stated that she was not to be given an epidural block at any point. She said that, even if she said in labour that she had changed her mind and was begging to be given an epidural, she must not have one. She was a lawyer. The ensuing labour was much more painful than she imagined possible. She requested an epidural block. The midwife and anaesthetist refused. She begged to be given one. The anaesthetist was worried that, once she was home, she would forget the severity of the pain and perceiving herself, in retrospect, to have been a failure in succumbing to having an epidural, sue the anaesthetist. She could, after all, produce the bit of paper written prior to labour, explicitly stating that she had said that she was not to be given an epidural block. In full view of the anaesthetist and midwife, the woman tore up her birth plan and told the anaesthetist to proceed. He did.

There are a number of issues to consider in this situation.

- If a woman changes her mind, and there is an extant birth plan, which clearly states she does not want to have epidural analgesia, some anaesthetists will decline to give an epidural block, saying she had exercised her prerogative of having choice and had stated she did not want to be given an epidural block. A pragmatic way around this, if asked to perform an epidural block in such a situation, is for the anaesthetist to speak to the woman and ascertain that there has been a genuine change of mind. The anaesthetist can ask the midwife whether, in her professional opinion, there has been a genuine change of mind and, if so, to document that fact in the notes, after which the anaesthetist can also write in the notes. If the obstetrician has been involved, perhaps encouraging an epidural block for obstetric reasons, then the obstetrician should also document the fact that the woman has agreed to be given an epidural block despite her birth plan. The woman herself can be asked to sign or initial the notes to the effect she has changed her mind. It is advisable that the anaesthetist has supporting documentation prior to performing the epidural block.

- Women should be allowed to change their minds and that change of mind should be acknowledged as genuine. Women, especially primiparous women, do not know how they will react to pain until they are experiencing it. Consequently, the moment of true informed consent could be construed as that moment in labour when they are feeling the pain[10].

- Birth Plans are not the same as Advanced Directives but are an indicator of a woman's wishes.

The situation in which a woman requests to have a Caesarean section for no medical reason is dealt with differently in different hospitals. Her reasons for such a request could be fear of labour, a desire not to risk the complication of stress incontinence, or for social reasons such as her partner being home briefly on leave from his job, or the organization of care for other children. Some NHS obstetricians can be persuaded in specific cases to perform an elective Caesarean section for social reasons but some refuse. It is the right of the woman to ask to be referred to another obstetrician, and the duty of the obstetrician to refer her to one, who may, or may not, consider her request favourably.

Women receiving private obstetric care should receive the same standard of clinical care as a woman under NHS care and may equally express a wish to have an elective Caesarean section. Wherever she chooses to deliver, the woman must be told in an unbiased manner the respective advantages, disadvantages, side-effects, and complications of both vaginal and operative delivery. She would have to accept that any non-negligent side-effect or complication that ensued was a result of her exercising her choice. With 'rights' come responsibilities.

An anaesthetist asked to anaesthetize a woman for an operation that is not medically necessary is placed in a difficult situation. Trainees may be placed in a particularly invidious position. If it is an elective procedure and the anaesthetist considers the operation not to be in the woman's best interests, the anaesthetist may wish to exercise his or her right to refuse. He or she is obliged to refer to another anaesthetist, who may or may not adopt a similar position.

There is always pressure on both anaesthetist and obstetrician when they have declined a woman her request of mode of delivery, and complications arise. A woman who has been denied her request and who goes on to suffer complications and side-effects from the mode of delivery that she did not want may make a complaint or may try to sue the obstetrician and anaesthetist. The fact that women have been empowered to exercise choice makes the obstetrician more inclined to grant her request. She is then less likely to be unhappy with her birth experience and will have less legitimate grounds for complaint if there is a complication, provided, of course, that there has been no negligence.

3.5

An anaesthetist was called to attend a 19-year-old woman in labour. She was a primiparous patient who was at term+5. Her cervix was 6 cm dilated. She had previously been under midwifery-led care. There was fetal distress. The obstetricians were in the room and said that there was profound fetal bradycardia and that the woman must have a Caesarean section immediately. Together with the midwives, they were wheeling the bed to the operating theatre. Her 20-year-old partner was very worried and asking what was going on. An obstetrician held a form in front of the woman and asked her to sign it. She refused. The obstetricians were shouting at everyone to hurry up. She arrived in theatre still not having signed the form. She continued to refuse to sign it. She would not let the anaesthetist insert an intravenous cannula and kept withdrawing her hand. The obstetrician was trying to hold her arm out forcibly so that the anaesthetist could insert an intravenous cannula. The midwife was saying that the fetal heart was still very slow. The obstetrician shouted louder, this time at the anaesthetist. The partner said he

3.5 *(continued)*

would sign the form for her. 'It is, after all, my baby too,' he said. The anaesthetist asked everyone to leave the vicinity or step back. He spoke to the woman who, despite his calming words and quiet explanation, still refused Caesarean section. The obstetrician tried again, with the same result. No Caesarean section was performed. The baby died.

This illustrates many points.

- Although approximately one in five women who give birth in England and Wales do so by Caesarean section, this lady was considered 'low risk' and was under midwifery-led care. The fact that she might require a Caesarean section, although always a possibility, had not been seriously considered and she was not psychologically prepared for such an eventuality.

- Consent, at least in the first instance verbal, should have been obtained in the delivery room prior to transferring her to theatre. Written consent is not strictly necessary but is considered good practice.

- Professionals who become outwardly distressed and start shouting are exhibiting behaviour that constitutes verbal assault.

- By holding her hand in *any* form of restraint, the obstetrician could be committing an assault which is against civil law and may be a criminal offence.

- The woman is the only person who can give consent.

- The partner has no legal rights concerning anything done to the mother even for the sake of the baby.

- The mother has total autonomy to refuse treatment and the baby *in utero* has limited legal rights.

- A child, if damaged, may subsequently bring an action against the mother for what happened when the child was *in utero*, for example, a child who suffers from cerebral palsy as a result of the choice made by the mother over mode of delivery may make a claim. The Civil Liability Act 1978 allows a child to bring a case against the mother if damage to the child was caused *in utero* by the mother's negligent actions.

- Information was given to the woman and the consequences of her decision made clear. She exercised her choice.

High-profile cases, like that of MB, have drawn the attention of the risks of not identifying in the antenatal period those women who are needle-phobic and arranging or not arranging either hypnotherapy or other counselling[5,9].

To state the obvious, by the time an anaesthetist sees an obstetric patient, she is already pregnant. It is extremely rare that a woman who is not pregnant is referred to see an anaesthetist to ascertain whether analgesia or anaesthesia may prove to be a problem during pregnancy. Preconception counselling is invariably the remit of the obstetrician or geneticist.

3.6

A single 23-year-old Para 1+2 was referred to the obstetric anaesthetists at 10 weeks' gestation. Her first pregnancy, from which she now had a 7-year-old child, had been when she was 16 years old. It had been a difficult pregnancy, with an early threatened abortion and bleeding at 20 weeks. During the pregnancy, a cardiac murmur had been diagnosed and a cardiology opinion was sought. An echocardiogram revealed moderate mitral stenosis with minimal regurgitation. There was mild pulmonary hypertension. She had gone into spontaneous labour at 32 weeks, delivering a small-for-dates baby who required artificial ventilation for a period and was nursed for five weeks in the Neonatal Intensive Care Unit. The child is profoundly deaf and has learning difficulties. The woman's condition improved post-partum and she was followed up by the cardiologists. She was advised that there was a risk to her life if she became pregnant again.

Two years later, she presented at 8 weeks' gestation. It was agreed by all parties that it was in the woman's best interests that the pregnancy be terminated. She had a surgical termination of pregnancy with no problems.

Six months later, she became pregnant again. She said that she felt guilty about agreeing to her termination on the previous occasion and would proceed with the pregnancy. She was monitored closely by the obstetrician and cardiologist. She was becoming increasingly breathless. She aborted the fetus at 18 weeks' gestation.

Having found a new and steady partner who had no children, she decided, against medical advice, to risk a further pregnancy. When seen by the anaesthetists at 12 weeks' gestation, she was already complaining of being very tired. She had a high BMI so she attributed her tiredness to being overweight and to the weather. The anaesthetists, obstetrician, and cardiologist held a multidisciplinary meeting to consider options and to plan how she should be managed through her pregnancy. She was determined to go on with the pregnancy. A repeat echocardiogram showed a marked deterioration and her pulmonary hypertension was much more severe.

She was seen weekly by the obstetrician, who was concerned by the lack of fetal growth. She required admission to hospital at 18 weeks' gestation because of increasing breathlessness and generally feeling unwell. She was advised that she should go to the tertiary centre. She refused as she was worried about her other child and it was a little distance away for people to visit.

She discharged herself after one week, to be readmitted with tightenings at 28 weeks' gestation. She was extremely dyspnoeic and her oxygen saturation on air was 89%. The safest thing was to allow her to go on and deliver with an epidural block using a low concentration of local anaesthetic with a high dose of opioid analgesic. Oxygen was given by a face mask. Fluid balance was strictly monitored.

She delivered a stillborn fetus. Syntocinon was given very slowly and was diluted twice. The auto-transfusion post-partum proved too great a stress to her already compromised circulation and she developed pulmonary oedema. Her trachea was intubated and her lungs were ventilated artificially in the Intensive Care Unit. Attempts were made to transfer her to a cardiac unit. She was too unstable, and died 12 hours after delivery.

Women who, 20 or 30 years ago, would have been told by the medical profession not to become pregnant because it would be an unacceptable risk to their own health are now exercising their choice and becoming pregnant.

The issues to consider here are as follows:

- The biological desire to procreate may be so strong in a woman that she will exercise her choice to become pregnant even if it puts her own life at risk.

- Anaesthetists are being presented with an increasing number of pregnant women who have cardiac problems, as some women are waiting until they are older to have children and are therefore potential sufferers from ischaemic heart disease. Women who had cardiac anomalies corrected at birth may decide that they will risk pregnancy. These are truly high-risk pregnancies.

- These women are a huge challenge to all the doctors and midwives involved and are an increased financial cost to the service.

- The first child was premature almost certainly because of the mother's pathology. The mother was prepared to risk not only her own life but also the possibility of having another child with potential pathology related to prematurity. That child might need a lifetime of care.

- Women who have one termination not infrequently become pregnant again soon after the termination. This is likely to be related to feelings of guilt.

- Referral to a tertiary unit would have been the optimal management. Hospitals which deal with greater numbers of more specialized cases build up collective experience and expertise.

- Good multidisciplinary management was provided throughout and all specialists communicated well to optimize her management.

- The decision had to be made about delivering the baby by Caesarean section or allowing her to have a vaginal delivery. She was unfit for a general anaesthetic. When regional anaesthesia is given in the presence of pulmonary hypertension, the anaesthetic has to be given very carefully to avoid hypotension.

- Drugs used in active management of the third stage can be dangerous in patients with cardiac disease and must be given slowly and in dilute form—if given at all. Ergometrine should be avoided[11,12]. A passive third stage risks post-partum haemorrhage.

- Cardiac disease is the second most common cause of maternal mortality[13].

- The fact that the woman became pregnant against advice, and chose to continue with the pregnancy against advice, does not allow the medical profession or the midwives to offer substandard care in any way and does not exonerate them from providing anything other than good practice in this situation. This woman put huge pressure on resources, namely time, expertise, and facilities. She exercised her choice which everyone, within the framework she dictated, respected. Unfortunately she paid the ultimate price for her decision, leaving a deaf child with learning difficulties to be looked after by foster parents.

- There is an increasing number of parturients who have a high body mass index (BMI). These women are at significant risk and present a huge challenge to midwives and medical staff.

3.7

A 22-year-old primiparous woman who had been referred to the obstetric anaesthetists at the time of booking, but who had failed to attend for either of the two appointments that had been offered to her, demanded to be given an epidural when she was admitted to the labour ward. She was Term +10. The reason for her original referral was that her BMI was 55. She weighed 145 kg, and she had a past history of backache. She had reluctantly agreed to induction of labour.

The first time that an anaesthetist saw this woman was on labour ward. She appeared to know nothing about what an epidural involved, she had not read the leaflet on pain relief in labour and was not listening to the anaesthetist telling her about the risks and complications. The anaesthetist asked the midwife to help to explain to the woman what was involved. The anaesthetist was not sure whether to proceed as he was not sure that the woman understood the risks and complications. The woman was becoming more distressed as the infusion rate of syntocinon was increased. The woman's mother, her birth partner, asked the anaesthetist to 'just get on with it'. The anaesthetist was not sure of the validity of the consent and asked the woman if she really did want to be given an epidural. Receiving just a nod, he proceeded.

It was a difficult epidural. The anaesthetist had to send to the operating theatre for a long Tuohy needle. He was unsuccessful. He called the consultant anaesthetist for assistance. The woman and her mother were getting angry. Eventually, the consultant managed to perform the epidural but the woman developed a unilateral block. Both anaesthetists tried all known manoeuvres to try to get an equal block, short of re-siting the epidural. They were unsuccessful. It was decided that she should use Entonox to help to provide pain relief.

The patient's cervix was 7 cm dilated when there was fetal distress. No one had told the operating theatre staff that she was over 135kg, the upper weight level for the operating table. The obstetricians said that there was no time to send to General Theatres for the table designed for people over 135 kg. The anaesthetists felt that it would be difficult to intubate her trachea and were reluctant to perform a general anaesthetic. She was demanding to be given a general anaesthetic. The obstetricians were impatient.

Because the epidural was unilateral, it was difficult to sit her up, so the decision was made to turn her on her side and try to insert a spinal needle and give a smaller dose as there was already some local anaesthetic in the epidural space and there was the risk of a high block. After much persuasion, she did turn on her side, when requested to do so, and a long spinal needle was inserted; a dose of 1.6 ml of hyperbaric bupivacaine was injected. The block was tested to T6 bilaterally to touch and T4 bilaterally to cold, and thought to be adequate. There was a good motor block.

After delivery of a 2,800-g baby with Apgar Scores of 7 at 1 min and 9 at 5 min, she said she had pain. Fentanyl was given. However, it was obvious that the degree of pain was unacceptable. She requested to be given a general anaesthetic. General anaesthesia was induced, but the anaesthetist could not insert an endotracheal tube.

3.7 *(continued)*

A failed intubation drill was instituted and fortunately a laryngeal mask could be inserted, through which her lungs could be ventilated. Although it was difficult for the surgeons to work when the suxamethonium wore off, because the abdomen rose and fell with respiration, oxygenation could be maintained with saturations about 92% and the operation was completed successfully.

Points for consideration are as follows:

- Obstetric anaesthetists are frequently confronted on the day of delivery with situations that have potential implications for patient safety. Ideally, an antenatal referral to the obstetric anaesthetists allows the woman to be seen, a plan made and documented, and the necessary equipment made available when the woman is admitted in labour. The obstetricians correctly referred her but the woman did not attend.

- There is always the risk that, if a woman suffers from a complication of a procedure such as an epidural, she claims afterwards that she had not been informed. Good documentation minimizes the consequences of that risk.

- It is important to tell women that, if they have had backache in the antenatal period, they are likely to have it after the delivery. Long-term postnatal backache is not likely to be due to the epidural[14].

- The anaesthetist proceeded because the woman was requesting an epidural, and the anaesthetist felt that, although the situation was not ideal, she had been told of the risks. There was doubt as to whether she totally understood all the risks. The anaesthetist had quite correctly documented that he had told her of the benefits, side-effects, and complications. For all elective and emergency procedures, a full list of all benefits, side-effects, and complications needs to be discussed with a woman, ideally before she is in pain and too distressed. Documentation of this discussion, timed, dated, and signed, should be written in the notes or on the anaesthetic chart.

- Equipment such as a long epidural needle was not readily available. This made an already difficult situation worse. Ensure before starting a procedure that the any necessary equipment is available.

- The anaesthetist was correct to call the consultant but maybe should have called for help earlier.

- As soon as the woman was admitted on to labour ward, operating theatre staff should have been informed so that a suitable operating table could be standing by in case operative delivery became necessary. If the midwives had not done this, then as soon as the anaesthetists were aware of her presence on labour ward, they, too, should have informed the operating theatre staff. There has been a claim when a parturient with a high BMI fell off an operating table which was not insured to carry a person of her weight.

- Although this epidural had been difficult, it may be argued that, as it had been recognized that it might be difficult to intubate her trachea, it would have been more appropriate to have tried to re-site the epidural when it was found to be providing a unilateral block, in case she required a Caesarean section. An inadequate epidural for labour will almost certainly be an inadequate epidural for an operative delivery. There are risks in inserting a spinal block when there is already local anaesthetic in the epidural space. In particular, there is a risk of a high block[15]. The anaesthetist did not want the complication of a high block as he did not want to have to try to intubate her trachea, so erred on the safe side by giving a small dose, which proved to be too small.

- The obstetricians were quite correctly concerned about the baby. Sometimes, however, they need reminding that the mother's safety and life come before those of the baby. It is unhelpful when they harass the anaesthetist, especially a trainee, in such a situation.

- The patient had been told that the block might not be adequate and there was the possibility of her requiring a general anaesthetic. The anaesthetist had tested the block with the different modalities of touch, pin-prick, and cold in an acceptable manner[16].

- The failed intubation drill was instituted and allowed the operation to continue, albeit with some difficulty, but ultimately with a successful outcome.

- Most of these problems were due to her high BMI. There is an urgent need for education, as obesity is already a serious problem. Not only are morbidity and mortality increased, but a woman with a high BMI puts a great strain on resources and challenges the skills of healthcare providers. A raised BMI in the non-pregnant population increases anaesthetic risk[17]. When the woman is pregnant, that risk is increased substantially[18,19].

- The Royal College of Obstetricians and Gynaecologists recommends that anaesthetists are notified of pregnant women whose BMI is over 35. In most hospitals in the United Kingdom, there are too many women in that category for the anaesthetists to see before admission to the labour ward.

Obstetric anaesthesia is a minefield for the uninitiated.

In summary

- A woman's choice has to be respected.

- Before consent for a procedure can be considered valid, it is vital to ensure that women have the necessary information and that they understand it.

- Good communications between midwife, obstetrician, and anaesthetist are essential.

- When there are high-risk women, the involvement of other medical professionals helps to improve outcome for both mother and child.

- Exchange of information is sometimes necessary with Social Services and the Trust solicitor.

References

1. The Abortion Act (1967).
2. Section 37, Human Fertilisation and Embryology Act (1990) (HFEA).
3. The Information Centre, Community Health Statistics. (2006). (www.ic.nhs.uk).
4. 'Changing Childbirth'. (1993). Government Report of Expert Maternity Group, Department of Health, London.
5. Cooper, G. M. and McClure, J. (2004). Anaesthesia. Why Mothers Die 2000–2002. Report on Confidential Enquiries into Maternal Deaths in the United Kingdom, p. 122. Royal College of Obstetricians & Gynaecologists, London.
6. *Gillick v. Norfolk and Wisbech Area Health Authority and another* (1985).
7. Family Law Reform Act (1969).
8. Kuczkowski, K.M. (2006). The safety of anaesthesia in pregnant women. *Expert Opinion on Drug Safety*, **5**(2), 251–64.
9. MB (Caesarean Section), *Re* (1997) 2 F.L.R. 426.
10. Scott, W. (1996). Ethics in obstetric anaesthesia. *Anaesthesia* **51**, 717–8.
11. Hart, K. (2006). Management of third stage of labour. *RCM Midwives*, **9.4**, 148.
12. Stevenson, J. (2005). The Bristol third–stage trial. *Midwifery Today International Midwife*, **73**, 41–3.
13. Malhotra, S. and Yentis, S.M. (2006). Reports on Confidential Enquiries into Maternal Deaths: management strategies based on trends in maternal cardiac deaths over 30years. *International Journal of Obstetric Anesthesia*, **15**, 223–6.
14. Russell, R., Dundas, R., and Reynolds, F. (1996). Long term backache after childbirth: prospective search for causative factors. *British Medical Journal*, **312**, 1384–8.
15. Gupta, A. (1996). Spinal anesthesia after failed epidural anesthesia. *Anesthesia and Analgesia*, **82**, 214–5.
16. Russell, I. F. (2004). A comparison of cold, pinprick and touch for assessing the level of spinal block at caesarean section. *International Journal of Obstetric Anesthesia*, **13**, 146–152.
17. Sjöstom, L. V. (1992). Mortality of severely obese subjects. *American Journal of Clinical Nutrition*, **55**, 216S-532S.
18. Hood, D. D. and Devan, D.M. (1993). Anesthetic and obstetric outcome in markedly obese parturients. *Anesthesiology*, **79**, 1212.
19. Rocke, D. A., Murray, W. B., Rant, C. P., *et al.* (1992). Relative risk analysis of factors associated with difficult intubation in obstetric anesthesia. *Anesthesiology*, **77**, 37.

Chapter 4

Emergency surgery

Bernard Riley

The National Confidential Enquiry into Perioperative Deaths (NCEPOD) published a report in 1997 in which emergency patients were defined as: '*Patients whose visit to the operating theatre was not foreseen but takes place as a result of illness or a complication requiring an urgent operation. These cases may have been admitted to hospital either electively or as emergencies. The operation may take place during an operating session scheduled primarily for elective surgery, scheduled primarily for emergencies, or in unscheduled sessions used for specific theatre cases, usually at short notice*'[1]. This report retrospectively examined the deaths of emergency patients following operations performed 'out of hours', i.e. between 18.01 h and midnight (evening) or midnight and 07.59 h (night-time), or operations performed on a Saturday, Sunday, or public holiday. The 1997 report was undertaken because previous NCEPOD studies had indicated that there appeared to be a disturbing number of deaths following operations performed out of hours. An analysis of over 50 000 cases in 355 NHS hospitals in 1995 and 1996 found that only 6.1% of weekday operations in the NHS were done out of hours but 93.4% of these were emergencies. Many of these procedures were carried out by trainee anaesthetists and surgeons, apparently without direct supervision. A total of 508 deaths were identified, of which 208 and 310 were subjected to detailed analysis of anaesthesia and surgery respectively. Seventy-one per cent of the deaths occurred following emergency admission, and co-morbidity was common, with 82% of patients classed as ASA grade 3 or higher. The report highlighted lack of preoperative preparation, low use of preoperative fluid resuscitation, infrequent objective assessment of cardiovascular function, and poor prophylaxis against thrombo-embolism. Suboptimal standards of care included delays in surgery, too junior levels of staff, poor interspeciality communication, and inappropriate operative procedures.

The finding of increased mortality in emergency surgical patients is not simply a British phenomenon. The Western Australian Audit of Surgical Mortality (WAASM) was established in 2001 to peer review all surgery-related deaths in Western Australia (WA)[2]. There were 876 deaths over 18 months; 669 (76%) followed an emergency admission, compared with 207(24%) following an elective admission. Interestingly, the proportion of deaths in which a deficiency of care was identified was significantly higher in elective admissions (67/207; 32%) when compared with emergency admissions (112/669; 17%). The risk of deficiency of care was 1.9 times higher in elective admissions than in emergency admissions.

Consent and emergency surgery

Although the increased risk of death or morbidity from emergency surgery *per se* is well documented, it is difficult to be certain that this is appreciated by either the patients or their relatives. If an emergency procedure is required on an unconscious patient, e.g. emergency decompressive craniotomy for intra-cranial bleeding, then there is no possibility of patient consent being obtained and, regardless of patient confidentiality issues, it would seem prudent to describe the planned procedures and the range of outcomes possible to the relatives. The relatives may be too distressed or preoccupied to understand a detailed prediction of outcome and in English law can give only their assent, rather than consent, unless appointed as a donee under the terms of the Mental Capacity Act 2005 (see Chapter 1). The ability to give consent may be considered to be dependent on various inter-related factors. (Box 4.1)

Box 4.1

Capacity—the ability/capacity to understand the information delivered
Disclosure—giving all the relevant facts
Comprehension—the individual must believe the facts and understand the options open to him
Self volition—the decision of the individual reached without coercion
Reflection—*appropriate* time to think about the decision and its implications

---

This paradigm poses particular problems in the emergency surgical patient. An unconscious patient is an obvious example in which there is no possibility of going through this process. However, in situations requiring emergency surgery, even where consciousness is preserved, the expectation that a patient will be able to perform these steps is flawed. Capacity and comprehension may be diminished by the effects of hypotension, hypoxaemia, hypercapnia, hypoglycaemia, hyperglycaemia, and the effects of analgesic drugs when present either singly or in combination on the brain function of the patient. All these factors may reduce the patients' ability to understand, believe, and retain information upon which they are expected to give informed consent. It is debatable whether such patients can be truly regarded as mentally competent. The law, however, is clear, with competency being assumed in all adults unless proven otherwise, and patients, thus have the right to refuse even life-saving emergency surgery or anaesthetic intervention should they so wish.

The very nature of the underlying problem and its description may cause problems, e.g. 'You have a ruptured abdominal aortic aneurysm and if we don't operate you will die'. Even allowing for an inability to understand medical jargon, the urgency of the situation certainly gives little or no time for reflection and could appear coercive. The time for detailed explanations to patients and relatives and the duration of resuscitation prior to surgery are also influenced by the urgency of the requirement for operation. The most commonly used descriptor for this urgency in the United Kingdom is the

Confidential Enquiry into Perioperative Deaths (CEPOD) Classification, and, in this chapter, 'emergency' surgery will be used to cover the following:

CEPOD 1 Emergency surgery within 1 h to save life or limb, e.g. ruptured abdominal aortic aneurysm

CEPOD 2 Urgent surgery within 24 h, e.g. limb fractures, bowel obstruction

Other components of the consent process aside, a patient with a CEPOD 1 emergency has less time to reach a conclusion compared to one with a CEPOD 2 condition.

Perhaps the most difficult component of the consent process is ensuring that the doctor gives all the relevant information to the patient. Should all risks, no matter how small, be described, or simply the more common risks? What constitutes low and high risk statistically may be of no interest to the patient or the relatives. The risk of death certainly is of interest. The difficulty in terms of the *Disclosure* component of the consent process described earlier in relation to emergency surgery is that precision in predicting death is very difficult to achieve. Furthermore, appropriate disclosure also necessitates communication of the risks associated with conservative treatment. It is certainly not always the case that choosing against surgery is guaranteed to mean loss of life, limb, or function.

While there may be common contributory factors to the increased risk of death in emergency over elective procedures, the magnitude of risk is to a large extent a function of the underlying disease process and the physical status of the patient. The most widely used categorization of physical status is the American Society of Anesthesiologists (ASA) grading system. There are five categories:

I Healthy patient

II Mild systemic disease with no functional impairment

III Moderate systemic disease, definite functional limitation

IV Severe systemic disease that is a constant threat to life

V Moribund patient, not likely to survive 24 h with or without operation

The addition of the postscript E indicates emergency surgery, e.g. ASA III E. The higher the ASA grade, the greater is the likelihood of perioperative mortality. The problem with the system is that it is open to subjective interpretation of clinical signs, with different anaesthetists allocating different scores to the same patient. This system of predicting risk of death is not sensitive or specific enough to be of use in quantifying risk for an individual patient. Other scoring systems have been developed in an attempt to make risk prediction more objective by basing the prediction on measured parameters. Broadly speaking, the greater the degree of variation from the normal range of physiological parameters, the sicker the patient and the greater the likelihood of death. Examples of such scoring systems include the Acute Physiology and Chronic Health Evaluation II (APACHE II) and the Physiological and Operative Severity for the eNumeration of Mortality and morbidity (POSSUM) scores[3]. The APACHE score (see appendix for descriptions of current severity scoring systems) is essentially an epidemiological tool for the critical care setting, which enables comparison of standardized mortality ratios between individual intensive care units (ICUs); it is not intended as a predictor of death for an individual patient. It has not been validated in the emergency surgical setting. Scoring systems such as POSSUM (see appendix for descriptions of current severity scoring systems) are directed mainly at surgical practice in that as well as physiological derangement. POSSUM takes the nature and complexity of the surgical procedure into account, together with intra-operative complications such as severe haemorrhage. Once again, POSSUM and its derivatives have been developed as audit tools for comparison of surgical unit performance rather than as predictive indices of an individual patient's risk of death. Both scoring systems are cumbersome and often involve the need to obtain results that would not form part of routine preoperative preparation. Furthermore, POSSUM requires data from the intra- and postoperative periods (such as blood loss, and return to theatre)and therefore cannot be used to describe preoperative risk directly. Despite these drawbacks, many surgical specialities now collect data for both APACHE II and POSSUM scoring and use the scores as part of individual risk assessment. More recently, Donati and colleagues[4] have described a relatively simple scoring system based on age, ASA grade, severity of surgery, and urgency of surgery,which performs as well as the more complex POSSUM system (see appendix for descriptions of current severity scoring systems) However, like most scoring systems, it has only a small number of patients in the high-risk groups; so the risks it provides are inevitably only estimates rather than concrete values.

Although the patients are ultimately giving consent to surgery, and 'formal consent' is therefore taken by the surgeon, many anaesthetists find themselves providing the information relevant to consent either for the surgeon or the patient and his or her family. Despite the relatively low risk of anaesthesia *per se*, the ultimate question still seems to remain: Is this patient 'fit for anaesthesia?' In order to answer this question honestly, anaesthetists must have some awareness of the significant risks faced by their patients.

Specific operative risk

There is a wide range of emergency surgery carried out from the relatively simple to the very complex. This section deals with some of the more common high-risk surgical procedures and aims to provide data on operative risk founded on accurate methodology. For these high-risk situations, various groups have attempted to provide specific scoring or prediction systems.

Ruptured abdominal aortic aneurysm

Factors affecting survival and mortality rate of patients who present with ruptured abdominal aortic aneurysms (RAAAs) have been studied extensively because the condition remains a relatively common life-threatening surgical emergency. In one study, the operative mortality of 84 patients at a small hospital during the period 1988 to 2003 was compared to the same hospital's results during 1983 to 1987. Overall mortality significantly decreased between the two time periods (62% to 44%). The mortality rate specifically associated with a free intraperitoneal rupture decreased significantly (97% to 63%), whereas mortality for those with retroperitoneal rupture was relatively unchanged. Patients at increased risk in the more recent series were those aged >70 years with a preoperative haemoglobin concentration of <10 g/dl, preoperative haematocrit of <0.28, and an initial emergency department systolic blood pressure of <120 mmHg. Type of rupture and preoperative haemoglobin concentration were the two factors most significantly associated with death[5].

While a small number of patents undergoing emergency surgery for repair of RAAA die during surgery of uncontrollable intra-operative haemorrhage or cardiac arrest, the majority survive to reach the ICU. Most of those who die in the ICU do so as the result of multiple organ failure. A retrospective study in the ICU of a Finnish university hospital to identify predictive factors for 30-day mortality after 48 h of maximal treatment in ICU after repair of RAAA between 1999 and 2003 reviewed 197 patients admitted as emergencies due to RAAA, of whom 138 survived for at least 48 h. Logistic regression analysis was used in an attempt to identify factors predictive of 30-day mortality. Thirty-day mortality of all RAAA patients was 46% (87/197), whereas the 30-day mortality for those survived for 48 h was 22% (31/138). Only organ dysfunction by Sequential Organ Failure Assessment (SOFA)score at 48 h, preoperative Glasgow Aneurysm Score, and suprarenal clamping during operation were independent predictors of death[6]. In the largest UK series, prospective postoperative APACHE II data were collected from patients undergoing AAA repair over a 9-year interval from 24 ICUs in the Thames region. A multilevel logistic regression model (APACHE-AAA) for in-hospital mortality was developed to adjust for both case mix and the variation in outcome between ICUs. A total of 1896 patients were studied, of whom 605 had an emergency repair. The in-hospital mortality was 46.9%. Four independent predictors of death were identified: age (odds ratio (OR) 1.05 per year increase), Acute Physiology Score (OR 1.14 per unit increase), emergency operation (OR 4.86), and chronic health dysfunction (OR 1.43). This study concluded that the APACHE II score seems to be to be an accurate risk-stratification model that could be used to quantify the risk of death after emergency AAA surgery[7].

The most recent advance in the emergency management of RAAA has been the introduction of endovascular aortic aneurysm repair (EVAR), which has been shown to offer decreased morbidity and mortality in elective repair. Although definitive studies regarding its use in emergencies are not yet available, early reports suggest that there may be no benefit of EVAR in ruptured aneurysm over conventional open approaches[8].

Cervical spine surgery

Acute cervical spinal cord compression is a major threat to life primarily as a result of rapid-onset respiratory failure. It may occur as a result of trauma, infection, myelopathy, atlanto-axial dislocation, and intramedullary or extramedullary tumour growth. Emergency surgery is often complex and prolonged, no more so than when combined anterior–posterior cervical spine surgery (CAP-CS) is required to deal with the underlying pathology. In addition to the risk of intra-operative spinal cord damage, there is a high risk of sudden loss of the airway during the immediate postoperative period. In a recent survey of 155 patients requiring emergency surgery, 7 of the 10 patients who needed CAP-CS surgery required emergency airway management in comparison with only 2 of the 155 patients who underwent other surgical approaches[9].

Cardiac surgery

Emergency cardiac surgery is often carried out under difficult circumstances either when myocardial infarction is ongoing or the myocardium is critically ischaemic in the presence of sepsis or thoracic aortic dissection. The Australasian Society of Cardiac and Thoracic Surgeons' (ASCTS) prospective database demonstrated a greatly increased risk of death for emergency procedures, e.g. valve replacement in the presence of sepsis, aortic arch dissection, or rescue coronary artery bypass grafting (CABG) following failed angioplasty, in comparison to their elective counterparts. Mortality rates increased from 1.8% for elective procedures to 4.1% for urgent and 24.6% for emergency or salvage operations[10]. Emergency operation is part of the Euroscore system for evaluating cardiac surgical risk and imparts approximately a 2% increase in early postoperative mortality[11].

Abdominal surgery

Emergency surgery for colorectal cancer is associated with high morbidity and mortality. One study of 107 consecutive patients undergoing emergency surgery for obstructing (78%) or perforating (22%) colorectal carcinoma from 1991 to 2002 found that major complications occurred in 70% and 34% of patients, respectively. The mortality rate was 15%. Age greater than 70 years (OR 14.1) and APACHE score ≥ 8 (OR 17.5) were independent risk factors for mortality. Major morbidity was predicted by ASA ≥ 3 (OR 3.3) and perioperative blood transfusion (OR 5.0)[12].

Similar data exist from other studies, Biondo and colleagues[13,14] reported a mortality rate of around 25% in patients with perforation of the left hemicolon, with reasonable prediction of mortality using either the Mannheim Peritonitis Index[15] or the Peritonitis Severity Score (see appendix). These scores use overlapping but distinct variables as shown in the table (see appendix). Komatsu and colleagues[16] found a similar mortality in their series, with a low preoperative pH, negative base excess (BE), low postoperative white blood cell count, low PaO_2/FiO_2 ratio, and poor renal output (24 h) all marking poor outcome.

Emergency surgery for colorectal carcinoma in the elderly is associated with high morbidity and mortality, with reported rates varying between 6% and 38% for emergency operations compared with 0.9% and 18% for elective operations in those over 70 years of age. The risk of postoperative death in patients aged over 80 years rises to 12–38% after emergency surgery, and 7.4–11.4% in elective cases[17].

The increased risk of complications associated with emergency surgery is not confined to malignant colorectal disease. Patients with diverticulitis are at risk of requiring emergency colectomy[18]. Age and recurrence characteristics can serve to predict the risk for adverse outcomes. In a series of over 25 000 patients, between 1987 and 2001, hospitalized for an initial episode of diverticulitis, around 20 000 were treated without an initial operation, 19% had recurrences, and 5.5% of patients had recurrent hospitalizations during which an emergency colectomy/colostomy was performed. The predicted probability of emergency colectomy/colostomy was highest in younger patients with multiple rehospitalizations[15]. Where stomas are performed as emergency procedures there are increases in morbidity and mortality[19].

The incidences of wound infection and anastomotic leak, following colorectal surgery involving formation of a primary anastomosis are influenced by the degree of urgency of the surgery. Sorensen and colleagues investigated variables predictive of surgical site infection and dehiscence of sutured tissue within 30 days after surgery using multiple logistic regression analysis on data from 4855 unselected patients undergoing open gastrointestinal surgery. Following elective operation, the incidence of tissue and wound complications was 6% compared with 16% in emergency surgery. These complications resulted in prolonged hospitalization in 50% of the patients and a 3-fold higher risk of re-operation though not increased mortality[20].

The factors responsible for increased mortality after emergency abdominal surgery are not clear, and it has even been suggested that gender differences related to immune system function may occur. However, a retrospective analysis of around 600 consecutive patients over 50 years old, who underwent emergency abdominal surgery showed that the overall 30-day mortality was 26%, with 74 (29%) males and 79 (24%) females dying within this period. The mortality rates were 25% in males and 10% in females after minor surgery, 26% in males and 23% in females after intermediate surgery, and 44% in males and 39% in females after major surgery. On univariate logistic regression analysis in males, increasing age ($P < 0.001$), severity of surgery, and seniority of anaesthetist were associated with increased risk of mortality. In females, however, only severity of surgery was associated with the risk of mortality[21].

Trauma surgery

Trauma constitutes the commonest cause for emergency surgery in the first three decades of life, with a second peak occurring in the elderly. Compared to a younger population, the treatment of older trauma victims is associated with higher mortality and morbidity. In one European study, data from over 400 multi-trauma patients, treated at a major urban trauma centre, were analysed retrospectively. Adults over 65 years of age were compared to younger patients (16–64 years). Despite similarity in injury severity and a comparable injury pattern, elderly multi-trauma patients had a higher rate of haemodynamic instability, required artificial ventilation of the lungs for a longer period (20 vs. 13 days), and had a higher mortality (53 vs. 27 %)[17,22].

One feature common to all age groups who sustain multiple traumas is the problem of missed injury. Patients who have sustained a life-threatening haemorrhagic injury may be resuscitated and taken to the operating theatre for control of haemorrhage prior to the identification of all the other injuries, which they have sustained. Often, injuries that are difficult to diagnose, e.g. ruptured diaphragm, are missed in the early stages of trauma management, and systems should be in place to identify those patients who have not undergone a full trauma primary or secondary survey[23]. This is particularly important in Critical Care Units following admission of trauma patients after operative treatment. The original notes, investigations, and imaging should be reviewed and a complete 'top to toe' examination of the patient carried out with new imaging or other investigations as required. This system of tertiary trauma survey decreases the incidence of missed injury[24].

By far the most common trauma surgical procedures associated with a high risk of morbidity and mortality are those employed for repair of fractured neck of femur. The population who sustain this injury is elderly with a median age of around 80 years, has multiple medical co-morbidities, and may have concomitant degrees of dementia which make informed consent difficult or impossible to obtain. Mortality at 30 days is approximately 10% in Europe[25]. In addition to the need to optimize medical therapy of concurrent medical disease, operative intervention must be undertaken as soon as possible to prevent deterioration, hospital acquired infection, or thrombo-embolic disease leading to increased morbidity and mortality.

Numerous factors have been associated with increased 30-day mortality in this population. POSSUM scoring does not work well in these patients to predict risk[26], but the Nottingham Hip Fracture Score (see appendix) predicts mortality reasonably accurately[27]. Although comorbidities predict risk of death, delaying surgery in an attempt to optimize the patient's condition probably does not improve outcome. One UK study examined in-hospital mortality and emergency readmission within 28 days. Nearly 130 000 admissions for fractured neck of femur with over 18 000 deaths in hospital (14.3%) in 151 hospitals were analysed. Delay in operation was associated with an increased risk of death in hospital. For all deaths in hospital, the odds ratio was 1.27 after adjustment for comorbidity (>1 day of delay compared to 1 day or less). Similar conclusions were reached from a preliminary meta-analysis of published trial data. Shiga and colleagues reported an increase in both 30-day and 1-year mortality for delays beyond 24–72 h (OR 1.44 and 1.33, respectively) [28]. There is inconclusive evidence regarding whether regional or general anaesthesia is associated with better postoperative outcome, though postoperative confusion may be less with spinal anaesthesia[29].

'High risk' patients

Despite the NCEPOD reports, the collection of data to identify and enable precise categorization of patients who are 'high risk' in terms of the probability of death has not been easy. Some data may be obtained by analysis of large databases collected for the purposes of audit and benchmarking of individual hospitals' performance in relation to case-mix corrected comparators. Deaths are most common in the population of older patients with co-existing medical disease who undergo complex surgery. Only limited data are presently available to describe this population. A recent UK survey has analysed the data on inpatient general surgical procedures and ICU admissions in 94 National Health Service hospitals between 1999 and 2004 collected by 2 national databases. High-risk surgical procedures were defined prospectively as those for which the mortality rate was 5% or greater. Of the 4 million surgical procedures, 70% were elective (0.44% mortality) and 30% emergency (5.4% mortality). A high-risk population of half a million patients was identified (mortality 12.3%), which accounted for 84% of deaths but for only 12% of procedures. In addition, this population had a prolonged hospital stay (median 16 days; interquartile range 9–29 days). Mortality following elective ICU admission was just over 10% compared to 29% for emergency admission. Among the ICU population, 41% of deaths occurred after the initial discharge from the ICU. The highest mortality rate (39%) occurred in the population admitted as emergencies to the ICU following initial postoperative care on a standard ward[29].

Having identified the high-risk group who died, it is possible to look at individual cases and identify any predictive variables. The ICNARC/CHKS data described earlier indicates age, co-morbidity, and surgical complexity as common patient factors, predictive of high risk, consistent with the data from Donati *et al.*[4]. On a smaller scale, another UK group has performed a retrospective cohort study of all non-elective general and orthopaedic surgical procedures performed in a 1-year interval in a district general hospital. They looked at over 1,800 patients who underwent urgent or emergency surgery in the year 2000. The case notes of those who died were reviewed and risk factors for mortality were examined using univariate and multivariate analysis. The mortality rates were 89/1869 (5%) at 30 days and 216 (12%) after 1 year. The high initial death rate continued for about 100 days after surgery. Increasing age, size of operation, and ASA grade were associated with a significantly higher risk of death at 1 year on multivariate analysis. The authors concluded that the high-risk group were patients aged over 50 years, of ASA Grade III or above, who needed major surgery; these patients had a 30-day mortality rate of 18%[30].

Perioperative optimization

The data detailed earlier allow anaesthetists to identify patients at risk, but the important question is whether anything can be done to mitigate this risk. Numerous studies have investigated the role of pre- and postoperative optimization of patients. The study from the United States by Rivers and colleagues demonstrated a survival benefit of aggressive emergency room resuscitation of patients with severe sepsis, although the applicability of this treatment to the less sick emergency patient is not clear[31]. Data for intra-operative optimization are scarce, although work by Sinclair[32] and Venn[33] suggested that length of hospital stay of patients undergoing operative repair of fractured neck of femur could be reduced by the use of intra-operative oesophageal Doppler or central venous pressure monitoring to guide fluid therapy. More recently, Pearse and colleagues demonstrated a reduction in complication rate and length of hospital stay using goal-directed therapy in the postoperative period in high-risk patients, although the majority underwent elective procedures[34]. In general, the evidence appears to favour perioperative fluid optimization[35,36].

Summary and conclusions

All the available research seems to agree that patients undergoing emergency surgical procedures have an increased risk of mortality and morbidity when compared to patients having elective procedures. There is no clear consensus as to why this occurs but audit data, particularly from the UK NCEPOD[1] and the Scottish Audit of Surgical Mortality[37] surveys, have highlighted problems, which despite the passage of time, seem to persist. The procedures are often performed by relatively junior medical staff, often not adequately trained or supervised. Inadequate preparation, resuscitation, and communication between teams may result in patients reaching the operating theatre in less than optimal physiological states. While delays in initiating or performing adequate resuscitation may cause a subsequent delay to the start of the operative procedure, these are often the result of failure in the system of delivery of health care. Not all hospitals provide 24-h access to fully staffed general or specialist surgical emergency operating theatres. Not all hospitals designate specialist consultant lead on-call surgical teams with no duties other than to be responsible for emergency admissions. Not all hospitals provide 24-h designated cover by consultant anaesthetists. Not all hospitals have appropriately staffed designated areas of increased levels of care, such as surgical high-dependency units, where patients may be admitted and resuscitated prior to surgery. This latter concept of 'pre-optimization' has been shown to be both cost-effective and to decrease perioperative mortality and morbidity[35].

References

1. Campling, E.A., Devlin, H.B., Hoile, R.W., Ingram, G.S., and Lunn, J.N. (1997). Who operates when? A report by the National Confidential Enquiry into Perioperative Deaths 1 April 1995 to 31 March 1996. NCEPOD, London.

2. Semmens, J.B., Aitken, R.J., Sanfilippo, F.M., *et al.* (2005). The Western Australian Audit of Surgical Mortality: advancing surgical accountability. *Medical Journal of Australia*, **183**, 504–8.

3 Copeland, G.P., Jones, D., and Walters, M. (1991). POSSUM: a scoring system for surgical audit. *British Journal of Surgery*, **78**, 355–60.

4. Donati, A., Ruzzi, M., Adrario, E., *et al.* (2004). A new and feasible model for predicting operative risk. *British Journal of Anaesthesia*, **93**, 393–9.

5. Stone, P.A., Hayes, J.D., AbuRahma, A.F., Jackson, J.M., Santos, A.N., and Flaherty, S.K. (2005). Ruptured abdominal aortic aneurysms: 15 years of continued experience in a Southern West Virginia community. Annals of Vascular Surgery, **19**(6), 851–7.

6. Laukontaus, S.J., Lepantalo, M., Hynninen, M., Kantonen, I., and Pettila, V. (2005). Prediction of survival after 48-h of intensive care following open surgical repair of ruptured abdominal aortic aneurysm. *European Journal of Vascular and Endovascular Surgery*, **30**(5), 509–15.

7. Hadjianastassiou, V.G., Tekkis, P.P., Goldhill, D.R., and Hands, L.J. (2005). Quantification of mortality risk after abdominal aortic aneurysm repair. *British Journal of Surgery*, **92**, 1092–8.

8. Hinchliffe, R.J., Bruijstens, L., MacSweeney, S.T.R., and Braithwaite, B.D. (2006). A Randomised Trial of Endovascular and Open Surgery for Ruptured Abdominal Aortic Aneurysm-Results of a Pilot Study and Lessons Learned for Future Studies. *European Journal of Vascular and Endovascular Surgery*, **32**(5), 506–13.

9. Terao, Y., Matsumot,o S., Yamashita, K., *et al.* (2004). Increased Incidence of Emergency Airway Management After Combined Anterior-Posterior Cervical Spine Surgery. *Journal of Neurosurgery Anesthesia*, **16**, 282–6.

10. Reid, C.M., Rockell, M., Skillington, P.D., *et al.* (2004). Initial twelve months experience and analysis for 2001-2002 from the Australasian Society of Cardiac and Thoracic Surgeons–Victorian database project. *Heart, Lung and Circulation*, **13**, 291–7.

11. Roques, F., Michel, P., Goldstone, A.R., and Nashef, S.A. (2003). The Logistic Euroscore. *European Heart Journal*, **24**, 882–3.

12. Alvarez, J.A., Baldonedo, R.F., Bear, I.G., Truan, N., Pire, G., and Alvarez, P. (2005). Presentation, treatment, and multivariate analysis of risk factors for obstructive and perforative colorectal carcinoma. *American Journal of Surgery*, **190**, 376–82.

13. Biondo, S., Ramos, E., Deiros, M., *et al.* (2000). Prognostic factors for mortality in left colonic peritonitis: a new scoring system. *Journal of The American College of Surgery*, **191**, 635–42.

14. Biondo, S., Ramos, E., Fraccalvieri, D., Kreisler, E., Rague, J.M., and Jaurrieta, E. (2006). Comparative study of left colonic Peritonitis Severity Score and Mannheim Peritonitis Index. *British Journal of Surgery*, **93**, 616–22.

15. Wacha, H., Linder, M.M., Feldman, U., Wesch, G., Gundlach, E., and Steifensand, R.A. (1987). Mannheim peritonitis index – prediction of risk of death from peritonitis: construction of a statistical and validation of an empirically based index. *Theoretical Surgery*, **1**, 169–77.

16. Komatsu, S., Shimomatsuya, T., Nakajima, M., *et al.* (2005). Prognostic factors and scoring system for survival in colonic perforation. *Hepato-gastroenterology*, **52**, 761–4.

17. Waldron, R., Donovan, I., Drumm, J., Mottram, S., and Tedman, S. (1986). Emergency presentation and mortality from colorectal cancer in the elderly. *British Journal of Surgery*, **73**, 214–6.

18. Anaya, D.A. and Flum, D.R. (2005). Risk of emergency colectomy and colostomy in patients with diverticular disease. *Archives of Surgery*, **140**, 681–5.

19. Harris, D.A., Egbeare, D., Jones, S., Benjamin, H., Woodward, A., and Foster, M.E. (2005). Complications and mortality following stoma formation. *Annals of The Royal College of Surgeons of England*, **87**, 427–31.

20. Sorensen, L.T., Hemmingsen, U., Kallehave, F., *et al.* (2005). Risk factors for tissue and wound complications in gastrointestinal surgery. *Annals of Surgery*, **241**, 654–8.

21. Harten, J., McCreath, B.J., McMillan, D.C., McArdle, C.S., and Kinsella, J. (2005). The effect of gender on postoperative mortality after emergency abdominal surgery. *Gender Medicine*, **2**, 35–40.

22. Aldrian, S., Nau, T., Koenig, F., and Vecsei, V. (2005). Geriatric polytrauma. *Wiener Klinische Wochenschrift*, **117**, 145–9.

23. Initial Assessment and Management. (1997). In: *Advanced Trauma Life Support for Doctors*, 6th edition, pp. 21–47. American College of Surgeons, Chicago.

24. Brookes, A., Holroyd, B., and Riley, B. (2004). Missed Injury in major trauma patients. *Injury, International Journal of the care of the Injured*, **34**, 407–10.

25. Fox, H.J., Pooler, J., Prothero, D., and Bannister, G.C. (1994). Factors affecting the outcome after proximal femoral fractures. *Injury*, **25**(5), 297–300.

26. Ramanathan, T.S., Moppett, I.K., Wenn, R., Moran, C.G. (2005). POSSUM scoring for patients with fractured neck of femur. *British Journal of Anaesthesia*, **94**, 430–3.

27. Maxwell, M.J., Moran, C.G., and Moppett, I.K. (2008). Development and validation of a preoperative scoring system to predict thirty-day mortality in patients undergoing hip fracture surgery. *British Journal of Anaesthesia*, **101**(4), 511–7.

28. Shiga, T., Wajima, Z., Imanaga, K., and Ohe, Y. (2007). Is operative delay associated with increased mortality of hip fracture patients? *Anaesthesiology*, **107**, A1828.

29. Parker, M.J., Handoll, H.H.G., and Griffiths, R. (2004). Anaesthesia for hip fracture surgery in adults. Cochrane Database of Systematic Reviews, Issue **4**. Art. No.: CD000521. DOI: 10.1002/14651858.CD000521.pub2.

30. Neary, W.D., Foy, C., Heather, B.P., and Earnshaw, J.J. (2006). Identifying high-risk patients undergoing urgent and emergency surgery. *Annals of The Royal College of Surgeons of England*, **88**, 151–6.

31. Rivers, E., Nguyen, B., Havstad, S., *et al.* (2001). Early goal-directed therapy in the treatment of severe sepsis and septic shock. *New England Journal of Medicine*, **345**, 1368–77.

32. Sinclair, S., James, S., and Singer, M. (1997). Intraoperative intravascular volume optimisation and length of hospital stay after repair of proximal femoral fracture: randomised controlled trial. *British Medical Journal*, **315**, 909–12.

33. Venn. R., Steele, A., Richardson, P., *et al.* (2002). Randomized controlled trial to investigate influence of the fluid challenge on duration of hospital stay and perioperative morbidity in patients with hip fractures. *British Journal of Anaesthesia*, **88**, 65–71.

34. Pearse, R., Dawson, D., Fawcett, J., *et al.* (2005). Early goal-directed therapy after major surgery reduces complications and duration of hospital stay. A randomised, controlled trial [ISRCTN38797445] *Critical Care*, **9**, R687-R693. (DOI 10.1186/cc3887).

35. Pearse, R.M., Rhodes, A., and Grounds, R.M. (2004). Goal-directed hemodynamic therapy in the ICU: Application and possible mechanism of therapeutic effect. In *Yearbook of Intensive Care and Emergency Medicine* (ed. J-L.Vincent). Springer Verlag, Berlin.

36. Kinsella, J. and Harten, J. (2001). Effect of perioperative fluid therapy on outcome following major surgery – a review of the evidence. *British Journal of Anaesthesia Bulletin*, **8**, 362–5.

37. Annual Report Scottish Audit of Surgical Mortality. (1999). http://www.sasm.org.uk/Reports/1999report/Finalreport1999.pdf (last accessed 13th January 2009).

Appendix

Donati risk score

Factor	Coefficient	Odds ratio
ASA	1.09	2.97 (1.73–5.11)
Age (per year)	0.03346	1.03 (1.003–1.07)
Severity		
Intermediate	0.5317	1.7 (0.936–3.09)
Major	0.6739	1.96 (1.04–3.7)
Mode		
Urgent	0.00477	1.005 (0.9–1.12)
Emergency	0.8163	2.26 (0.799–6.41)
Constant	–8.087	

Source: Donati, A., Ruzz, M., Adrario, E., *et al.* (2004). A new and feasible model for predicting operative risk. *British Journal of Anaesthesia*, **93**, 393–9. With permission.

Note: Risk of mortality is given by: Risk of death = $1/(1+ e^{(-X)})$ where X = (Sum of coefficients – 8.087).

POSSUM score

	Score			
Variable	1	2	4	8
1. Age (yrs)	<60	61–70	>71	None
2. Cardiac signs	No failure	On cardiac drugs or steroid	Oedema Warfarin	Raised JVP
Chest radiograph	Normal	None	Borderline cardiomegaly	Cardiomegaly
3. Respiratory signs	Normal	SOB on exertion	SOB stairs	SOB rest
Chest radiograph	Normal	Mild COAD	Moderate COAD	Any other change

(continued) POSSUM score

Variable	Score 1	2	4	8
4. Systolic Blood Pressure (mmHg)	110–130	131–170 100–109	>171 90–99	— <89
5. Pulse rate (bpm)	50–80	81–100 40–49	101–120	>121 <39
6. Glasgow Coma score	15	12–14	9–11	<8
7. Serum urea (mmol/l)	<7.5	7.6–10	10.1–15	>15.1
8. Serum Na (mmol/l)	>136	131–135	126–130	<125
9. Serum K (mmol/l)	3.5–5	3.2–3.4 5.1–5.3	2.9–3.1 5.4–5.9	<2.8 >6
10. Haemoglobin (g/100ml)	13–16	11.5–12.9 16.1 to 17	10–11.4 17.1 to 18	<9.9 >18.1
11. WBC (x10⁹/l)	4–10	10.1–20 3.1–3.9	>20.1 <3	
12. ECG	Normal		Atrial fibrillation (rate 60–90)	Any other change

Note: Points are given for each datum according to the table; JVP—jugular venous pressure; SOB—shortness of breath; COAD—chronic obstructive airways disease; WBC—white blood count.

Operative severity score

Variable	Score 1	2	4	8
Magnitude	Minor	Intermediate	Major	Major +
Number of operations within 30 days	1	No score	2	>3
Intra-operative blood loss	≤100 ml	101–500 ml	501–999 ml	≥1000 ml
Peritoneal soiling (General)	None	Minor (serous fluid)	Local pus	Free bowel contents, pus or blood
Contamination (Orthopaedic)	None	Incised wound	Minor contamination or necrotic tissue	Gross contamination or necrotic tissue
Presence of malignancy	None	Primary only	Node metastases	Distant metastases
Timing of operation	Elective	No score	Emergency (<48 h) Resuscitation possible	Emergency (<6 h) Immediate surgery

Note: Risk of mortality is given by: Predicted mortality rate $= 1/(1 + e^{(-X)})$, where $X = (0.13 \times$ sum of physiologic score$) + (0.16 \times$ sum of operative score$) - 7.04$.

Note: The modification for orthopaedics is an alternative score for soiling.

Mannheim Peritonitis Index

Factor	Score
Age >50 years	5
Female sex	5
Organ failure	7
Malignancy	4
Preoperative duration of peritonitis >24 h	4
Origin of sepsis not colonic	4
Diffuse generalized peritonitis	6
Exudate	
Clear	0
Cloudy, purulent	6
Faecal	12

Source: From Wacha, H., Linder, M.M., Feldman, U., *et al.* (1987). Mannheim peritonitis index – prediction of risk of death from peritonitis: construction of a statistical and validation of an empirically based index. *Theoretical Surgery*, **1**, 169–77. With permission.

Peritonitis severity score

Factor	PSS		
	1	**2**	**3**
Age (years)	≤70	>70	—
ASA grade	I–II	III	IV
Preoperative organ failure	None	—	One or more organ
Immunocompromised	No	Yes	—
Ischaemic colitis	No	Yes	—
Peritonitis stage	1–2	3–4	—

Source: From Biondo, S., Ramos, E., Deiros, M., *et al.* (2000). Prognostic Factors for Mortality in Left Colonic Peritonitis: A New Scoring System. *Journal of The American College of Surgery*, **191**, 635–42. With permission.

APACHE II

Factor	Acute physiology score								
	4	3	2	1	0	1	2	3	4
Core temp (°C)	>41	39–40.9		38–38.9	36–38.4	34–35.9	32–33.9	30–31.9	<29.9
Mean arterial pressure (mmHg)	>160	130–159	110–129		70–109		50–69		<49
Heart rate (bpm)	>180	140–179	110–139		70–109		55–69	40–54	<39
Respiratory rate (bpm)	>50	35–49		25–34	12–24	10–11	6–9		<5
Oxygen delivery (ml/min) (If $FIO_2 \geq 0.5$)	>500	350–499	200–349		<200				
PaO_2 (kPa) (if $FIO_2 < 0.5$)					>9.3	8.1–9.3	7.3–8.0	<7.3	
arterial pH	>7.7	7.6–7.69		7.5–7.59	7.3–7.49		7.25–7.3	7.15–7.2	<7.15
Serum sodium (mmol/l)	>180	160–179	155–159	150–154	130–149		120–129	111–119	<110
Serum potassium (mmol/l)	>7	6–6.9		5.5–5.9	3.5–5.4	3–3.4	2.5–2.9		<2.5
Serum creatinine (µmol/l)	≥305	170–304	130–169		54–129		<54		
Haematocrit (%)	>60		50–59.9	46–49.9	30–45.9		20–29.9		<20
White cell count (10^9/l)	>40	20–39.9		15–19.9	3–14.9		1–2.9		<1
Glasgow Coma Score	Score = 15–actual GCS								

Age points

Age	Age score
<44	0
45–54	2
55–64	3
65–74	5
>75	6

Chronic health points

History of organ insufficiency preceding current admission	Chronic health score
Non-operative patients	5
Emergency operative patients	5
Elective operative patients	2

Note: Crude mortality is given by: Predicted death rate $= e^{(X)}/(1 + e^{(X)})$, where X = Total APACHE II score $- 0.146 - 3.517$.

Note: The crude mortality can be adjusted according to admission diagnosis and urgency.

Nottingham hip fracture score

Variable	Value	Odds ratio	NHFS score
Age	66–85 years	4.34	3
	≥86 years	7.28	4
Sex	Male	1.66	1
Admission Hb	≤10 g/dl	1.55	1
MMTS	≤6 out of 10	1.577	1
Living in an institution	Yes	1.508	1
Number of co-morbidities	≥2	1.63	1
Malignancy	Yes	1.76	1

Source: Maxwell, M.J., Moran, C.G., and Moppett, I.K. (2008). Development and validation of a preoperative scoring system to predict thirty-day mortality in patients undergoing hip fracture surgery. *British Journal of Anaesthesia*, **101**(4), 511–7.

Note: Risk of mortality is given by: 30 day mortality (%) $= 100/ 1 + e^{(4.718 - (NHFS/2))}$, where NHFS is the sum of the ascribed points.

Chapter 5

Critical care

Adam C March & Robert J Winter

The treatment of patients in intensive care units involves a multidisciplinary approach, with communication between medical professionals, the patient's family, and most importantly, when possible, the patient. Problems may arise when patients are unable to express their own wishes either as a direct result of their illness, or secondary to medical interventions such as tracheal intubation and sedation. In these circumstances, the process of gaining consent for treatment can be challenging if not impossible, and often results in the patient losing the ability to exert the right to autonomy. At such times, carers and healthcare professionals must make decisions based on their patient's 'best interests'. However, determining a patient's 'best interests' can be equally challenging and can create disagreement between doctors and family members when deciding upon the most appropriate course of medical therapy. Resolution of these issues can provide doctors with a wide range of ethical dilemmas, many of which can be emotive in nature.

This chapter aims to address the ethical and legal principles involved in gaining informed consent from patients treated in intensive care units. It will also discuss some of the key issues surrounding good practice in circumstances in which patients lack the capacity to give consent. Many of these factors are considered in the recently formulated Mental Capacity Act 2005[1], which came into force in 2007, with the intention of protecting individuals who lack the capacity to make their own decisions. It contains guidance for those who are responsible for the care of incapacitated individuals and gives legal powers to prosecute those who abuse their position of trust.

The principles of consent in those who possess capacity

The concept of consent can be viewed as a legal and ethical process formulated by society to respect the autonomy of its citizens[2]. Respect for patient autonomy forms the heart of good medical practice and never before have its medico-legal implications been so important. Legally, treatment without consent can result in negligent practice ending in a charge of battery and assault against the medical practitioner. Ethically, gaining informed consent implies that respect has been shown to the patient's belief-forming systems and that their autonomy has been respected. In order to be legally valid, consent must be given *voluntarily*, by an *appropriately informed* person who can be shown to possess the *capacity* to make a reasoned decision[3]. This applies to treatment provided by every healthcare service involved in the multidisciplinary approach to treating patients in the intensive care unit and thus encompasses therapy administered by nursing staff, physiotherapists, radiologists, pharmacists, and dieticians, in addition to doctors[4]. In 2008, the GMC produced updated guidelines on consent for medical professionals entitled 'Consent: patients and doctors making decisions together.'[5]. This provides an ethico-legal framework to follow when seeking consent from a patient.

Capacity

The key concept behind acquiring informed consent is the possession of capacity. Patients must be shown to possess capacity in order to be competent to make reasoned decisions. The definition of capacity is given by the High Court in the case *Re C (Adult: Refusal of Treatment)* [1994] 1 All ER 819. This relates to the treatment of a schizrenic patient who refused treatment for a gangrenous foot believing that it was better to die with both feet than to live with one. The test used in this case to determine the capacity of C has become known as the Re C Test and has three components, all of which need to be satisfied. Firstly, the patient must *understand and retain* all the information given relating to the decision to be made. Furthermore, the patient must *believe* the information and be able to *weigh it up* in order to balance any risks against the benefits of treatment on the basis of his or her own specific needs[3].

It can be seen that gaining consent for treatment in the intensive care unit has the potential to provide clinicians with challenging problems. Within an intensive care environment, patients vary widely in their cognitive ability. Patients who possess capacity pose relatively few problems as adequate communication can occur between the doctor and patient, facilitating information exchange and the satisfaction of the necessary criteria. However, the majority of critically ill patients are not competent to make such decisions, or there may at least be doubts about their mental capacity in relation to the decision-making process. These are the patients in whom the right to autonomy is lost, making them vulnerable to the imposed unwanted wishes of a third party in a position of power.

The mental capacity act and consent in those who lack capacity

The Mental Capacity Act 2005[1] was formulated to protect the rights of those who lack the capacity to make their own decisions. At its heart is the primary goal of endeavouring to respect the autonomy of individuals as far as possible. It came into force in 2007 in England and Wales; Scotland has its own Adults with Incapacity Act, 2000[6]. The act applies to everyone over the age of 16 and covers a broad spectrum of situations, ranging from everyday choices such as what to eat and wear through to important decisions concerning financial issues, housing, and medical treatment. The act clarifies confusion which existed about who can make these decisions and how the decisions should be made. In doing so, it not only protects vulnerable people but also the carers and professionals charged with the responsibility of looking after them. It also enables people to plan ahead for a time when they may lose capacity.

The Mental Capacity Act is based on a set of five key principles:

- A presumption of capacity—every adult has the right to make his or her own decisions and must be assumed to have the capacity to do so unless it is proved otherwise;
- The right for individuals to be supported to make their own decisions—people must be given all appropriate help before anyone concludes that they cannot make their own decisions;
- Individuals must retain the right to make what might be seen as eccentric or unwise decisions;
- Best interests—anything done for or on behalf of people without capacity must be in their best interests;
- Least restrictive intervention—anything done for or on behalf of people without capacity should be the least restrictive of their basic rights and freedoms.

It can be seen that the Act therefore has great relevance for the treatment of incapacitated patients in the intensive care unit and its contents should be familiar to all those who work within a critical care environment. The following sections aim to clarify the process of providing treatment to those who cannot consent, as the law and practice surrounding these issues can be complex.

Consent Form 4

When treatment is required to be given to a patient who is unable to consent, the following two criteria must be satisfied:

- The patient must lack the capacity ('competence') to give or withhold consent to the procedure and
- The procedure must be in the patient's best interests.

These two criteria form the basis of the National Health Service's 'Consent Form 4; Form for adults who are unable to consent to investigation or treatment'. Consent Form 4 provides a framework to ensure that the correct assessment of each patient is made prior to the initiation of treatment[4]. It requires four principal sections to be completed and signed by the health professional proposing the procedure, and includes a space for the identification and signature of a second person if required.

The four principal sections are:

A. Details of the procedure or course of treatment proposed.
B. Assessment of the patient's capacity.
C. Assessment of the patient's best interests.
D. Involvement of the patient's family and others close to the patient.

Details of the procedure or course of treatment proposed

Within the intensive care environment, critically ill patients often require multiple, relatively invasive procedures to be performed as part of their ongoing diagnostic and therapeutic care. Many of these interventions pose significant risk of injury and would thus warrant the completion of Consent Form 4 (e.g. percutaneous tracheostomy insertion). However, it would be unreasonable to expect a form to be filled out for every minor intervention (e.g. each time suctioning was performed). The form is therefore directed at procedures in which documentation of the decision-making process is deemed to be important. Most practitioners view these as interventions with potentially serious side-effects. However, this view is open to much individual interpretation and currently no guidelines exist as to which procedures warrant the completion of Consent Form 4.

All medical interventions have a risk–benefit ratio unique to the individual situation. Competent patients make decisions based on the level of perceived significance placed on factors on each side of the equation. Deciding on how much information to disclose to a patient can be difficult and the legal position with regard to information disclosure in the United Kingdom is moving away from the 'reasonable doctor' standard founded on the *Bolam* principle (*Bolam v Friern Hospital Management Committee* [1957] 1 WLR 582) towards the 'reasonable patient' standard proposed by *Lord Scarman* in *Sidaway* (*Sidaway v Board of Governors of Bethlem Royal Hospital and the Maudsley Hospital* [1985] 1 AC 871). The doctor must now disclose any information that they believe *the patient* would consider 'significant'[7]. With this in mind, it may be prudent to complete a Consent Form 4 for any procedure in which the risks, no matter how small, might be significant to the patient.

Assessment of patient's capacity

Many patients in the intensive care unit are often presumed to lack capacity either as a direct result of their medical condition (e.g. cerebral contusion) or secondary to the influence of medical interventions such as sedation with hypnotic agents. By losing capacity, patients lose their right to autonomy. This is such a fundamental right that both the GMC[5] and Mental Capacity Act[1] stipulate that every individual should have the right to make his or her own decisions and must be presumed to have the capacity to do so unless proven otherwise.

In order to possess capacity, the Mental Capacity Act states that an individual must satisfy all of the following criteria:

1. The person must comprehend the information given to them relevant to the decision. Information must be provided at a level appropriate to the person's level of understanding to ensure appropriate comprehension.

2. The person must be able to retain this information long enough to be able to make a decision.

3. The person must be able to use the information in order to reason the consequences of treatment choices.

4. The person must be able to communicate his or her decision.

The first three criteria apply to many patients in an intensive care unit. The fourth applies to circumstances in which a patient may possess metal capacity but lacks the physical ability to express a decision (e.g. locked in syndrome). Each test must be 'decision specific' and therefore has no bearing on the individual's general decision-making ability at that time or in the future. By ensuring this, the Act covers individuals in whom loss of capacity is partial (a person may lack capacity in relation to one matter but not in relation to another), and/or temporary (those in whom capacity fluctuates).

The Mental Capacity Act stipulates that loss of capacity must be secondary to an 'impairment of, or disturbance in, the functioning of the mind or brain'. This is termed the 'diagnostic test' and encompasses common conditions encountered in the intensive care unit such as traumatic brain injury and pharmacologically induced states of coma. However, no single diagnosis can confer an automatic presumption of lack of capacity, and thus any neurological impairment resulting in loss of cognitive function can satisfy the earlier definition. Regardless of the aetiology, the Act states that when significant treatment decisions have to be made, all possible attempts must be undertaken to establish capacity thereby enabling the patient to be included in the decision-making process.

This may necessitate interventions such as temporary withdrawal of sedation or the use of alternative methods of communication (e.g. picture boards/sign language). Information provision should be pitched at a level which the patient can understand, with lay terms being used whenever it is felt necessary. Nationally or locally produced information booklets published with diagrams, large print documentation, and printed even in Braille, can be employed to aid this process, as can the use of translators, whenever a language barrier exists. However the information is transferred, it is the responsibility of the doctor to assess the patient's level of comprehension and rectify any areas of misunderstanding. In many cases, these attempts fail. If so, there should be clear documentation indicating that adequate capacity could not be achieved despite the best efforts to do so.

If doubt exists about the capacity of the patient to give consent, a second opinion should be sought in the form of an experienced colleague or a psychiatric review. In very problematic cases, legal advice should be obtained. The Mental Capacity Act facilitates this with the formation of the Court of Protection, to which all cases of indeterminate capacity can be referred for resolution. Full documentation explaining the reasons behind any decisions made regarding the possession of capacity should be recorded at each stage of the decision-making process within the patient's medical record.

Often, the possession of capacity fluctuates during the course of a patient's illness. If a patient is predicted to regain capacity at any point, then decision-making should be postponed if possible until that time. In addition, any decision made while the patient was previously competent should be reviewed before embarking on further courses of treatment, in an attempt to ensure that the management is, as far as possible, consistent with the views expressed by the patient at that time. Whether deemed to be competent or not, patients should be consulted about their treatment preferences as far as is reasonably possible in all circumstances except coma.

Assessment of patient's best interests

Any decision taken for an incapacitated patient should be done in their 'best interests'. This is viewed as a fundamental concept which must be upheld at all times, thus reinforcing its current position in common law. No legal definition of 'best interests' exists, as each case has its individual merits but the Mental Capacity Act does state that its determination requires 'all relevant circumstances to be considered' and that no conclusions should be made on the basis of 'potentially unjustified and prejudicial assumptions' such as the patient's age, appearance, or condition. At present, practice is governed according to the *Bolam* principle, which dictates that the doctor has to make decisions in accordance with those which would be reached by a responsible and competent body of medical professionals. The GMC[5] stipulates that, when deciding what options are in a patient's best interests, the following should be considered:

- which options for treatment would provide overall clinical benefit for the patient
- which option, including the option not to treat, would be least restrictive of the patient's future choices
- any evidence of the patient's previously expressed preferences, such as an advance statement or decision
- the views of anyone the patient asks you to consult, or who has legal authority to make a decision on their behalf, or has been appointed to represent them
- the views of people close to the patient on the patient's preferences, feelings, beliefs and values, and whether they consider the proposed treatment to be in the patient's best interests
- what you and the rest of the healthcare team know about the patient's wishes, feelings, beliefs and values.

The key concept here relates to the fact that a patient's best interests do not necessarily relate to their medical best interests. Doctors often feel the need to act in their patient's '*medical* best interests', and in doing so, allow their actions to become paternalistic in nature. Many other factors constitute a patient's best interests, including their ethical, moral, and religious values, all of which the doctor can never fully comprehend. Occasionally, these interests may conflict with one another, with only the patient being in a position to decide which one, if any, carries the greater significance. When the patient is unable to communicate these wishes, the obligation to consult widely with family and friends forms an extremely important step in determining the patient's best interests[8]. In addition, whenever an incapacitated patient is admitted to the intensive care unit, relatives or friends should be asked about the existence of an advance decision.

Advance decisions   An advance decision (advance directive, living will) is a method by which competent individuals can indicate their preferred treatment choices at a potential future time of incapacity. There are numerous clauses that need to be satisfied for advance decisions to be valid. A person must be eighteen years of age or older and must be competent (i.e. possess capacity) at the time the decision is made. The decision has to be made voluntarily by a fully informed individual and must specify clearly the treatment that is being refused and in what particular circumstances this may apply. If all these criteria are satisfied, a competent adult patient's anticipatory refusal of consent remains legally binding even if the patient subsequently becomes incompetent (*HE v NHS Trust A and AE* [2003] EWHC (Fam), a case concerning refusal of blood transfusion).

Advance decisions become invalid when there is evidence to suggest that the individual's actions or beliefs have become inconsistent with those previously stated. This may indicate that the person has changed their mind since making the advance decision. They are also not applicable if the person is judged to possess capacity at the time that treatment is being proposed. If the advance decision is applicable, all treatment decisions must fall within the criteria stipulated. However, it should not be implemented if it is felt that the individual had not anticipated the specific situation which has arisen and that, if the person had anticipated it, the decision would have been altered.

Further rules apply to advance decisions in which patients refuse treatment that is necessary to sustain life. In these circumstances, advance decisions are not valid unless they are verified by a statement which specifically confirms that the decision is to apply even if life is at risk. The decision must be presented in writing and must posses sa witnessed signature. It is apparent that advance decisions can be subject to variable interpretation, and if any doubt arises as to their existence, validity, or applicability, then the Court of Protection should be consulted to resolve the issue. In the meantime, action may be taken to prevent the death of the individual or to prevent serious deterioration in the patient's condition until such time that the matter is resolved.

Involvement of the patient's family and others close to the patient

It is the duty of the decision maker to elucidate as much information as possible about the patient's feelings, beliefs, and values, to try to establish, if possible, what decision the patient would have made if competent. Attempts should be made to determine the patient's past and present wishes through communication with everybody involved in the patient's welfare. Examples may include the patient's wishes regarding organ transplantation in the event of brainstem death or relating to cardiopulmonary resuscitation in the event of a cardiac arrest. The opinions of carers and family members on such matters must be determined and the Mental Capacity Act gives them the right to be consulted. In addition, discussions facilitate information transfer between the family and doctor, helping to build trust within the professional/family relationship. Full documentation must always be recorded about relevant discussions held with family members.

Proxy consent

Once a patient is deemed to lack capacity, consent to treatment cannot be given. Under previous legislation, nobody could give proxy consent on behalf of a mentally incapacitated patient[7] (*F v. West Berkshire Health Authority* [1989] 2 All ER 545). However, the Mental Capacity Act has introduced a system in which other individuals can be authorized to give proxy consent: Lasting Power of Attorneys (LPA) and Independent Mental Capacity Advisors (IMCA). The Act allows an individual, whilst competent, to appoint an attorney (LPA) to act on his or her behalf in the event that the capacity to make decisions is lost. LPAs replace the previous system of 'Enduring Power of Attorney (EPA)' and expands surrogate decision-making powers to encompass, for the first time, decisions relating to health and medical welfare (including decisions about life-sustaining treatment). Any attorney appointed is duty-bound to act in the patient's best interests and can act only within any limitations stipulated within the LPA document itself.

Some patients who lack capacity will have no friends or family to support them during times when serious medical treatment decisions are required. These patients are particularly vulnerable and, as a consequence, the Mental Capacity Act created a new role tasked with the provision of their support—the IMCA. Once appointed, the IMCA should support the patient as far as possible to participate in the decision-making process. He or she should elucidate, if possible, the patient's feelings, values, and beliefs; should represent the patient's views; and should evaluate all relevant treatment options with the patient's best interests in mind.

Special circumstances

Organ donation

In England, Wales, and Northern Ireland, the code of practice surrounding consent for the donation of organs, tissue, and cells for transplantation is governed by the legal framework stipulated in the Human Tissue Act 2004[9] (similar laws exist in Scotland and are covered by the Human Tissue (Scotland) Act 2006[10]). Within the intensive care unit, this framework is most relevant to potential organ donors who have fulfilled the criteria for brainstem death and whose situation is encompassed in the section dealing with deceased donation. The Act stipulates that 'where an adult has, whilst alive and competent, consented to one or more of the scheduled purposes taking place after their death, then that consent is sufficient for the activity to be lawful'[9]. This is a departure from previous legislation whereby organ donation could only proceed if it was the wish of the potential donor's relatives.

Consent for organ donation can be registered by potential donors through the NHS Organ Donor Register, their will, or in other legal documents such as advance decisions. These sources should always be checked by trained individuals such as the transplant co-ordinator, so that the existence of any prior consent relating to tissue donation can be determined. If prior consent to tissue donation is found, the family should be notified of the deceased person's wishes and the subject of organ donation should be discussed. If objections are raised by the family, they should be sensitively encouraged to accept the deceased person's wishes and should be informed that they have no legal right to veto or overrule those wishes. However, each case is individual and there may be situations in which donation is deemed to be inappropriate despite the expressed wishes of the deceased.

If prior consent to organ donation does not exist, a combined, planned approach by clinicians and the transplant co-ordinator should be made to discuss the option of organ donation with the deceased individual's family. The objectives of such an approach are to elucidate the wishes of the deceased person, if possible, and to establish any thoughts and feelings regarding potential tissue donation held by the family. If the deceased has nominated a person to deal with the use of the body after death, that individual can give proxy consent for tissue donation in the event of the deceased individual's wishes not being known. If a nominated representative does not exist and the deceased has not indicated a wish for or against tissue donation, the act states that 'consent can be given by a person who was in a "qualifying relationship" immediately before the death of the individual in question'[9].

The use of experienced transplant co-ordinators working in combination with medical staff has been shown to increase the rates of consent given by family members for tissue donation. Consequently, transplant co-ordinators should always be involved in the consent-gaining process and should play an integral role in any approach made to families regarding the emotive subject of potential tissue donation from a deceased loved one.

Emergencies

In emergency situations, the patient may lack the capacity to consent to treatment as a result of severe injury or unconsciousness. This is one of the few situations in which treatment can be undertaken without consent, provided that the treatment is limited to what is immediately necessary to save life or avoid significant deterioration in the patient's health. In these cases, it would be reasonable to expect a doctor to initiate treatment based upon an assessment of what the patient's wishes would be if in a position to provide informed consent (*predictive consent*). An example would be that of a patient who presents to hospital in status epilepticus and who requires tracheal intubation in order to provide adequate airway protection and ventilation.

Research in patients who lack capacity

Research into the effects of new drugs and new treatment strategies often takes place within the intensive care environment. Normally, informed consent would be sought from competent patients prior to enrolment in a clinical trial, but this is often impossible in a population of patients who frequently lack capacity. In order to address this, the Mental Capacity Act sets out clear parameters for research. In summary, it states that research on incapacitated patients can be carried out lawfully only if a Research Ethics Committee deems that the trial is necessary, safe, and relates to the patient's condition. Taking part in the trial must provide a potential benefit to the patient which should outweigh any associated risks or complications and any medical intrusion should be kept to the minimal amount possible.

The Act also stipulates that carers and family members must be consulted and agree that the patient would want to participate in the trial, prior to inclusion in any study. They should be provided with all relevant information regarding the proposed research, enabling them to make an informed decision based on what they feel the patient's wishes would be. At any point, if the patient indicates unwillingness to take part in the trial or shows resistance towards any planned interventions, participation in the trial must cease immediately except where what is being done is intended to protect him from harm or to reduce or prevent pain or discomfort[11]. Similarly, if any nominated deputy or attorney feels that the patient would not want to take part in the trial, the researcher must ensure that the individual is not enrolled at any point.

Applying to the court

Disputes can sometimes arise between the wishes of medical professionals and those of the family and carers regarding what constitutes a patient's best interests. In such cases, the opinion of an experienced colleague should be sought. When a dispute that cannot be resolved arises, it may become necessary to apply to the newly formed Court of Protection to seek a legal opinion. The Court of Protection regulates the way in which the Mental Capacity Act works in law and is the final arbiter on problematic cases in which conflict cannot be resolved. The GMC guidelines recommend that the Court's approval should be sought whenever a patient lacks capacity to consent to a non-therapeutic or controversial medical intervention such as withdrawal of life support from patients in persistent vegetative states. An individual found guilty of ill-treatment or neglect of any person who lacks capacity is liable to a prison sentence of up to five years.

Conclusion

Gaining informed consent for medical interventions forms one of the cornerstones of good medical practice. It ensures that the patient's right to autonomy is respected and, in doing so, empowers the patient to make treatment decisions that satisfy his or her individual belief systems. The key component behind attaining consent is the possession of capacity and nowhere is this more important than in critically ill patients treated in intensive care units. Critically ill patients should always be presumed to possess capacity until it is proven otherwise; consequently, all possible means to establish capacity must be taken for decision-making purposes. If a patient is shown to lack capacity, all decisions made on his or her behalf must be in the patient's best interests, and doctors are duty-bound to consult widely in their attempts to achieve this. Occasionally, disagreement occurs between the wishes of medical professionals and those of the

Case study

The following is a common scenario witnessed on the intensive care unit and serves as an example to highlight some common problems surrounding gaining consent in this often challenging population of patients. It also underlines many of the aforementioned principles that should be followed when attempting to consent such patients.

A previously fit and well 32-year-old female was admitted to hospital following a collapse at home. On hospital arrival, she had a Glasgow Coma Score (GCS) of 3/15 necessitating tracheal intubation in the emergency department for airway protection and control of ventilation. CT scan of her head revealed an extensive subarachnoid haemorrhage with associated hydrocephalus, for which an extra-ventricular drain was inserted in theatre. Postoperatively, she was admitted to the intensive care unit for continuing ventilatory and cardiovascular support and neurological assessment. Twelve hours following admission, sedation was stopped with the aim of assessing neurological function. Once off sedation for 24 h, the patient's GCS remained low, only increasing to a maximum of 5/15. Her blood pressure and heart rate also became problematic, rising to a systolic value in excess of 230 mm Hg and 150 beats per min, respectively. Sedation was recommenced in order to regain control, and a second sedation hold was performed the following day. This time the GCS rose to 7/15 before gross agitation with associated hypertension and tachycardia ensued. Again, sedation had to be restarted, and the decision to perform a percutaneous tracheostomy on day five was made

Case study *(continued)*

to facilitate weaning from ventilatory support and provide airway protection. In this situation, how should consent be gained and what are the surrounding ethical issues?

Consent is sought for tracheostomy insertion as potentially serious complications can arise during the procedure. The Mental Capacity Act states that every patient should be considered to possess capacity unless proven otherwise. However, in this scenario, it is clear that the patient lacks capacity to give informed consent as a result of brain injury and sedative drug administration. This has been demonstrated on two separate occasions by the failure of the patient to regain full consciousness despite two sedation holds. The reason why capacity has been lost should be clearly documented in the medical notes, as should any efforts made to restore it such as, in this case, the sedation holds. The patient has therefore lost her right to autonomy as she is unable to express her own wishes and the decision to proceed with tracheostomy insertion is now based upon what constitutes the patient's best interests. The concepts of beneficence (doing good) and non-maleficence (not doing harm) now become important factors in a risk-benefit analysis of the procedure. On one hand, a tracheostomy will hopefully facilitate weaning from ventilatory support, thus reducing the risk of ventilator associated pneumonia, whilst improving cardiovascular stability off sedation and risk of further intracranial haemorrhage. On the other, the risks of life-threatening haemorrhage, pneumothorax, tracheal injury, and infection are all significant and potentially catastrophic. Again, in this situation, the Mental Capacity Act advises clinicians to 'consult widely'. The procedure should therefore be discussed with family members and next-of-kin in order to ascertain what the patient would have wanted in this situation. Discussion also allows the family to raise any concerns regarding the procedure and will hopefully result in a consensus decision on the proposed course of action.

A Consent Form 4 for those patients who are unable to give consent will need to be completed in this scenario, prior to proceeding with tracheostomy insertion. This ensures that the above processes have been followed and that the reasons why capacity is lacking are documented along with any efforts made to restore it. It also has a section relating to communication with the family although the final decision to proceed rests ultimately with the clinician

family and friends concerning what factors are in an individual's best interests. Good communication can help to resolve many of these issues, but sometimes this is not possible. In such circumstances, the Court should be consulted to give legal guidance as to the most appropriate way to proceed. The Mental Capacity Act 2005 provides a statutory framework to guide decision-making on behalf of those who lack the capacity to do so.

References

1. Department for Constitutional Affairs. The Mental Capacity Act 2005. http://www.opsi. gov.uk/acts/acts2005/ukpga_20050009_en_1 (last accessed 10th December 2008).

2. White, S. and Baldwin, T. Consent. (2004). In *Legal and Ethical Aspects of Anaesthesia, Critical Care and Perioperative Medicine*, pp. 49–72, 1st edition. Cambridge University Press. Cambridge.

3. Brooks, A., Girling, K., Riley, B., and Rowlands, B. (2004). Ethics in Critical Care. In *Critical Care for Postgraduate Trainees*, pp. 161–6, 1st edition. Hodder Arnold. London.

4. The Process of Consent within the Intensive Care Unit – Draft Proposals for Consultation. http://www.ics.ac.uk/icmprof/downloads/Consent%20Document%20For%20Website.pdf

5. General Medical Council. Consent: Patients and doctors making decisions together. (2008). http://www.gmc-uk.org/guidance/ethical_guidance/consent_guidance/index.asp (last accessed 10th December 2008).

6. Adults with Incapacity (Scotland) Act 2000. http://www.opsi.gov.uk/legislation/scotland/ acts2000/asp_20000004_en_1 (last accessed 10th December 2008).

7. British Medical Association. Report of the Consent Working Party, March, 2001. http://www.bma.org.uk/ap.nsf/Content/Reportoftheconsentworkingparty (last accessed 10th December 2008).

8. Consent for Anaesthesia, Revised Edition (2006). Association of Anaesthetists of Great Britain and Ireland, London, 2006.

9. Human Tissue Authority. Code of Practice – Donation of organs, tissue and cells for transplantation. http://www.hta.gov.uk/guidance/codes_of_practice.cfm (last accessed 10th December 2008).

10. Human Tissue (Scotland) Act 2006. http://www.opsi.gov.uk/legislation/scotland/acts2006/ asp_20060004_en_1 (last accessed 10th December 2008).

11. Mental Capacity Act 2005, Section 33(2)(a). http://www.opsi.gov.uk/acts/acts2005/ ukpga_20050009_en_3#pt1-pb8-l1g30 (last accessed 10th December 2008).

Legal cases

Bolam v. Friern Hospital Management Committee (1957) 1 WLR 582.

Sidaway v. Board of Governors of the Bethlem Royal Hospital and the Maudsley Hospital (1985) 1 All ER 643/871.

ReC (adult: refusal of treatment) (1994) 1 All ER 819.

F. v. West Berkshire Health Authority (1989) 2 All ER 545.

Chapter 6

High-risk patients

Simon J Howell

Patients frequently perceive anaesthesia and surgery as being fraught with risk. It is a testament to modern medical techniques that, in many cases, this is not true. Elective minor and intermediate surgery in healthy patients is now remarkably safe. The risk of death during such surgery is a small fraction of 1% and is difficult to quantify. Forrest and colleagues reported a mortality rate of 0.11% and a combined death, myocardial infarction, and stroke rate of 0.15% amongst 17 201 patients recruited into the 'Multicenter study of General Anesthesia'[1]. Unfortunately, not all patients are low risk. The patient with significant co-morbidity may be at substantially increased risk. Major operations such as those for cancer of the stomach or operations on the aorta are hazardous. Urgent surgery is more dangerous than elective surgery. This chapter deals with identifying high-risk patients and communicating this risk to the patient. Generic issues of risk communication are dealt with in detail in Chapter 2.

Even in this era of evidence-based medicine, there is much in the care of the high-risk patient that remains a matter for clinical judgement rather than clinical guideline.

Modern major surgery can be very complex indeed: modern anaesthesia and critical care equally so. It is difficult, if not impossible, for even the most experienced clinician to understand fully every aspect of the care of a patient, with several co-existing diseases, who is to undergo a major operation such as a gastrectomy. Before presenting the risks and benefits of an operation to the patient, the anaesthetist and surgeon may have to discuss these between themselves. There is no shame in seeing and assessing a patient and concluding the first interview with, 'I need to discuss your case with my colleagues and then we can advise you further.' The clinician must not be afraid of saying truthfully that it is very difficult to estimate just how risky surgery will be in a particular case and that the best that can be offered is a rough estimate.

These complexities, daunting for the clinician, can be overwhelming for the patient. The doctor must resist the temptation to share every detail of risk assessment with the patient. The aim should be to present a clear summary of risks and benefits and an estimate of how these balance out. This information should be given in a measured fashion and notice taken of the patient's responses, body language, and apparent understanding. A recited litany of the dangers of surgery may let the doctor feel that his or her duty has been done while doing little service to the patient. Time is needed for what is said to sink in, and we strive to achieve this counsel of perfection against the demands for efficiency that are part of every modern health service. When possible, it may be wise to invite the patient to go away and consider what has been said and return to discuss it further on another occasion.

Quantifying risk

At first sight it would seem simple to know how dangerous an operation is. For most major operations, there are published case series reporting death rates and major complication rates. For example, Bayly et al., in a study conducted for the Vascular Anaesthesia Society of Great Britain and Ireland, reported that the in-hospital mortality rate in a series of patients undergoing aortic surgery was 7%[2]. A moment's reflection will make it clear that there is a broad range of risk concealed within this figure. The regression analysis of data from this study suggested that the expected mortality for a man aged less than 64 years undergoing elective aortic aneurysm repair is 4.4%. In contrast, for a woman aged over 74 years undergoing aortic surgery for occlusive disease, the estimated mortality was approximately six times higher. For the 85-year-old patient who has had two previous myocardial infarctions, one of which was followed by heart failure, has an exercise tolerance of a few steps and has renal impairment, the risk of death following aortic surgery may be greater still. Patients vary, and there is no 'one size fits all' estimate of operative risk.

Risk scores

Clinical risk-scoring systems represent an attempt to address the problem of estimating perioperative risk in different patients. Amongst the best known are those that provide an estimate of the risk of perioperative cardiac complications. Lee Goldman described the eponymous Goldman Risk Score in 1977[3]. This was constructed from a statistical analysis of the incidence of perioperative cardiac complications in 1001 patients. Nine cardiac risk factors found to be associated with perioperative cardiac complications were allocated a score (Table 6.1). By totalling up the risk score for a patient, the clinician can estimate the risk of perioperative cardiac complications. Despite being carefully and thoughtfully constructed by one of the pre-eminent researchers in this field, the Goldman Risk Score proved far from perfect and illustrates many of the difficulties that beset clinical risk scoring. The score was constructed by noting the presence or absence of over 50 different cardiac risk factors in each of the 1,001 patients. Patients were followed up after surgery, and the occurrence of cardiac complications was recorded. A complex statistical technique was used to identify those risk factors associated with cardiac complications. The stronger the association, the higher was the points score awarded to the risk factor. All this sounds simple enough. However, the statistical power of a study of this type depends not on the number of patients studied but on the number of complications that occurred. To be statistically robust, the study should include at least 10, and ideally 20, patients who suffered a complication for each factor that is in the final risk index[4-6]. Fifty-eight patients in Goldman's study suffered cardiac complications and nine risk factors are included in the final index. With just over six risk factors per complication, the model is statistically weak. Furthermore, Goldman and his colleagues attempted to study a very large number of risk factors at the outset, many of which were related to each

Table 6.1 The Goldman risk index

Class	Point total	No or only minor complications number(%) (*n*=943)	Life-threatening complications number(%) (*n*=39)	Cardiac deaths number(%) (*n*=19)
I (*n* = 537)	0–5	532(99)	4(0.7)	1(0.2)
II (*n* = 316)	6–12	295(93)	16(5)	5(2)
III (*n* = 130)	13–25	112(86)	15(11)	3(2)
IV (*n* = 18)	>26	4(22)	4(22)	10(56)

Note: **Criteria**	**Points**
History	
Age >70 years	5
Myocardial infarction in previous 6 months	10
Physical Examination	
Third heart sound (S3) or jugular venous distension	11
Important valvular aortic stenosis	3
Electrocardiogram	
ECG: premature atrial contractions or rhythm other than sinus	7
>5 premature ventricular contractions per minute at any time before surgery	7
General Status	
$PaO2<60$ mmHg (8.0 kPa) or $PaCO2>50$ mmHg (6.7 kPa)	3
$K^+<3.0$ mmol.L^{-1} or $HCO_3^-<20$ mmol.L^{-1}	
Blood urea nitrogen >50 mg.dL^{-1} (18 mmol.L^{-1})	
Creatinine >3.0 mg.dL^{-1} (260 μmol.L^{-1})	
Abnormal serum glutamic oxalacetic transaminase (aspartate aminotransferase or AST)	3
Signs of chronic liver disease	
Patient bedridden from non-cardiac disease	
Operation	
Intrathoracic, intra-abdominal or aortic surgery	3
Emergency operation	4

other and therefore not independent. For example, the presence of a third heart sound, the presence of crepitations in the lung fields, evidence of cardiomegaly on chest X-ray, and a number of other risk factors are all potential evidence of heart failure, but each was awarded a score. While these may seem to be damning criticisms of this risk index, it should be borne in mind that at the time that it was produced it was the most rigorous study of perioperative cardiac risk available and it represented a significant advance.

There have been a number of large studies that have attempted to refine or improve upon the Goldman Risk Score[7,8]. It has now been superseded by the Revised Cardiac Risk Index Score, which was published in 1999; Goldman was one of the authors[9]. This score was derived from a study of over 2893 patients and validated in a study of a further 1422 patients. It includes the risk factors listed in Table 6.2. Each is allocated one point, and the sum of the points gives an estimate of perioperative cardiac risk. It is more robust than the original Goldman Risk Score because it was derived from a larger cohort of patients with a larger number of cardiac events. In addition, the authors took a more general approach in their definition of cardiac risk factors. For example, the perioperative risk associated with the individual symptoms and signs of

Table 6.2 The Lee risk index

Revised cardiac risk index class	Number of risk factors	Cardiac event rate in the validation cohort of the study population $n=1,422$ events/population	Risk of cardiac complications rate (95% confidence interval) (%)
I	0	2/488	0.4 (0.05–1.5)
II	1	5/567	0.9(0.3–2.1)
III	2	17/258	6.6(3.9–10.3)
IV	3 or more	12/109	11(5.6–18.4)

Note: Risk Factors
High-risk type of surgery
History of ischaemic heart disease
History of congestive heart failure
History of cerebrovascular disease
Preoperative treatment with insulin
Preoperative serum creatinine >2.0 mg.dL^{-1} (177 μmol.L^{-1}).

congestive heart failure, such as the presence or absence of a third heart sound, was not studied. Instead, congestive heart failure itself was examined as a risk factor. The Revised Cardiac Risk Index indicated that the two major cardiac pathologies, ischaemic heart disease and congestive heart failure, increase perioperative cardiac risk and it is further increased by a history of cerebrovascular disease, the presence of renal impairment or diabetes and by major surgery, and allows an estimation to be made of the magnitude of the increased risk.

The perfect risk tool would allow the clinician to dichotomize risk. It would give the patient a 95% risk of a major complication or a 95% chance of surviving without mishap. Such tools do not exist. Scores such as the Revised Cardiac Risk Index can take account only of common diseases and common situations. Individual patients are far more complex and frequently have other co-existing diseases that have not been included in the risk calculation. Risk scores are useful epidemiological and audit tools. If a surgeon and anaesthetist operate on 100 patients who have a 10% risk of complications, and 10 of those patients suffer a complication, the team is performing as expected. However, within those 100 patients will be individuals with a risk of greater than 10% and others with a risk of less than 10%. The doctor should not depend on statistics alone but also trust his or her own judgement and experience.

Preoperative testing

We rely on clinical tests to give us more information about perioperative risk. Much has been written about the lack of value of preoperative tests in low-risk patients with little or no co-morbidity. Despite the limitations of the recent National Institute of Clinical Excellence report on this topic, tests such as the ECG and blood tests are usually normal in the healthy patient and offer little additional information[10,11]. High-risk patients often have extensive co-morbidity, and the results of preoperative investigations are more likely to be abnormal. This may help the doctor to gauge the severity of the co-existing disease, but the value of such results should not be overstated. Patients with a history of previous myocardial infarction and left ventricular impairment may have a grossly abnormal ECG with deep Q waves and T-wave flattening or inversion. It is rare to find an abnormal echocardiogram in a patient with a normal ECG. In contrast, the patient with a previous extensive left ventricular infarction and severe left ventricular dysfunction may have only relatively minor changes in the ECG[12]. Perioperative screening tests can add information but they are often difficult to interpret. An abnormal test may indicate an increased likelihood of suffering a mishap but it is not a certain predictor of complications. A patient with a normal test is unlikely to suffer major complications, but not every patient with an abnormal preoperative test will suffer a related complication. This is illustrated in Table 6.3.

Major surgery is a source of major physiological stress[13]. One of the limitations of routine preoperative tests is that they test the body 'at rest' rather than under conditions of stress. Tests such as the exercise ECG, dobutamine stress echocardiography, and cardiopulmonary exercise testing examine the responses of the respiratory and cardiovascular systems to an increasing work load. Their use is advocated in guidelines such as those of the American College of Cardiology/American Heart Association for the assessment of perioperative cardiac risk[14]. It is suggested that selected patients who have a major risk factor for perioperative cardiac complications, who have a limited or unknown exercise tolerance, and are scheduled to undergo major surgery should be subjected to preoperative stress testing. The limitation of such tests is that negative results are far more informative than positive ones. A patient with a negative stress test is unlikely to suffer perioperative cardiac complications. The negative predictive value of the test is high. Although patients with a positive test are more likely to suffer a perioperative cardiac complication, the positive predictive value of the test is not great, ranging between 10 and 20% in various studies[14]. Even aggressive preoperative cardiovascular assessment can leave the clinician facing considerable uncertainty.

Table 6.3 An example to illustrate the relative positive and negative predictive values of a hypothetical preoperative test. The numbers in the table are numbers of patients. A population of 10000 patients is assumed. Ten percent of these patients suffer a postoperative complication. The hypothetical preoperative test is abnormal in a significant proportion of the population, in this case almost 30%. In this high-risk population, 10% of patients suffer a postoperative complication

		Postoperative complication	No postoperative complication	Totals
Preoperative test	Positive	950	2000	2950
	Negative	50	7000	7050
	Totals	1000	9000	10000

Note: Sensitivity of test = 950/1000 = 95%.

Note: Specificity of test = 7000/9000 = 77%.

Note: Positive predictive value of test = 950/2950 = 32%.

Note: Negative predictive value of test = 50/7050 = 99%.

Modifying risk

When faced with a high-risk patient, the obvious question is what can be done to reduce the risk of perioperative complications? It is comparatively easy to suggest that the patient's medical treatment should be optimized. It is certainly appropriate to rectify any major deficiencies in the treatment of cardiac or respiratory disease. For example, patients who have severe angina or heart failure, or poorly controlled reactive airways disease, should be referred for treatment. However, modifying medical treatment frequently comes at the price of delaying surgery. Many high-risk patients have complex medical problems and have been receiving treatment for many years. Their medical condition, although not perfect, may be the best that can be achieved.

On occasions, aggressive efforts to reduce perioperative risk can be detrimental to the patient. There is evidence that prior coronary revascularization in patients with ischaemic heart disease results in a reduced risk of perioperative cardiac complications from non-cardiac operations[15,16]. It is therefore tempting to refer patients with coronary artery disease who need non-cardiac surgery for prior coronary angioplasty or bypass grafting. The problem with this approach is that it involves exposing the patient to a series of procedures, each with its own risk. The patient needs to undergo coronary angiography and then prophylactic coronary artery bypass grafting before finally undergoing the major non-cardiac surgery that was originally planned. The combined risk of these three procedures often outweighs the risk of simply proceeding with surgery and accepting the risks associated with the co-existing coronary artery disease. There are a number of studies and analyses which indicate that prophylactic coronary revascularization, while superficially attractive, is not in the patient's best interests[17]. Coronary revascularization should be performed only if indicated for the patient's underlying heart disease[18]. Generally, patients should not be subjected to interventions in preparation for surgery unless it can be demonstrated that these will have a positive effect on the patient's prognosis.

Weighing risk and benefit

Occasionally, treatment for the patient's underlying medical condition may increase the risks associated with surgery. An example of this is the use of anti-platelet drugs such as aspirin and clopidogrel in patients with coronary artery disease. A number of studies have shown that these drugs are associated with an increased risk of surgical bleeding[19,20]. However, there is evidence that discontinuing aspirin in patients with active coronary artery disease may increase the likelihood of cardiac death[21]. While there are limitations in the evidence, the available data suggest that aspirin should be discontinued only when there is a serious risk of morbidity or mortality from perioperative bleeding, such as in neurosurgery[22].

This dilemma is even more pronounced in patients who have undergone coronary artery angioplasty by stenting. Patients who have undergone recent coronary artery stenting, especially with drug-eluting stents, are at greatly increased risk of myocardial infarction if operated on within three months of the coronary intervention[23]. Surgery in these circumstances is best avoided, but sometimes has to be performed. These patients are often treated with both aspirin and clopidogrel. There is little or no direct evidence to guide the clinician as to what to do in these circumstances, and the best course of action currently is a matter of clinical judgement[24].

Uncertainty and indecision

The pros and cons of high-risk surgery are complex and challenging for both doctor and patient. The patient must be told about the main risks associated with anaesthesia and surgery but should not be swamped with a surfeit of information. If there are two or three possible courses of action, both doctor and patient may need time to make a decision as to which is the best choice, and either may change their mind at a later date.

These dilemmas are illustrated by the procedure of endovascular aortic stenting. An abdominal aortic aneurysm may be repaired by open surgery or by the percutaneous insertion of a stent graft into the aorta under X-ray control. Endovascular aortic stenting carries some immediate risk and has a 30-day mortally of between 1 and 2%[25]. However, the short-term risks of aortic stenting are much less than those of open aortic repair, which has a perioperative mortality of approximately 7%[2]. Against this must be set the differing long-term prognoses of the two procedures. Patients who undergo open surgery need have little concern about the future integrity of their aortic graft; graft rupture and the development of further aneurysmal disease are well described but are relatively uncommon. In contrast, stent grafts may become displaced within the aorta and need regular monitoring with either CT or ultrasound scanning. It is common for the patient to have to undergo further procedures and to have further devices placed in the aorta to deal with problems with the initial stent graft. Young patients and those with aortic anatomy unsuited to stent grafting are generally advised to undergo open repair. Older patients, especially those with significant co-morbidity, are generally advised to undergo stent grafting if this is possible[26]. In many cases, the best choice is far from clear, and doctor and patient are faced with a difficult decision to be made on limited information. It is not surprising that some patients and surgeons reverse their initial decision.

The position in patients who have an abdominal aortic aneurysm and who are not fit for open aortic repair is even more challenging. Here, the choice is between no treatment and hoping that the aneurysm does not rupture, or inserting an aortic stent graft, which carries some initial risk, and sentences the patient to a lifetime of graft surveillance with possible revision procedures if required. Of course, doing nothing does not imply that the patient should be neglected. The patient should receive optimal medical therapy for the coexisting disease that has made him or her unfit for open surgery. The patient lives with the possibility that the abdominal aortic aneurysm may rupture at any time; if this happens, the patient is less likely to survive. However, if the patient has rejected insertion of a stent, the immediate risks of a procedure for stent insertion are avoided, and the patient may live for several years without being troubled by the aortic aneurysm, and may die of another cause. This is another circumstance in which the best course of action is not clear.

The EVAR 2 (Endovascular Aortic Repair 2) study was conducted to guide clinicians as to the best course of action in these patients. High-risk patients considered unfit for open aortic repair were randomized to either aortic stenting or best medical treatment[27]. During the study and follow-up periods, over a quarter of the 172 patients randomized to medical treatment subsequently underwent either aortic stenting or open repair. Of these, 30% received surgery because of patient preference, and 30% received surgery for unrecorded reasons, possibly because of surgeon preference.

These protocol violations significantly weaken the statistical power of the study, biasing it against EVAR and making it more difficult to judge the true value of this treatment. In human terms, they represent an unsurprising and understandable response on the part of the doctor and the patient. Clinical trials are conducted from a position of equipoise. We are uncertain which treatment is best and assume that both are equally good. A trial is conducted to test this assumption, and patients are allocated to one or other treatment by random chance. In this study, the patients were asked to accept random allocation to either an endovascular aortic repair or no active surgical treatment. Faced with the threat of aortic rupture, it is perhaps unsurprising that some patients who were randomized to medical treatment alone (and their doctors) chose to break with the random allocation prescribed by the study and to undergo aortic repair. Even if there is no proof that having an aortic repair improves survival, the possibility of sudden death in the absence of surgical treatment may persuade patients to have an aortic stent graft inserted rather than to do nothing.

End–of-life decisions

Even in the best hands, some high-risk patients undergoing major surgery suffer major complications, have a protracted stay on the Intensive Care Unit, and die. Modern intensive care can support failing organ systems for many days. The dilemma for the intensivist is to decide if such treatment offers the patient the opportunity to recover or is merely deferring inevitable death, while adding to the patient's burden of suffering and loss of dignity. These are complex decisions that have been reviewed in detail elsewhere and will not be discussed in detail here[28,29]. It is appropriate that such decisions are informed by the patient's opinions. It is often too late to seek the patient's views if the immediate postoperative course has been stormy. It is certainly correct to warn the high-risk patient scheduled for elective major surgery that treatment in the Intensive Care Unit may be required after the operation. It may be appropriate to seek the patient's views on how he or she would wish to be cared for if a major complication develops. It is not appropriate to dissuade the patient from having potentially life-saving surgery by overplaying the prospect of dire complications. All medical interventions carry some risk. The risks associated with taking a simple analgesic tablet are very small, whereas those of major cardiovascular or gastrointestinal surgery may be considerable. One of the burdens of medical practice is the danger of doing harm. This is a burden that the doctor must carry and not transfer to the patient. It is entirely appropriate that patients should be told about the hazards that they face, but a 10% risk of major complications, while daunting, implies a 90% chance of successful surgery and good outcome. It behoves us not to forget this.

Urgent and emergency surgery

Patients undergoing urgent or emergency surgery are often at high risk of serious complications. Conditions such as faecal peritonitis or intestinal obstruction cause severe physiological derangement and may require urgent surgical intervention. All reasonable efforts should be made to resuscitate the patient and to correct disorders of fluid and electrolyte imbalance. However, it may be impossible to restore physiological normality completely until the underlying disease is treated and it is inappropriate to delay surgery while futile attempts are made to achieve normal blood test results. The clinician needs to find an appropriate balance between making the patient as well as is possible prior to surgery and not allowing inappropriate delays.

For patients undergoing urgent surgery, the opportunities for preoperative assessment and investigation may be limited. The pressure to proceed places constraints on the consent procedure. There should certainly be time to explain the operation to the patient and the family but there may not be time for a period of detailed reflection before surgery must proceed. These difficulties may be confounded by the fact that the patient's illness may limit the ability to understand fully the information that has been given.

In the case of a patient suffering life-threatening haemorrhage or other catastrophic events, only the briefest of explanations is possible before taking the patient to the operating theatre. The greatest difficulty here lies if the patient refuses treatment. A hypotensive, bleeding patient may have cerebral ischaemia and may not be behaving rationally. However, a patient who has undergone multiple previous operations may have made a considered and rational decision not to undergo further treatment. It is important to speak to those who have been involved in the care of the patient and to have a competent colleague examine the notes while simultaneously make rapid preparations to go to the operating theatre. If the patient has made a considered and clearly documented decision not to have further treatment, this decision must be respected. If not, and if it may be possible to save the patient's life and achieve a good outcome and good quality of life, then every effort should be made to do so.

The elderly patient with a hip fracture

It is well recognized that frail, elderly patients immobilized by a hip fracture are at high risk of developing hypostatic pneumonia and death, if surgery is not undertaken. Surgical fixation of the fractured hip allows the patient to be mobilized, and greatly improves the prognosis. It also relieves the pain associated with the fracture. However, many of these patients are frail and extremely elderly, with a number of co-existing diseases. The hip fracture may have been caused by a fall precipitated by a medical event such as a myocardial infarction or stroke. In some cases, the patient is suffering from dementia and is not in a position to give consent.

Fractured neck of femur is a preterminal event in a substantial proportion of patients. Foss and Kehlet reported a 30-day perioperative mortality rate of 13% for patients undergoing surgery for hip fracture. The authors suggested that between 25 and 50% of these deaths were unavoidable and perhaps only 25% of the causes of death were amenable to treatment[30]. Nevertheless, it is appropriate, whenever possible, to fix the broken hip surgically, both to give the patient some chance of recovery and for analgesia. The anaesthetist and surgeon are therefore faced with the need to obtain consent in a frail, high-risk patient who may have a very poor prognosis.

It is important that the implications of surgery and of not proceeding with surgery are discussed with the patient and with the family. Time should be taken to determine if the patient is mentally competent. It should not be assumed that old age equates with dementia and a loss of autonomy. It may be difficult to communicate verbally with a very deaf patient, and alternative means of communication should be explored before deciding that the patient is not competent. Consent should be obtained by experienced members of staff, and the discussion with the patient and the final decision should be carefully documented. If it is decided that the patient is not competent to make a decision regarding surgery, this should be recorded. If an advocate has been appointed under the Mental Capacity Act, then third party consent should be sought. If not, Consent Form 4 should be used if it is thought that surgery is in the patient's best interests (see Chapter 5).

When to say no

In some circumstances, the risks of surgery may be high and the benefits very limited. While obtaining consent to carry out high-risk surgery can be difficult, persuading the patient that nothing can be done may be even more challenging. It may be inappropriate to operate on a patient who has widespread cancer and is unlikely to survive for more than a few weeks or months, but inactivity in the face of impending death can be difficult for the patient to bear. These patients deserve just as much time and explanation as those who are going forward to surgery.

Summary

Obtaining consent for surgery in the high-risk patient can be fraught with difficulty. The magnitude of the risk faced by the patient can be difficult to gauge. There may be a number of therapeutic options and the best choice may not be obvious. The patient may need time to consider what he or she is being told, and both the patient and doctor may change their minds at a later date. In urgent or emergency surgery the risks may be high but there may be limited time for obtaining consent. As with consent in general, the doctor should be open with the patient, and the discussions surrounding consent should be clearly documented. It is important not to lose sight of the fact that high-risk surgery can yield great benefits that make the risks worth taking. It is the duty of the doctor to weigh up the risks and benefits and to share this information with the patient. It is entirely appropriate for the doctor to suggest the correct course of action. Indeed it is an abdication of medical responsibility to leave the patient to make a difficult decision without guidance.

References

1. Forrest, J.B., Cahalan, M.K., Rehder, K., *et al.* (1990). Multicenter study of general anesthesia. II. Results. *Anesthesiology*, **72**, 262–8.
2. Bayly, P.J., Matthews, J.N., Dobson, P.M., Price, M.L., and Thomas, D.G. (2001). In-hospital mortality from abdominal aortic surgery in Great Britain and Ireland: Vascular Anaesthesia Society audit. *British Journal of Surgery*, **88**, 687–92.
3. Goldman, L., Caldera, D.L., Nussbaum, S.R., et al. (1977). Multifactorial index of cardiac risk in noncardiac surgical procedures. *New England Journal of Medicine*, **297**, 845–50.
4. Concato, J., Peduzzi, P., Holford, T.R., and Feinstein, A.R. (1995). Importance of events per independent variable in proportional hazards analysis. I. Background, goals, and general strategy. *Journal of Clinical Epidemiology*, **48**, 1495–501.
5. Peduzzi, P., Concato, J., Feinstein, A.R., and Holford, T.R. (1995). Importance of events per independent variable in proportional hazards regression analysis. II. Accuracy and precision of regression estimates. *Journal of Clinical Epidemiology*, **48**, 1503–10.

6. Peduzzi, P., Concato, J., Kemper, E., Holford, T.R., and Feinstein, A.R. (1996). A simulation study of the number of events per variable in logistic regression analysis. *Journal of Clinical Epidemiology*, **49**, 1373–9.

7. Detsky, A.S., Abrams, H.B., Forbath, N., Scott, J.G., and Hilliard, J.R. (1986). Cardiac assessment for patients undergoing noncardiac surgery. A multifactorial clinical risk index. *Archives of Internal Medicine*, **146**, 2131–4.

8. Larsen, S.F., Olesen, K.H., Jacobsen, E., *et al.* (1987). Prediction of cardiac risk in non-cardiac surgery. *European Heart Journal*, **8**, 179–85.

9. Lee, T.H., Marcantonio, E.R., Mangione, C.M., *et al.* (1999). Derivation and prospective validation of a simple index for prediction of cardiac risk of major noncardiac surgery. *Circulation*, **100**, 1043–9.

10. Reynolds, T.M. (2006). National Institute for Health and Clinical Excellence guidelines on preoperative tests: the use of routine preoperative tests for elective surgery. *Annals of Clinical Biochemistry*, **43**, 13–6.

11. The use of routine preoperative tests for elective surgery. (2003). In *National Institute for Clinical Excellence*.

12. Manes, C., Pfeffer, M.A., Rutherford, J.D., *et al.* (2003). Value of the electrocardiogram in predicting left ventricular enlargement and dysfunction after myocardial infarction. *American Journal of Medicine*, **114**, 99–105.

13. Desborough, J.P. (2000). The stress response to trauma and surgery. *British Journal of Anaesthesia*, **85**, 109–17.

14. Eagle, K.A., Berger, P.B., Calkins, H., *et al.* (2002). ACC/AHA Guideline update for perioperative cardiovascular evaluation for noncardiac surgery–Executive Summary. A report of the American College of Cardiology/American Heart Association Task Force on Practice Guidelines (Committee to Update the 1996 Guidelines on Perioperative Cardiovascular Evaluation for Noncardiac Surgery). Available from: http./www.acc.org/clinical/guidelines

15. Eagle, K.A., Rihal, C.S., Mickel, M.C., Holmes, D.R., Foster, E.D., and Gersh, B.J. (1997). Cardiac risk of noncardiac surgery: influence of coronary disease and type of surgery in 3368 operations. CASS Investigators and University of Michigan Heart Care Program. Coronary Artery Surgery Study. *Circulation*, **96**, 1882–7.

16. Foster, E.D., Davis, K.B., Carpenter, J.A., Abele, S., and Fray, D. (1986). Risk of noncardiac operation in patients with defined coronary disease: The Coronary Artery Surgery Study (CASS) registry experience. *Annals of Thoracic Surgery*, **41**, 42–50.

17. Fleisher, L.A., Skolnick. E.D., Holroyd, K.J., and Lehmann, H.P. (1994). Coronary artery revascularization before abdominal aortic aneurysm surgery: a decision analytic approach. *Anesthesia and Analgesia*, **79**, 661–9.

18. McFalls, E.O., Ward, H.B., Moritz, T.E., *et al.* (2004). Coronary-artery revascularization before elective major vascular surgery. *New England Journal of Medicine*, **351**, 2795–804.

19. Kapetanakis, E.I, Medlam, D.A., Boyce, S.W., *et al.* (2005). Clopidogrel administration prior to coronary artery bypass grafting surgery: the cardiologist's panacea or the surgeon's headache? *European Heart Journal*, **26**, 576–83.

20. Nielsen, J.D., Holm-Nielsen, A., Jespersen, J., Vinther, C.C., Settgast, I.W., and Gram, J. (2000). The effect of low-dose acetylsalicylic acid on bleeding after transurethral prostatectomy--a prospective, randomized, double-blind, placebo-controlled study. *Scandinavian Journal of Urology and Nephrology*, **34**, 194–8.

21. Collet, J.P., Montalescot, G., Blanchet, B., *et al.* (2004). Impact of prior use or recent withdrawal of oral antiplatelet agents on acute coronary syndromes. *Circulation*, **110**, 2361–7.

22. Burger, W., Chemnitius, J.M., Kneissl, G.D., and Rucker, G. (2005). Low-dose aspirin for secondary cardiovascular prevention - cardiovascular risks after its perioperative withdrawal versus bleeding risks with its continuation - review and meta-analysis. *Journal of Internal Medicine*, **257**, 399–414.

23. Kaluza, G.L., Joseph, J., Lee, J.R., Raizner, M.E., and Raizner, A.E. (2000). Catastrophic outcomes of noncardiac surgery soon after coronary stenting. *Journal of the American College of Cardiology*, **35**, 1288–94.

24. Spahn, D.R., Howell, S.J., Delabays, A., and Chassot, P.G. (2006). Coronary stents and perioperative anti-platelet regimen: dilemma of bleeding and stent thrombosis. *British Journal of Anaesthesia*, **96**, 675–7.

25. Endovascular aneurysm repair versus open repair in patients with abdominal aortic aneurysm (EVAR trial 1): randomised controlled trial.(2005). *Lancet*, **365**, 2179–86.

26. Cronenwett, J.L. (2005). Endovascular aneurysm repair: important mid-term results. *Lancet*, **365**, 2156–8.

27. Brown, L.C., Epstein, D., Manca, A., Beard, J.D., Powell, J.T., and Greenhalgh, R.M. (2004). The UK Endovascular Aneurysm Repair (EVAR) trials: design, methodology and progress. *European Journal of Vascular and Endovascular Surgery*, **27**, 372–81.

28. Rubenfeld, G.D. (2004). Principles and practice of withdrawing life-sustaining treatments. *Critical Care Clinics*, **20**, 435–51.

29. Fassier, T., Lautrette, A., Ciroldi, M., and Azoulay, E. (2005). Care at the end of life in critically ill patients: the European perspective. *Current Opinion in Critical Care*, **11**, 616–23.

30. Foss, N.B. and Kehlet, H. (2005). Mortality analysis in hip fracture patients: implications for design of future outcome trials. *British Journal of Anaesthesia*, **94**, 24–9.

Chapter 7

Children

Oliver R Dearlove

During recent decades, the shift in children's healthcare towards one based on a close and continuous involvement of the child's family has become commonplace in the Western world. When a child is ill, the family is always affected; it is the family that is the constant in a child's life. It is therefore important that a good parent–professional relationship develops at all levels of healthcare involving a child. However, allowing children the freedom to participate in the decision-making process is fraught with ethical and legal dilemmas. For sick children and anxious parents, the dilemmas also involve the clinician, who must act in the best interests of his patient.

The law has long presumed that children and young people do not have the capacity to make important decisions, thus denying them their rights to self-determination; parents and doctors have traditionally made most medical decisions for and on behalf of children in their care. More recently, the introduction of family-centred approaches to healthcare accommodate and respect the complex nature of parent–child relationships and the dependence and vulnerability of the child and his developing morality and capacity for decision-making. Nevertheless, it is most often the doctor and the parent who determine the child's role in decision-making, thus excluding the child from involvement at the first hurdle. The decision is therefore parent-centred and not patient-centred.

The case of *Gillick v West Norfolk and Wisbech Area Health Authority*[1] established in England that children under 16 years of age could give legally effective consent to medical treatment, independent of their parents' wishes, provided that they had sufficient understanding and intelligence. However, the legal and ethical concept of the 'best interests of the child' is vague and open to manipulation and abuse, and the legal right to refuse care still eludes children and young people. Although a young person may have full capacity to understand the nature and purpose of a proposed procedure and the consequences for him, he may nevertheless be overruled in his decision or have been denied the opportunity to share in decision-making in the first place. Although the standard of reasonableness is used in law, young people are seldom deemed reasonable when they disagree with their doctors and parents.

In 2004, in a report compiled from 59 separate reports by voluntary bodies and statutory organizations and published for the Commission for Health Improvement[2] Peter Boylan stated that: 'young people felt that they had the right to participate in decisions about their treatment rather than being passive recipients of care, that they were unhappy with the lack of communication, and that they did not think that they were sufficiently involved in the decision-making process'. The developing autonomy of children has increasingly being recognized in medical decision-making. In assessing competency in young people aged 9 to 21 years of age, Weithorn and Campbell showed that 14-year-olds do not differ from adults, and children as young as 9 years of age are capable of making reasonable preferences regarding treatment[3]. Most teenagers who want to, are capable of making reasoned decisions about their care[4], and the average 14-year-old may be in a better position to make informed rational decisions than his parents. Conversely, Priscilla Alderson has demonstrated that the exclusion of a child from the decision-making process, particularly as a result of parent–doctor collaboration, is likely to cause resentment or reduced trust[5].

Society generally accepts that the parent and doctor will act in the child's 'best interest', and in the absence of any evidence to the contrary, a doctor should assume that a parent has his child's best interests at heart. When the child is not judged to be competent or to have legal rights, the parents are most often obligated to act as proxy decision-makers and the law[6] confers on the parent this right regardless of the child's maturity. In distinct contrast, on the turn of a birthday, an 18-year-old adult's ability to reason is not called into question and his competence is extremely unlikely to be challenged, regardless of the decision he chooses to make. Furthermore, regardless of his previous dependence on his parents, they have no rights in respect of treatment decisions he makes, unless he invites them into the decision-making process. The competent adult may therefore define his own concept of best interests even if they appear to be irrational and out of synchrony with others or with the rest of the society. Young people appear to be disadvantaged; they may not be consulted or given choices and often others choose for them. This has been described as a licence 'to bulldoze children into treatment regardless of their personal wishes, fears, or capacity to understand the implications of their decisions'[7]. English law appears to be at variance with European and international law, which emphasizes the right of every child to self-determination, dignity, respect, non-interference, and the right to make informed decisions[8].

Increasingly, however, it is being recognized that children and young people have a lot to contribute to decision-making. Involving young people helps to protect their integrity, shows them respect and trust, and facilitates honest and open communication. This enables children to have some control over their care and contributes to the development of their personal autonomy.

Beauchamp and Childress suggest that, for proxy decision-making, the following abilities are required to make reasoned judgements: adequate knowledge and information, emotional stability, and a commitment to the incompetent patient's interest that is free of conflicts of interest and free of controlling influence by others who may not act in the patient's best interest. But parents are not infrequently in a position of anxiety and distress that they too may not have full capacity to make important decisions for their child.

Scenario 1

A sturdy 14-year-old sports playing teenager landed heavily so that a sharp fencing upright pierced his axilla but missed all important structures such as the brachial plexus. The child was placed first on an operating list starting at 09.00 h after a period of starvation from the time of his admission in the early hours of the morning. The anaesthetic might be complicated by the wood which was sticking up vertically and pointing towards his face. The mother had parental authority of the child. The father was also present. The child was clearly Gillick competent. The mother stated that the father did not have power to consent at all to the anaesthetic or operation whereas the father was offering to write his name on the consent form. The child's sister was also present. Everyone chipped in. The mother was insisting that she alone could consent to surgery on her son. The mother went on to say how disturbed she was at the media interest. Photographs had been taken with permission at another hospital, she told us, but it was not clear who had possession of the photographs and which of the three have given permission for the photographs to be taken. The media were inquiring and might have been offering to pay for some photographs, which were in fact published later that day. It was not clear if the mother had consented to their release. The conclusion drawn by the clinician was that all parties should sign the consent form for the operation. Separate consent was drawn up for clinical photographs that the anaesthetist took. The anaesthetist checked that previous photographs had been validly consented to by the mother. It was these photographs, which were later published. The child made a good postoperative recovery. The child was given control of the digital images and the issues of his fee for publication was not pursued.

Discussion

The end-point and the focus for all concerned should be twofold: prevention from harm and the successful treatment of the patient. Secondary issues concern ownership and rights to photographs. Assuming that this patient has the capacity to consent, it should be with his understanding of the nature and purpose of treatment and its potential consequences, both good and bad, and hopefully with the co-operation of his parents. However, the seriousness and urgency of this situation is likely to limit his and his parents' capacity for decision-making. Even though time has been allowed to elapse between the patient presenting as an emergency and being prepared for surgery, psychological trauma and accompanying anxiety and discomfort in patient and parents may have diminished only marginally.

The law expects that someone, normally the patient, has capacity to consent. The law may be explicit about who has the right to consent and in what circumstances, but seldom does it anticipate and regulate the unique circumstances faced by clinicians throughout their professional lives. In this situation, it should not be assumed that patient or parents have the capacities to make fully informed decisions about treatment and care.

In this scenario, there appears to be excessive focus on who has the 'right' to sign the consent form, which is exacerbated by tension between all involved. This is complicated by arguments regarding 'rights' to ownership and publication of photographs.

The child may understand fully the nature of his injury and the proposed surgery, but may not comprehend the risks associated with anaesthesia. He therefore will not be competent to decide for himself and will need the help of others to guide and share in the decision-making process. Consent is not about the signature but about a patient, parent or guardian giving permission for the doctor to provide treatment. Further, this permission should result from the patient and parents being appropriately informed and that the risks and benefits of the procedure are presented and understood. If the child in this scenario has capacity to consent, then with his permission, or at his request, the parents may be informed of his condition and treatment plan.

How is the clinician so sure that the young man is 'clearly Gillick competent'? In more normal, controlled healthcare environments, should he and his parents have experienced them, decisions will have been made in consultation with his clinician and between him and his parents. It would be very unusual for him to act in isolation of his parents unless he was familiar with the healthcare environment and his own health problems. However, this situation is far from normal or controlled. There is nothing to indicate that this patient or his parents are familiar with a healthcare environment. In such unfamiliar territory, the parents would be expected to be anxious, upset, and even confused, and the patient more so because of tiredness, pain, analgesics, and starvation.

One of the most troubling aspects of this case is the 'argument' concerning photographs, which may have caused the patient undue stress and anxiety. This was introduced during the preoperative interview and may have allowed all involved to become distracted from the purpose and process of consent and details of the treatment. Images taken by clinicians in the course of their work are the property of their employer. They should be taken only for the purposes of facilitating care. With the patient's permission, they may be used for educational and teaching purposes in the future. Patients may request copies of such photographs, but may have to pay a small amount for them.

This case illustrates the difficulties faced in obtaining valid consent in emergency situations. In similar situations, doctors may need to speak privately with young patients to ascertain the level of their capacity for decision-making about different aspects of their care.

Scenario 2

A 10-year-old suffered a severe head injury in another part of the city. Scans showed a collection of blood within the brain, and the child was referred to a specialist centre for emergency drainage. The child arrived in a poor clinical condition and was pushed from the receiving bay directly into the operating theatre. A mature 17-year-old teenage boy who identified himself as an older brother had driven in behind the ambulance. The anaesthetist told him that the child was an emergency and that he wished to anaesthetize without further ado in order to save her life. The teenager stated that he was not able to consent on behalf of his sister and that he should therefore wait for the parents, who were driving more slowly to the hospital. The young adult then burst into tears. The child was anaesthetized and operated on. She did well postoperatively.

Discussion

This case illustrates the problems that may often arise when other family members are asked to assent to care. The anaesthetist wished to indicate clearly that consent was not necessary for an operation in order to save life, but the explanation was interpreted as a request for consent. In the midst of the family crisis, the request that he understand what was going on and why was hopelessly confused as a request for permission to operate on a dying sibling.

The clinician's duty of care to the patient in this regard is clear. The need for a skilled and experienced clinician communicator is essential but, even when one is available, such confusion may arise from time to time. While the parents' presence may have allayed their son's trauma, they too would have been presented with the same information. They too may have been equally fraught with tears, upset, and anxious.

Consent is neither necessary nor important in such emergency circumstances but skilled communication is. Indeed, some attempts to obtain consent or assent for treatment may be unethical because they result in harm to that relative. Such 'harm' is described earlier. Nevertheless, skilled communication is always essential, and more so when the trauma and urgency of care are immediate and life-threatening. However, patients have the right and the need to know about care and treatment received after the event. Commonly, trainee anaesthetists, and others ill-equipped to handle these problems, are faced with having received little or no training or directly supervised experience in communicating bad news to patients and relatives. Equally commonly, language and culture barriers between patient, relative, and doctor prevent adequate information exchange, in addition to exacerbating poor communication.

Scenario 3

A child has a complex disease, and the medical team decides that lumbar puncture, skin biopsy, and the taking of venous blood for laboratory measurements should be undertaken under general anaesthesia. The ear, nose, and throat (ENT) consultant will assess the airway, and a general surgical consultant will perform cystoscopy. This is all to be performed in one operating session on a Thursday morning. The team's junior doctor protests that the clerking of the patient has no educational value for her, and she cannot take consent for lumbar puncture as she has not been assessed as competent to perform the procedure. She refuses to seek consent for any form of anaesthesia. The team's registrar therefore undertakes this task. The ENT team agrees to seek separate consent for the airway assessment. The procedure goes ahead even though the general surgeon is detained at another hospital, because the rest of the team are present. The remainder of the procedures are performed, and the junior doctor who is giving the anaesthetic shows the haematology trainee the technique of lumbar puncture but refuses to give or check any drug given. The child is wheeled into the recovery room without having had the cystoscopy because the general surgeon is still absent. In the recovery room, it is found that the patient's records indicate that the child has had a skin biopsy but should have had a muscle biopsy. The ENT surgeon insists he is not in charge.

Discussion

In England, the Department of Health (DH) guidelines recommend that there should be a unified consent form including permission for anaesthesia, and that the anaesthetist should visit the patient for discussion, which is recorded in the notes. Anaesthetists' professional bodies guide them on the standards of care which patients should expect: amongst others in preoperative assessment, aspects of communication, provision of information, and obtaining consent. Consultants and trainees should be familiar with each others' responsibilities regarding clinical supervision.

Of fundamental importance to patient safety is good teamwork. In this scenario, the absence of all of the abovementioned factors has put this patient's safety in jeopardy, and resulted in the need for further procedures under another general anaesthetic.

The case illustrates many challenges that are faced in multidisciplinary team work. These have the potential to fragment care to such a degree that the team fails to manage patient-centred care effectively. Various members of the team have agreed to perform procedures for which consent is necessary and which they will obtain. For a raft of procedures, there may be two or three consent forms. This not only goes against DH guidance but will result in several visits and form-filling for doctors and patient/parent. This example illustrates how the doctor in charge may vary depending on where the child is in the patient journey. No single lead clinician appears to have oversight of the child's treatment. The physician requesting the procedures does not appear to have made adequate arrangements for the patient's care and assumptions are made that everything will fall into place without this coordination. Neither does their appear to be any concern for the fact that trainee doctors may be performing procedures in which they are inexperienced and which require direct supervision.

There appears to have been ample time to arrange for the coordination of all necessary procedures and investigations and for parent and child to be given all the information necessary to consent to this package of care.

If the child was knowledgeable about the condition and old enough to understand, he should have been given the opportunity to know about all the procedures, and in particular their benefits and the risks, in addition to the benefits and risks associated with the general anaesthetic. Assumptions are all too often made about competency based on age alone, and this is misleading. For many children with chronic or long-term conditions, competencies are many but not necessarily complete, and therefore assumptions should not be made. For example, a 12-year-old child with a chronic condition may be an expert in his own condition and its problems and have full capacity to understand the nature and purpose of investigations alongside the consequences of not going ahead. Nevertheless, he may never have experienced a general anaesthetic and therefore the anaesthetist must be sure that the understanding of this and its relative risks is also satisfactory in order for consent to be valid. Children as young as 8 years of age may be fully involved in decision-making processes concerning their care. In contrast, an apparently intelligent 16-year-old young person may have great difficulty weighing up such decisions or even contemplating the decision-making process at all.

Children are inquisitive by nature. They are open to learning about themselves from being very young and teachers often say they are a delight to teach up to the age of 8 or 9 years because they absorb a considerable amount of information in such an enthusiastic way. Children must never be denied the right to ask questions and be given appropriate and honest answers—these enable normal human social and psychological development. It is therefore essential that it is the child, not the parent, who is the centre of the discussion; this means speaking to the child in the presence of the parent, not the parent in the presence of the child. If the child is not satisfied with answers, he almost invariably asks why?—what does that mean?—and so on. Children tend to stop asking when they have received enough information. Children are very perceptive of withholding of information and inevitably mistrust those who do so and are found out. This is likely to have long-term damaging consequences for a child, particularly one who is dependent on continuing care. Therefore, care, skill, time, and effort must always be taken to communicate with a child or young person.

From the parents' perspective, where are the parents? Has the nature and purpose of the investigations been explained? When and how? If the decision to go ahead with these procedures was reached in advance, it is essential that this is properly communicated to all concerned, including the parents. Is information explained in a way that is appropriate for a parent to give valid consent? If circumstances change, child and parent should be informed. Have the child and the parent been informed of the possibility that another general anaesthetic will be necessary if all investigations are not carried out together? Should consent for surgery and investigations be separate from consent for anaesthesia? When a patient or carer gives permission for treatment, they do so as a result of receiving sufficient information in a timely and sensitive manner and being given time to query and reflect on that information; the adequacy of information should be based on what the patient wants and ought to know, not on what the doctor deems appropriate. Consent is invalid if information is withheld and if, by commission or omission, the patient or parent is misled or misinformed. Nevertheless, this should not suggest that each procedure requires a different consent form. Trusts require forms to be completed, signed, and filed at management's convenience rather than for patient's needs and wants. The essential element is in *what* is communicated and recorded, not on *whether* or *how* it is recorded. The importance of consent for anaesthesia should not be underestimated, as in this case, the procedures will not go ahead with it.

Should a doctor seek consent for procedures in which they have insufficient skills and knowledge? An anaesthetist may have sufficient knowledge and experience to inform a patient about general anaesthesia but may have no experience of caring for children. Alternatively, he may be unable to be understood because of a poor command and clarity in spoken English in the local dialect. If a doctor fails to communicate effectively, it is unlikely that valid consent can be obtained.

Does a doctor have the right to decline a delegated task on the basis that it has no educational value? Doctors in training are employed to provide a service to the NHS: training and service delivery are inextricably linked. It is unethical for a doctor to refuse care and assessment of a patient, merely because it is of no educational value or interest to that doctor. Educational value is gained by experiential learning within a supervisory framework, and this is applied and relearned over a lifetime of care.

Are junior medical staff appropriately led and supervised? The magnitudes of the problems of communication in this case are brought into stark relief when one considers the following:

- The doctors do not appear to relate well to each other.
- There appears to be no adequate communication with child or parents.
- The doctors are poorly led and guided, and unsure of their responsibilities.
- The patient has undergone general anaesthesia and is taken to the recovery room before the completion of all necessary investigations, necessitating another anaesthetic in the near future.

Of particular concern in this case is that, because of poor clinical governance and leadership, there has been a failure to carry out the necessary care for this child. Cystoscopy has not been performed, and a skin biopsy has been taken instead of a muscle biopsy. What degree of harm will result from communicating (or not communicating) to the patient and the parent the need to for a further general anaesthetic to perform these procedures? There may be a complete loss of trust between patient, parent, and clinical team. Parents, like their children, are reliant on a continuing relationship with clinicians and should be able to trust that their professionalism and integrity remain intact.

Scenario 4

A Congolese refugee presents to the cardiology department of the hospital. The child has had an operation for cyanotic congenital heart disease at a European Hospital elsewhere in the European community; the details are unknown. The child has presented for assessment for further surgery, and cardiac catheterization is planned. The father and cousin are in attendance, and the uncle speaks English. There is no bed at present in the cardiology ward and the cardiologist is in transit from a hospital in another city. The anaesthetist's visit for pre-anaesthetic assessment proceeds in private with the cousin translating, but it is obvious that the translations are being truncated. The pre-interventional work-up is uneventful. It is pointed out that the bed is being made ready, and the cardiologist is delayed. The uncle has to go to work in 2 h. Later, after the child has been anaesthetized and cardiac catheterization has been carried out uneventfully, the father complains that he has not had enough time to discuss the procedure with the cardiac team.

Discussion

It is not uncommon for doctors to find themselves in situations where a relative interprets and translates for a patient. In this scenario, father and child are in a strange country and unfamiliar environment. The anaesthetist is unlikely to obtain a good medical history and this has potential consequences for the care of the patient, and for the father, who shows his unhappiness about the amount of information he has received regarding his daughter's care. The father probably knows a lot about his daughter's previous medical care, but is unable to convey this information to the hospital staff, even though he knows it is relevant to the present condition and treatment.

When a friend, community elder, or family member is involved in translation for patients, they are more likely to interpret and translate unreliably and inaccurately than is an independent interpreter. The translator may have a poor grasp of English, may not understand the nature and purpose of treatment offered, and may lack understanding of the full implications of what is being said. Additionally, there is a strong temptation to act as an advocate to represent what the interpreter regards as the patient's views, and the interpreter may use his own values and judgements to determine how risks and benefits of what is being proposed are expressed to the patient and parent. Sometimes, usually with the best of intentions, a relative acting as an interpreter may mislead or misinform the patient to achieve what he considers to be in that patient's best interests.

In contrast, independent translators are equipped to relay questions and concerns in a way in which the patient expresses them, and then to interpret the doctor's answers accurately. This information exchange should be objective, honest, and free from bias: an uphill challenge for a relative who may be emotionally involved with the patient. Furthermore, it is the most appropriate method of obtaining a good medical history and valid consent. There is no doubt that NHS trusts are continually challenged to anticipate such needs. But if the family is already known to the general practitioner or the hospital, there should be no excuse for substituting family members for an independent translator, other than in an emergency situation.

Even very young children can be quite traumatized by anaesthesia and surgery, something that may only manifest itself when entering the operating theatre suite or in the postoperative period. This is likely to be more problematic if the parent and child lack understanding of their environment. People are at their most vulnerable when under stress. The stress of serious illness creates in most of us an inability to understand or comprehend what clinicians perceive as even the most basic medical information. Patients value time to reflect on what is said and to ask questions or seek clarification regarding medical jargon and complicated procedures, something which is difficult to achieve without professional translation services.

It would appear, therefore, that the best and safest care in this case is underpinned by professional translation services. However, translation services are costly. The result is that many NHS services do not provide independent translation services unless requested by patients. The fact that the anaesthetic pre-assessment and cardiac catheterization was uneventful is no justification for the failure to ensure adequate pre-interventional assessment and provision of appropriate information. Clinicians and managers who pay lip service to the needs of such vulnerable people would do well to reflect by putting themselves in this parent's position. The parent was entitled to a full consultation and explanation, with appropriate interpreter facilities.

Scenario 5

A 14-year-old child has a hernia, which had previously been incarcerated and so it is advised that the child should have an operation. The parents consent to the procedure on his behalf, according to the hospital protocol. He is pathologically afraid of all things to with anaesthesia. He says that he is well aware of the necessity for the operation and consents to that but asks for help in coping with the stress of the operation and anaesthetic. He does not wish to see an anaesthetist before the procedure but states that he has confidence in a play-specialist. A social contract is presented for agreement with the anaesthetist of do's and don'ts, which are agreed. Intravenous access is to be gained on the ward by the nursing intravenous team. Everyone agrees that an oral premedicant should be prescribed but it has a disgusting taste and he spits it out. Thirty minutes after he is sent for by the operating theatre staff, he is to be seen with the play specialist in the main corridor. An hour later, he is back in the anaesthetic room having briefly visited 15 min previously. As soon as the induction drug is given, he insists that he wants to go home. He falls asleep and the operation is carried out uneventfully.

Discussion

Because the child's parents have consented to the procedures, it is lawful for the hospital staff to carry out the procedure. Nevertheless, it is now not usual practice to proceed with the operation if the child is refusing consent and is more than 10–12 years of age.

The issue here is that the child has said that he wishes to have the operation and so consents, but behaves as if he has not consented. A social contract is constructed with a person he trusts, but by spitting out the premedication, the contract is almost immediately broken.

Everyone agrees that forcing the child to have the treatment, which might have been a commonplace solution 15 years ago, is not appropriate to the circumstances today. Some of the surgical team state that the child is really refusing and quite extensive hospital resources are being used to convert a 'no' to a 'yes'. They say that the child's refusal should be respected.

There must be some underlying reasons for this child's 'pathological' dislike of all things anaesthetic. Is this a 'pathological' or 'psychological' dislike; the former might indicate to the clinical reader that this patient is an awkward, self-centred attention seeker. The latter may indicate that this child needs help to overcome a complex problem. It will only be when an appropriate expert assessment is made of this child's underlying anxiety that help and preparation for surgery can begin.

Ethical issues continue to tax clinicians in the 21st century. The plethora of advice, which is based on previous mishaps or difficulties encountered with technological advances, may not equip clinicians to help them overcome issues that occur much more commonly.

References

1. AC 112 (1986).
2. Boylan, P. (2004). Children's voices project. Feedback from children and young people about their experience and expectations of health care. www.chi.nhs.uk/childrens_voices/index.shtml
3. Weithorn, L. A. and Campbell, S. B. (1982). The Competency of Children and Adolescents to Make Informed Treatment Decisions. *Child Development*, **53**(6), 1589–98.
4. Sanci L. A., Sawyer, S. M., S-L Kang, M., Haller, D.M., and Patton, G.C. (2005). Confidential Health Care for Adolescents: reconciling clinical evidence with family values. *Medical Journal of Australia*, **183**(8), 410–4.
5. Alderson, P. (1993). Children's consent to surgery. Open University Press, Buckingham, p. 9.
6. In England Northern Ireland and Wales a parent may consent for a child up to age 18. Re MB (an adult: medical treatment) [1997] 2 FLR 426 (CA).
7. Shield, J. P. and Baum, J. D. (1994). Children's Consent to Treatment. *British Medical Journal*, **308**, 1182–83.
8. Alderson, P. (1993). European charter of children's rights. *Bulletin of Medical Ethics*, 12.

Chapter 8

Incapacity: learning impaired, dementia, mental, and emotional disturbance

Stuart M White

Consent is a moral concept that reflects the respect given by society towards the autonomy of its citizens. In clinical practice, consent allows an autonomous patient to define and protect his or her own interests and to control bodily privacy[1].

However, there is a large and increasing number of patients who do not possess the ability to make autonomous healthcare decisions, in that they lack the capacity to think, decide, and act on the basis of such thought, independently and without hindrance by others. Such patients are commonly encountered in anaesthetic and critical care practice—for example, the demented geriatric patient requiring operative fixation of a fractured neck of femur, the majority of interventions administered to intensive care patients, the semiconscious inebriate requiring anaesthesia for computed tomography of the head, followed by operative drainage of a traumatic intracerebral haemorrhage, and the emergency resuscitation and continuing care of a variety of medical, surgical, and obstetric patients.

Yet adult patients who lack legal capacity still require health care, whether it is necessary to alleviate their condition or to prevent further deterioration. If incapacitated patients are not able to participate in directing their own treatment, of necessity it falls to others—usually doctors, occasionally judges or relatives—to make treatment decisions on the patients' behalf. This requires that such proxy decision makers to refer to some putative but transparent set of values when deciding what is best for the patient.

The aim of this chapter is to describe what the common law is, with regard to medical decision-making on behalf of adults who lack capacity, and to describe how this has been superseded by statutory legislation in the form of the Mental Capacity Act 2005, brought in to further protect incapacitated patients, and enforced from October 1st 2007, in England and Wales.

The common law relating to adults without capacity

In law, consent is a device that protects the autonomy of a patient from interference by another party. Any doctor, for example, may be liable in battery if he or she administers a treatment to a patient without obtaining valid consent.

Under common law, consent to medical treatment is judged valid if it is given voluntarily by an appropriately informed, *competent* patient[2]. Refusals of medical treatment are accorded similar legal status, provided that the patient is appropriately informed, competent, and acting voluntarily[3].

Every adult is presumed to have the capacity to consent to medical, surgical, or dental treatment, unless that presumption is disproved[4].

A patient lacks capacity/competence if unable to make a decision whether to consent to, or refuse, treatment. The index legal case in this instance is that of *Re C*[5]. C, a 68-year-old chronic paranoid schizophrenic (and convicted murderer) detained at Broadmoor psychiatric hospital, developed gangrene of the right lower leg. His surgeon strongly suggested C undergo a below-knee amputation as a curative treatment. C contested that he would rather 'die with two feet than live with one', but consented to local debridement and skin grafting. C's solicitor requested an undertaking from the hospital that they would not amputate in future, in view of C's repeated refusals. The hospital sought the court's guidance as to whether C was competent to refuse amputation. Justice Thorpe decided that C was indeed competent to make contemporaneous refusals of treatment. In deciding, the judge recognized a three-stage test of competency used by a forensic psychiatrist involved in the case, in order to determine C's competency. This test has subsequently become the legal standard of competence with regards consent, such that a patient is declared competent to consent or refuse treatment if:

- They can take in and retain the information provided (particularly with relevance to the consequences of their decision);
- They can believe the information;
- They can weigh that information, balancing risks and needs, when considering their decision.

A subsequent decision in the Court of Appeal in the case of *Re MB*[4], omits the necessity of believing the information. Essentially then, patients are competent if they can understand and remember the information provided to them, and can use the information in order to decide on the course of treatment (if any) that they wish to undertake.

The decision made by the patient does not have to be sensible, rational, or well-considered, although an irrational decision which is at odds with the information provided or based on beliefs not widely held by society might indicate that the patient is suffering from mental illness[6].

It should be noted, however, that mental illness *per se* does not automatically render a patient incapable of making decisions about medical treatment, although mental illness may impair a patient's capacity to provide valid consent for treatment. According to Section IV of the Mental Health Act, 1983 (with regard to the recently published Mental Health Act 2007), compulsory treatment without consent may be provided for the mental disorder from which the patient is suffering (s.63). Nevertheless, consent (and/or a second opinion) is still required for the administration of electroconvulsive therapy (ECT)(s.58) or psychosurgery (s.57).

The competence of a patient is a question of fact—the patient is either competent to decide or incompetent. The more serious the decision to be made, the proportionately greater the level of capacity is required[3].

In clinical practice, a third group of patients may be identified—those with fluctuating levels of competence. It is often difficult to determine whether such patients are in fact competent. Furthermore, such patients may be subject to pain, anxiety, stress, or the secondary cerebral effects of systemic disease. However, these factors do not necessarily render patients incompetent. In her judgement of *Re MB*[4], concerning a needle-phobic 23-year-old who refused intravenous access for caesarean section, Dame Elizabeth Butler-Sloss noted that 'although confusion, shock, fatigue, pain, or drugs may completely erode capacity', those concerned must be satisfied 'that such factors are operating to such a degree that the ability to decide is absent'.

That said, the law is clear: competent adult patients may consent to or refuse any and all treatments, at any time. The question that then becomes obvious is, what is the legal mechanism that allows medical treatment to be provided for adults who lack the capacity to decide for themselves? Furthermore, who makes the decision on behalf of the patient without capacity?

These questions have relevance to a sizeable—and growing—number of patients. A significant proportion of the UK population lacks the capacity to make decisions about their personal, financial, or medical affairs. Their incapacity may be predictable (e.g. Alzheimer's disease, Huntington's dementia), permanent (e.g. perinatal brain damage or persistent vegetative state), or temporary (e.g. unconsciousness following intoxication with drugs or alcohol, head injury, or during general anaesthesia). In the United Kingdom, approximately 7 50 000 people have dementia, 1.5 million have some form of learning disability, and 1 20 000 have ongoing problems as a result of severe brain injury. Seventy percent of weekend accident and emergency patient episodes (1 million cases annually) are related to alcohol intoxication[7].

Until recently, the common law has been very clear—no other person (including the courts, relatives, those with legal powers of attorney or any health professional) may consent to medical treatment for an adult without capacity. However, the courts have stated that doctors have a legal duty to administer treatment to adults without capacity providing that the treatment is *necessary* and in the *best interests* of the patient, such that instigating or continuing treatment under these circumstances would not constitute a battery. It should be noted that 'best interests' are more than just 'medical best interests', and represent a sum assessment of the patient's wider welfare (e.g. previous wishes, family wishes, quality of life, etc.).

It is usually the doctor who decides whether the patient is competent (i.e. can understand, remember, and use information to make a decision), although a secondary opinion from a colleague (usually a psychiatrist) or from the courts may be sought in equivocal cases. The doctor must be prepared to justify his decision to the court if asked to do so. Courts remain the final arbiters for determining capacity, and for deciding whether an adult without capacity should receive treatment or not, when there is disagreement.

Bournewood

However, a recent decision by the European Court of Human Rights (ECtHR) in the case of *HL v UK*[8] (the '*Bournewood*' case) has challenged the 'best interests' principle, and may have significant implications for the anaesthetic and intensive care management of hospitalized patients without capacity.

In 1997, Mr L, a 49-year-old with severe autism, was informally detained in his own 'best interests' at Bournewood Hospital, under the common law doctrine of necessity. He did not resist detention. His carers contested unsuccessfully in the High Court that his detention was unlawful. The Court of Appeal overturned that decision, but the House of Lords unanimously found against Mr L.

The ECtHR, however, found that Bournewood Hospital *had* unlawfully deprived Mr L of his liberty, in contravention of Article 5(1) of the European Convention of Human Rights, because the doctors treating him 'exercised complete and effective control over his care and movements', even though the doctors claimed that the treatment was necessary and in his best interests.

Effectively, therefore, adult patients without capacity may not be detained in hospital purely because their doctors deem continuing treatment necessary and in the patients' best interests. However, the judgement does not imply that doctors should not initiate or continue to provide necessary emergency medical care to incapacitated patients in their best interests.

An estimated 22 000 'Bournewood' patients are resident in NHS hospitals[9], lacking legal capacity but complying with treatment provided in their best interests, who are effectively not allowed to leave hospital, and have no recourse to legal review of their detention.

These patients are commonly encountered in anaesthetic practice (e.g. patients with severe learning difficulties who require dental treatment, brain-damaged patients who require gastrostomy, and demented patients who require semi-elective orthopaedic procedures) and are subject to 'complete and effective control over their care and movements' when they are admitted to NHS hospital wards. This is particularly the case when they are admitted to intensive care or high-dependency facilities, where a degree of chemical or physical restraint may be required to facilitate certain procedures, such as mechanical ventilation.

The ECtHR decision has forced the UK government to instigate a consultation process aimed at producing legislation to protect these vulnerable patients, over and above the protection afforded by the Mental Capacity Act 2005 (see below).

Although the ramifications of *HL v UK* are still unclear, anaesthetists and intensivists should be aware that if they continue with procedures that might deny a patient without capacity their liberty (e.g. sedation to prevent a patient leaving their bed, premedication that facilitates transport to theatre, and interhospital transfer of a recovering patient due to bed shortages), particularly if those procedures are opposed by relatives or friends of the patient, their employers may be exposed to the risk of costly litigation under the Human Rights Act 1998[10].

Problems with the common law relating to adults without capacity

Whereas the law sees only black and white, medicine tends to deal in shades of grey. Although the legal system is used to determine specific answers to questions concerning legal capacity, there is little in the way of concrete advice on how to establish capacity—determination is usually made on a subjective basis by doctors according broadly with the three-stage test described in *Re C*. Furthermore, there is concern that since the introduction of the Human Rights Act 1998, public authorities and their employees (including doctors) are at risk of litigation if they fail to recognize their statutory duty towards the individual, competent or otherwise.

Adults has capacity if they can understand and remember the information presented to them, and use it to arrive at a decision. A number of questions arise from this statement. What do they have to understand—everything, the 'important bits' or broadly what is being suggested? Is their understanding dependent on their intelligence, psychological or psychiatric function, or social factors, such as their education? What about the role of communication—different languages, the doctor–patient interaction (what the doctor says is not necessarily what the patient hears), deafness, and speaking difficulties? Furthermore, do patients therefore lack competence if they are unable to remember part or all of what they are told? Several studies have shown that surgical patients remember less than 10% of what they are told more than 24 h later. Finally, should patients be considered incompetent if they refuse to make a choice, or defer the choice back to the doctor ('Do what you think is best, doc'), or to a relative?

If patients fall into one or more of these categories, then they are at risk of having their autonomy overruled, and decisions about medical treatment made for them in their best interests. Given that the provisions of the Human Rights Act 1998 are very much geared towards the protection of individual autonomy, the UK government has been recently compelled to introduce an important new piece of legislation, the Mental Capacity Act 2005, in order to clarify the law safeguarding decision-making by others on behalf of mentally incapacitated adults.

Case study

The mental capacity act 2005[11]

With a few notable exceptions, the Mental Capacity Act 2005 ('the Act') is simply a statutory formalization of the common law in the area of capacity for decision making. The Act received Royal Assent on 7th April 2005, and was fully enforced on 1st October 2007.

The Act is founded upon a considerable amount of background input, from, amongst others, the Law Commission (Report No. 231 [1995] *Mental Incapacity*[12]), the government themselves (*Who decides? Making decisions on behalf of mentally incapacitated adults* [1997][13] and *Making Decisions* [1999][14]), and a Joint Committee of both Houses of Parliament, all with the aim of improving the legal protection afforded to those over the age of 16 in England and Wales who lack (or may in future lack) the ability to make decisions for themselves about medical, personal, or financial matters.

The Act itself is separated into three parts. Part 1—'Persons who lack capacity'— explains the principles underlying the Act, the definition of incapacity, the role of Lasting Powers of Attorney and court-appointed deputies, the law concerning advanced decisions, and the legal conditions required for involving incapacitated adults in research. Part 2 describes the institution and operating procedures of a Court of Protection, to whom applications and referrals are made concerning adults without capacity. Part 3 deals with miscellaneous and general matters.

Section 1 of the Act states the five principles on which the rest of the Act is based, whilst Sections 2–7 clarify some of the definitions used in Section 1. Broadly, three concepts are outlined in the following paragraphs.

(i) Adults have capacity unless proved otherwise

Section 1[(2)] states the first principle, that '*A person must be assumed to have capacity unless it is established that he lacks capacity*', which reflects the common law position. Section 2[(1)] states that, '*a person lacks capacity ... if at the material time he is unable to make a decision for himself ... because of an impairment, or a disturbance in the functioning, of the mind or brain*'. Essentially then, all adults (or at least anyone over the age of 16 under this Act) must be assumed to be competent to make decisions about their treatment, unless they are manifestly unable to make a decision at the time they are required to do so. The Act does not expressly prescribe *when* consent should be sought from a patient or an assessment of their capacity made; in theory, patients may give consent at any time prior to an intervention (i.e. even in the anaesthetic room directly prior to induction), provided that they are able to make that decision, although in elective situations, it remains good practice to allow patients time to reflect on the information provided to them[(15)].

The Act helpfully attempts to define what is meant by an inability to make decisions, by restating the two-stage test of capacity from *Re MB*, namely that the person should be able to *understand* and *remember* the information relevant to the decision, and *use* that information to arrive at a decision. The capacity of patients is therefore a question of fact, albeit based on the balance of probabilities—they can either understand/remember/use the information given to them, in which case they have capacity and can provide valid consent or refusal, or they cannot, in which case they lack capacity (and cannot consent or refuse an intervention).

The Act does not attempt to describe either the extent or the standard of information that should be given to patients, merely that the information should be '*relevant to the decision*'. However, the Act is explicit in pointing out that the information must always contain '*information about the relatively foreseeable consequences of deciding one way or another or failing to make the decision*'.

(ii) Patients must be given a reasonable chance to demonstrate their capacity

The second and third principles, respectively, state that, '*A person is not to be treated as unable to make a decision unless all practicable steps to help him to do so have been taken without success*', and '*A person is not to be treated as unable to make a decision merely because he makes an unwise decision*'. In addition, s.2(3) notes that '*a lack of capacity cannot be established merely by reference to: (a) a person's age or appearance, or (b) a condition of his, or an aspect of his behaviour, which might lead others to make unjustified assumptions about his capacity*'. In terms of anaesthetic practice, therefore, anaesthetists must not assume that patients lack capacity because, for example, (i) they are patients in the intensive care unit, (ii) they have received sedation or premedication, (iii) they are subject to restraint under the Mental Health Act 1983, (iv) they are acting irrationally, or have consumed alcohol, (v) they are refusing what appears to be sensible treatment, (vi) they are very elderly, or residents of a care home/nursing home, or (vii) they are otherwise unable to communicate their decisions or questions verbally.

The Act obliges doctors to make reasonable efforts to provide information for patients with questionable capacity, in order that they can decide their own treatment. This may require the anaesthetist, for example, to use simple language or pictures to explain an intervention, and to provide the means whereby patients can express their wishes non-verbally (letter charts, keyboards, blinked yes/no answers). Even then, if the communicated decision appears unwise or potentially life-threatening, a patient should not be declared incapable, although declaratory relief from the courts may be required in such circumstances.

(iii) The treatment of adults without capacity must be in their best interests

Principles 4 and 5 state, respectively, '*An act done, or a decision made, under this Act for or on behalf of a person who lacks capacity must be done, or made, in his best interests*', but '*Before the act is done, or the decision is made, regard must be had to whether the purpose for which it is needed can be as effectively achieved in a way that is less restrictive of the person's rights and freedom of action*'. In other words, the medical treatment of adults without capacity must be both *necessary* and in the patient's *best interests*; it remains to be seen whether the decision in *Bournewood* will affect these principles.

Anaesthetists are therefore obliged to take into consideration more factors than merely what is medically best for the patient when determining best interests, including:

(a) Whether the patient may, in time, recover capacity, and be able to determine his or her own treatment.

(b) The wishes of the patient, either in written form or through consultation with relatives, or Lasting Powers of Attorney.

(c) When determining best interests, a decision to withdraw or withhold life-sustaining treatment must not be taken with the intention of bringing about a patient's death. The presumption of the Act is that it is always in the best interests of the patient for his or her life to continue, although this presumption may receive less weight in any decision about best interests if prolonged intervention would be considered unnecessarily burdensome, for example, in someone with a terminal condition.

Lasting Powers of Attorney (LPAs)/Court-Appointed Deputies (CADs)

Perhaps the greatest change in the common law position comes with the statutory recognition of these agents. Until the Act was enforced in 2007, it was the case that no one could consent or refuse medical treatment on behalf of an adult without capacity, treatment being decided by the doctors on the basis of the patient's best interests.

The Act has created new law, in that a proxy decision-maker may be appointed by the patient (in the case of LPAs) or by the Court of Protection (in the case of CADs), in order to consent or refuse treatment on behalf of the patient in the event of incapacity (as well as managing their property and affairs).

In general, the donees (i.e. those people appointed by the patient) of an LPA will be created by a competent adult patient who is expecting to lose capacity in the future (e.g. patients with Huntington's chorea, who may develop dementia). CADs may be appointed by the court for adult patients who have never had capacity, or who have never appointed a donee of an LPA. The donees and deputies must themselves be over 18 years of age, and competent to make decisions on the patient's behalf (i.e. must understand, remember and use the information given to them), and are only empowered if the patient lacks capacity at the material time that a decision needs to be made. A future return of the patient to capacity (e.g. after intensive care treatment for an exacerbation of a medical condition) relieves the donee/deputy of their proxy powers. More than one donee/deputy may be appointed per patient and these may act independently, together, or both in some instances. Donees or deputies may not subtend their powers to other individuals, and may have their powers revoked either by the patient, if he regains the capacity to make such a decision, or by the court, if the donee/deputy is acting illegally or contrary to the best interests of the patient.

The authority invested in a donee/deputy extends to giving or refusing consent to the carrying out or continuation of a treatment by a doctor, excepting treatment that is life-sustaining, or considered inappropriate by the doctors for that patient. The donees of an LPA *may* refuse life-sustaining treatment, but only if the patient had specifically (and probably explicitly or in writing) authorized the donee to do so. Court-appointed deputies, however, cannot make decisions about life-sustaining treatment.

A new public body, the Public Guardian, will act as the registering authority for LPAs and CADs, and will supervise deputies. Although unclear, it seems that a person will not be able to function as the donee of an LPA unless registered with the Public Guardian.

A new Court of Protection has jurisdiction relating to the whole Act and is the final arbiter for capacity matters. The Court of Protection may be asked for a declaration if there is disagreement between either professionals or donees/deputies, or between professionals and donees/deputies about proposed medical treatment for an adult without capacity. The Court can also be approached to clarify the details of an LPA, for example, with reference to specific refusals of life-sustaining treatment.

One further actor that may be encountered by anaesthetists is the Independent Mental Capacity Advocate (IMCA). An IMCA is someone appointed by an 'appropriate authority' (the Secretary of State for Health, with regard to medical matters) to support an adult without either capacity or any representative. The role of an IMCA is to indicate to decision-makers (for example, CADs or doctors themselves) the person's wishes, feelings, beliefs and values, and to provide information about all factors that are relevant to the decision. An IMCA can challenge the decision-maker on behalf of the person lacking capacity, if necessary. However, an IMCA *cannot* make decisions themselves about medical treatment on behalf of an adult without capacity.

Advanced decisions to refuse treatment

Under common law (*Re AK*[16]), anticipatory refusals of treatment by adult patients (over the age of 18) are held to be legally valid if:

- A refusal of treatment is clearly established (e.g. the patient refuses blood transfusion even if it is clinically indicated).
- At the time of the decision, the patient is competent, adequately informed, and makes the decision voluntarily.

- The decision is intended to apply in the circumstances that subsequently arise (e.g. cardiopulmonary resuscitation should be attempted if the patient is involved in a road traffic accident, but not if the same patient requires ventilation in the intensive care unit as a consequence of future motor neurone disease).

These conditions form the statutory basis of advance decision-making under the Mental Capacity Act. Doctors are bound to comply with an advance decision if the decision is both valid and intended to apply in the circumstances. The Act refers to refusals of treatment; it is clear that it is not the intention of the act to allow patients to demand specific treatments should they lose their capacity in future.

Advance decisions are not valid if they are withdrawn by a competent patient, superseded by power invested in the donee of an LPA, or manifestly contrary to the expressed wishes of a patient (although the opinion of the Court of Protection should probably be sought in the last two instances). An advance decision must specify the treatment that is to be refused; this can be expressed in medical language or lay terms, as long as it is clear what is meant.

Advance decisions may be given orally or in writing. However, decisions that concern life-sustaining treatment must be given in writing and signed by the patient, or by another person in the patient's presence, and witnessed by a third person, who must countersign the statement. Such statements must include an explicit refusal of life-sustaining treatment even if the patient's life is at risk.

Time permitting, doctors should make reasonable efforts to ascertain the existence or provisions of an advance statement if they are informed of its existence. Emergency treatment should not be delayed if there is doubt about the existence or provisions of an advance directive.

Doctors who treat someone in contravention of a valid, applicable advance decision may be subject to a claim for damages for battery or to criminal liability for assault. Similarly, doctors may become liable in negligence if they withhold treatment according to an invalid advance decision, unless they can prove that they had reasonable grounds for believing that the decision was valid and applicable.

Doctors who have a conscientious objection to what is proposed in an advance decision must continue to provide necessary emergency medical treatment (unless proscribed under the advance decision), but should refer the patient to another doctor for continuation (or withdrawal) of treatment.

In summary, a significant legal shift with regards to medical decision-making on behalf of adults without capacity has taken place with the enforcement of the Mental Capacity Act 2005. A greater degree of statutory protection is now afforded to these patients, compared to that given through the previous common law, with far greater possibilities for proxy representation being made by friends and relatives of the patient, and appointees of the court. This is likely to curtail the unanimous authority in decision-making that clinicians previously possessed. This should not be viewed as an unwarranted challenge to medical professionalism. Treatment decisions involving adults without capacity are often the most difficult we face, and greater recognition of third-party input, as well as complying with professional guidelines[15,17,18], can only benefit the continuing treatment of such vulnerable patients.

Summary

Consequences of the Mental Capacity Act 2005[19,20]:

- The Act came into force in October 2007
- It applies to anyone aged 16 or over in England and Wales
- It represents a statutory codification of the common law:
  - Consent to, or refusal of, medical treatment is legally valid if it is given voluntarily by an appropriately informed, competent (capacitant) patient
  - Every adult is presumed to have capacity, unless that presumption is disproved
  - efforts must be made to help all patients to express their opinions
  - Patients lack capacity if their doctor (usually) decides that they are unable to understand and use relevant information when choosing whether to consent to, or refuse, treatment
  - Mental illness does not automatically mean that a patient lacks the capacity to consent to or refuse medical or surgical treatment
  - Temporary factors (e.g. pain or drugs) may completely erode capacity, but must be operating to such a degree that the ability to decide is absent
  - No other person may consent to medical treatment for an adult with capacity
  - Treatment for adults without capacity may be administered providing it is *necessary* and in the *best interests* of the patient
  - 'Best interests' are more than just 'medical best interests'
  - Anticipatory refusals of treatment by adult patients are legally valid if at the time of the decision, the patient is competent, adequately informed, and makes the decision voluntarily, a refusal of treatment is clearly established, and the decision is intended to apply in the circumstances that subsequently arise
- Lasting Powers of Attorney (LPA):
  - May be granted to a donee by a competent patient who predicts future incompetence
  - Must be registered with the Public Guardian
  - May make proxy decisions about medical treatment in the patient's best interests
  - May refuse life-sustaining treatment for the patient, provided that the patient has specifically empowered them to do so in writing
- Court-appointed deputies (CAD):
  - Are appointed by the Court of Protection and registered with the Public Guardian, if no LPA has been created
  - May make proxy decisions about medical treatment in the patient's best interests
  - May not refuse life-sustaining treatment

Case Illustrations

Case 1. An elderly, demented patient who requires surgery

Ada, who is 94, demented and living in a nursing home, has fallen out of bed and fractured her right neck of femur, necessitating operative repair. Her son, Bertie, has power of attorney, and refuses to sign a consent form, allowing the surgery to continue, because he says that his mother never would have consented to surgery if she knew in advance that she would be in such a physical and mental condition. How should the clinician proceed in this instance?

Discussion

This, as many readers may have experienced, is a variation on a very common problem encountered in anaesthetic practice, namely who has the authority to make decisions about treatment that is in a patient's best interests.

In order for Ada to provide consent for surgical fixation of her fractured neck of femur, she would have to do so voluntarily, based on the information provided her about the nature, purpose, risks, and benefits of treatment. She would also require the capacity to make such a decision, such that she would have to understand and remember the information provided, and use it to come to a decision. It is unlikely (although not impossible) that her dementia, particularly in light of her age, will render her competent to make this decision.

Nevertheless, a decision is required concerning surgical intervention. Under the Mental Capacity Act 2005, it is clear that any such decision should be made in Ada's best interests. In the author's experience, it is usually considered that surgical fixation is necessary and preferable to non-operative care in these instances, for the purposes of pain relief and patient mobility/pressure care. However, remembering that 'best interests' are not necessarily the same as 'medical best interests', it is important to ascertain whether there are extenuating circumstances in Ada's case, that might mean that non-operative care is preferable.

In this case, Ada's son Bertie would appear to provide strong evidence that his mother would not have wanted the proposed surgery. The law, which was relatively clear until October 2007, (i.e. that no one could consent or refuse treatment on behalf of an incapacitated adult) is now less certain. Bertie's refusal to sign the consent form, although legally irrelevant, reinforces the evidence about his mother's wishes, and should be taken seriously into consideration when arriving at a decision about Ada's best interests.

Nevertheless, in the absence of an advanced decision, or without input from an LPA, a CAD, or an IMCA, it remains up to the doctors treating Ada to decide what is in her best interests, albeit they must take a wide view, and be able to justify their decision to the courts. However, in light of the enforcement of the Mental Capacity Act 2005, it would seem prudent to consult the Court of Protection through the hospital's lawyers, in advance of any decision. Professional guidelines highlight the necessity of communication with friends and relatives of the patient, in order to ascertain any wishes and feelings that the patient may have previously expressed.

Bertie may be able to consent or refuse treatment on behalf of Ada, because he has power of attorney over his mother's affairs, but only if he had been specifically authorized to do so (i.e. in writing) as the result of a competent decision made by Ada, and was registered with the Public Guardian as the donee of a Lasting Power of Attorney (LPA), as described by the Mental Capacity Act 2005. His previous power of attorney is not transferable for the purposes of medical decision-making under the new Act, and given that Ada lacks the capacity to newly appoint him as the donee of an LPA, he will continue to be unable to direct her medical treatment.

Case 2. An unconscious 42-year-old with a living will

Jane, 42, has Huntington's disease. Having seen her father die with the condition as a child, she is understandably nervous about developing the end stages of the disease. She does not want to be treated if dementia eventuates, and writes a living will forbidding cardiopulmonary resuscitation (CPR) if it is ever needed in future. A week later she is severely injured in a road traffic accident, and is rushed to hospital, accompanied by her husband, Mark. During CPR, the Accident and Emergency doctor finds a copy of the living will in her purse, but decides that Jane doesn't intend that CPR shouldn't be attempted under the current circumstances, also noting that the will does not appear to have been witnessed. Unfortunately, Jane suffers severe hypoxic brain damage, requiring prolonged ventilation. She develops ventilator-associated pneumonia, and bed sores, which break down, requiring surgical debridement. During the procedure, she has an asystolic arrest. Despite CPR, Jane dies.

Discussion

What are the legal issues raised by this case?

Huntington's disease (HD) is an incurable, inherited disorder, whose signs and symptoms develop progressively from the 4th to 5th decade, resulting in premature death some 15–20 years after onset of the symptoms. Dementia is inevitable, and manifests as early onset behavioral changes, followed by impaired intellectual function, and memory disturbances.

Living wills (also known as advanced decisions or anticipatory refusals) are legally binding, provided that they are made voluntarily by a competent adult (over the age of 18), based on information provided about the likely consequences of treatment refusal, and are clearly intended to apply under the circumstances that subsequently arise.

Given her age and the nature of her disease, it would be pertinent to ascertain whether Jane was in fact competent to formulate her advanced decision, such that she could understand, remember, and use the information pertaining to the risks and consequences of her refusal. A lack of witnesses to her decision would not necessarily invalidate the living will.

Accepting that she is competent, the question then arises as to exactly what treatment she is refusing, and under what circumstances. Until the living will was discovered, of course, it was the duty of the doctor to administer all necessary emergency treatment. Given the timescale, it can be assumed that if she was competent to make a living will, she cannot be assumed to have dementia a week later, and therefore, on discovering the living will, the accident and emergency doctor may be correct in disregarding her advanced decision if he thought it was only intended to apply in the case of her developing dementia. Clinically, it is also professionally difficult to stop CPR on an ostensibly fit person, on the basis of an uncorroborated refusal of treatment.

Conversely, it could be argued that Jane has expressly forbidden CPR, and therefore her doctor has committed a battery in carrying out the procedure. This would be a decision for the courts to decide in hindsight.

Further information as to what Jane might have wanted could be gleaned from her husband Mark, although the ultimate decision concerning ongoing treatment rests with her doctor.

The statutory basis for advanced decision-making under the Mental Capacity Act 2005 follows the common law. However, decisions relating to life-sustaining treatment must be written and signed by the patient (or by another person in the patient's presence), and countersigned by a third person (such as a solicitor). A refusal of life-sustaining treatment—even if the patient's life is at risk—must be explicitly stated.

Since the enforcement of the Mental Capacity Act 2005, it may be that Mark might have a role to play in determining whether CPR should have been continued in the first instance, but only if he had been created the donee of Jane's Lasting Power of Attorney, and Jane had explicitly authorized him to make proxy decisions about life-sustaining treatment. Even in these circumstances, it would be sensible to consult the Court of Protection through the hospital's lawyers.

Jane's subsequent treatment is more contentious. Ventilation for hypoxic brain damage would appear to be outside the remit of her living will, but could be considered as proscribed treatment within the spirit of Jane's intentions (i.e. that life-sustaining treatment should not continue after her irreversible loss of capacity). Further treatment should be decided on the basis of necessity, in Jane's best interests, and it could be strongly argued that Jane's best interests would be best served by discontinuing treatment. Given that treatment in this instance may be considered futile, given the nature of her cerebral damage, the doctors might be right to consider the withholding or withdrawal of life-sustaining therapy at any point after initial CPR. Certainly, any conflict between the doctors, Mark and any other relatives would best be referred to the courts for a decision.

References

1. White, S.M. and Baldwin, T.J. (2003). Consent for anaesthesia. *Anaesthesia*, **58**(8), 760–74.
2. White, S.M. and Baldwin, T.J. (2004). Consent. In *Legal and Ethical Aspects of Anaesthesia, Critical Care and Perioperative Medicine*, pp. 49–71. University Press, Cambridge.

3. *Re T (adult: refusal of treatment)* (1992) 4 All ER 649.

4. *Re MB (an adult: medical treatment)*(1997) 38 BMLR 175 (CA).

5. *Re C (adult: refusal of medical treatment)* (1994) 1 All ER 819 (Fam Div).

6. *St Georges NHS Trust v S* (1998) 3 All ER 673 (CA).

7. Cabinet Office. Prime Minister's strategy unit. March [2004). *Alcohol harm reduction strategy for England*. http://www.cabinetoffice.gov.uk/strategy/work_areas/alcohol_misuse. aspx (last accessed 1st December 2008).

8. *HL v United Kingdom*, Application no 45508/99, decision of 5 October 2004. http://www. echr.coe.int/Eng/Press/2004/Oct/ChamberjudgmentHLvtheUK051004.htm (last accessed 1st December 2008).

9. Department of Health. March (2005). *'Bournewood' consultation. The approach to be taken in response to the judgment of the European Court of Human Rights in the "Bournewood" case*. HMSO London.

10. White, S.M. and Baldwin, T.J. (2002). The Human Rights Act, 1998: implications for anaesthesia and intensive care. *Anaesthesia*, **57**(9), 882–8.

11. White, S.M. and Baldwin, T.J. (2006). The Mental Capacity Act, 2005. Implications for anaesthesia and intensive care. *Anaesthesia*, **61**(4), 381–9.

12. The Law Commission. (1995). *Mental Incapacity*. Report No. 231. HMSO, London. http:// www.lawcom.gov.uk/summary_recommendations.htm (last accessed 1st December, 2008).

13. Lord Chancellor's Department. (1997). *Who decides? Making decisions on behalf of mentally incapacitated adults*. http://www.dca.gov.uk/menincap/meninfr.htm (last accessed 1st December, 2008).

14. Lord Chancellor's Department. (1999). *Making Decisions. The Government's proposals for making decisions on behalf of mentally incapacitated adults*. Cm. 4465. The Stationary Office, London.

15. Association of Anaesthetists of Great Britain and Ireland. (2006). *Consent for Anaesthesia*. http://www.aagbi.org/pdf/Consent.pdf (last accessed 1st December, 2008).

16. *Re AK (Adult patient)(Medical treatment: consent)* (2001) 1FLR 129.

17. Department of Health. (2001). *Reference Guide to Consent for Examination or Treatment*. http://www.dh.gov.uk/en/Publicationsandstatistics/Publications/ PublicationsPolicyAndGuidance/DH_4006757 (last accessed 1st December 2008).

18. General Medical Council. (2008). Consent: patients and doctors making decisions together. GMC, London, UK.

19. Department for Constitutional Affairs. *The Mental Capacity Act 2005*. http://www.opsi.gov. uk/acts/acts2005/ukpga_20050009_en_1 (last accessed 1st December 2008).

20. Department for Constitutional Affairs. *Mental Capacity Act 2005. Code of Practice*. http://www.justice.gov.uk/guidance/mca-code-of-practice.htm (last accessed 1st December 2008).

Chapter 9

Clinical research, audit, and training

Elizabeth A Flockton & Jennifer M Hunter

The twentieth and even the twenty-first centuries have seen major advances in clinical medicine. As we continue to push forward 'the frontiers of science', the expectation of our patients to have a longer and improved quality of life increases at a rate that outstrips these advances. The demand for biomedical research to develop treatments for disease or to improve upon existing therapy has never been greater.

Medical research is not a recent phenomenon. In the first century AD, Aulus Cornelius Celsus described in *De Medicina* various surgical procedures, such as removal of cataracts and treatment of bladder stones, and gave detailed notes on the preparation of ancient remedies including opioids. Celsus is credited as being one of the forefathers of human experimentation[1]. In *De Medicina*[1] he wrote, 'It is not cruel to inflict on a few criminals sufferings which may benefit multitudes of innocent people through all centuries.' How unacceptable such an approach would be today.

In our desire to increase the understanding of the aetiology and pathogenesis of disease, we have, on occasion, overlooked the principle of *first do no harm*. Recent history is littered with examples of mistreatment and abuse committed in the name of medical research. Perhaps the most notorious were the medical experiments conducted by the Nazis upon civilians and prisoners of war between 1939 and 1945, including infection with epidemic jaundice and spotted fever, and exposure to seawater, high altitude, freezing, and mustard gas. We can also find examples closer to home. For almost a century, the British Raj sent political prisoners to a penal colony in the Andaman Islands where they were subjected to secret pharmaceutical trials undertaken by British army doctors[2]. In the United States, the Tuskegee syphilis study sought to determine the course of untreated syphilis. The participants were all African–American males who, believing they were receiving an adequate level of care, were not given penicillin and suffered the debilitating effects of the disease[3]. History has demonstrated the need to establish a code of practice governing the conduct of clinical trials, to prevent such inhumanities occurring again.

The aims of the various sections of this chapter are to describe the ethical principles and the codes of conduct governing clinical research; to discuss the necessary steps involved in setting up a clinical trial; to detail the role of the ethics committee; and to discuss the issues surrounding informed consent for clinical trials. Some case scenarios will be introduced to test the research principles described. The final part of the chapter explores the difficulties associated with obtaining consent from patients for training of non-medical staff, medical students, and trainee anaesthetists in the perioperative period, and particularly while the patient is unconscious.

Many of the issues relating to informed consent for clinical research are addressed long before an investigator attempts to recruit a patient to a clinical trial. Codes of conduct have been developed with the primary intention of protecting patients.

Codes of conduct

The Nuremberg Code was the first document to cover the ethical conduct of clinical research involving human subjects[4]. It was written in 1949 in response to the atrocities committed by the Nazis during the Second World War. There have since been documents addressing the perceived deficiencies in the Nuremberg Code, of which the Declaration of Helsinki[5] and the Good Clinical Practice Guidelines[6] are the most widely adopted.

The Declaration of Helsinki

The World Medical Association adopted the Declaration of Helsinki in June 1964 and all its subsequent amendments, the final one being in 2000[5]. The declaration is a statement of ethical principles to guide medical research involving human subjects, including research on identifiable human material or identifiable data. This specification means that audit involving identifiable patient data has to be submitted to an ethics committee for independent review.

The basic principles laid down in the Declaration relate to the responsibilities of physicians towards their subjects and the conduct of clinical research to an acceptable scientific standard. Its major points are as follows:

- Medical research must conform to accepted scientific principles and be based on a thorough knowledge of the scientific literature. The design and performance of each experimental procedure should be clearly formulated in an experimental protocol that has been submitted to, and approved by, a specially appointed ethical review committee.

- Every medical research project should be preceded by an assessment of predictable risks in comparison with foreseeable benefits to the subject or others, and should only be conducted if the importance of the objective outweighs the risks. Physicians should not engage in research involving human subjects unless they are confident that the risks involved have been assessed and can be appropriately managed. Physicians should cease investigation if the risks outweigh the benefits or if there is conclusive evidence of positive results.

- Each potential subject must be informed of the aims, methods, anticipated benefits, and potential risks or discomfort entailed in the research project as well as any conflicts of interest, institutional affiliations, and sources of funding for the researcher. The research population should have a reasonable likelihood of standing to benefit from the results of the research.

- It is the physician's responsibility to protect the life, health, privacy, and dignity of the subject. The subjects must be both volunteers and informed participants in the research project. The subject should be informed of the right to abstain from participation in, or to withdraw from, a study at any time without reprisal. The physician should obtain the subjects' freely given informed consent, preferably in writing.

♦ For research subjects who are legally incompetent, or who are physically or mentally incapable of giving consent, or where the subject is a minor, informed consent must be obtained from the legally authorized representative. When a legally incompetent subject is able to give assent, this must be in addition to the consent of the legally authorized representative. In general, these groups should not be included in research unless it is necessary to promote the health of the group being represented, or where the condition preventing informed consent being given is a desirable characteristic of the study population.

♦ Researchers have a responsibility to publicize, or make publicly available, the results of their research. They are obliged to preserve the accuracy of their results and to report both positive and negative findings. In the publication, the investigators should declare any sources of funding, any affiliations, and any conflicts of interest. Research that is not conducted in accordance with the principles laid down in the Declaration of Helsinki should not be published.

♦ A physician may combine medical research with medical care when the research is justified by its potential prophylactic, diagnostic, or therapeutic value. In this situation, there are additional standards that apply to protect patients who are research subjects. These standards are that the benefits and risks of a new method should be tested against the best existing method, or placebo, if no proven method exists; that, at the study conclusion, every patient who participated in the study should be assured of access to the best method identified in the study; and that the physician should ensure that the patient understands which aspects of his care are related to the study. A patient's refusal to participate in a study should not be allowed to impact on the patient–physician relationship.

The principles in the Declaration of Helsinki are to be adhered to in conjunction with specified national and international ethical, legal, and regulatory requirements for research on human subjects. These national requirements should not be allowed to impair the protection for human subjects laid down in the declaration.

Case Scenario: 1

A 45-year-old male presents to his general practitioner with a six-month history of shortness of breath, cough, and haemoptysis. Systemic enquiry reveals a 3-stone weight loss over 6 months, and clinical examination shows enlarged cervical lymph nodes. His medical history is of high alcohol intake, heavy cigarette smoking, and chronic schizophrenia. He has had repeated hospital admissions following suicide attempts and self-harm, one episode being within the previous two weeks. He is taking multiple antipsychotic medications but has poor symptom control. He is seen at a rapid access clinic for suspected lung malignancy, where investigations show an inoperable lung carcinoma with liver and lymph node metastases. He is referred to the oncologists and is reviewed at the oncology clinic by a specialist registrar. The registrar assesses the patient as meeting the inclusion criteria to enter a randomized controlled trial of standard therapy versus a new chemotherapy regimen. He discusses the options with the patient, obtains consent, and proceeds to recruit him to the trial.

Question: Is this patient in his right mind and thus able to give informed consent?

Comment: Although the subject may meet the inclusion criteria for the trial, and hence be eligible for recruitment, his psychiatric history brings into question his mental capacity to give informed consent. His recent hospital admission following a self-harm episode suggests that he may not have the capacity at this time point to consent to study participation. It may be wise not to recruit the patient to the clinical trial but to give him standard management. It would be acceptable to recruit him only if the clinical trial was investigating a new treatment for refractory schizophrenia. In this situation, it would be necessary to obtain consent from a legally authorized representative as well as assent from the patient.

Good clinical practice guidelines

The International Conference on Harmonization of Technical Requirements for Registration of Pharmaceuticals for Human Use developed the Guidelines for Good Clinical Practice (GCP) in 1996[6]. The conference was organized by the regulatory authorities of the European Union, United States, and Japan. GCP is an international quality standard governing the design, conduct, recording, and reporting of trials involving human subjects. This standard is unified for the European Union, United States, and Japan. It allows data from a trial in one country to be accepted by the regulating authorities of another country; it also ensures credibility of data obtained from a trial.

The principles of GCP can be divided broadly into those governing ethical principles and those governing scientific quality. The ethical principles are similar to those discussed earlier. Indeed, GCP specifies that the trial should be conducted in accordance with the principles laid down in the Declaration of Helsinki. The principles relating to scientific quality are:

- There should be adequate clinical and non-clinical information available on an investigational product to support the proposed trial. The design of the trial should be scientifically sound and should be described in a clear, detailed protocol that has received approval from an independent ethics committee.

- The trial should be conducted according to the protocol that has received ethics committee approval. An appropriately educated, trained, and experienced individual must undertake each task.

- Information obtained from a clinical trial should be recorded and stored in such a manner as to allow accurate reporting, interpretation, and verification of the data as well as protecting the privacy and confidentiality of the subjects.

- Investigational products should be manufactured, handled, and stored according to good manufacturing practice and used only as specified in the approved protocol.

- There should be a quality control system ensuring that the quality of each step of the trial is reaching an acceptably high standard.

Planning a clinical trial

The aims of this section are to consider the key stages involved from posing the research question to commencing the trial. To doctors who are new to clinical research, the greatest challenges are likely to be posing a research question and developing a trial that is compliant with the Declaration of Helsinki, GCP Guidelines, and UK regulations. However, this is just the beginning of the long process necessary to gain approval by the authorities that regulate research, without which a clinical trial cannot commence.

Phases of a clinical trial

In respect of potential new drugs, there are typically four phases to the clinical development programme. The phases occur in a sequential fashion with subsequent phases not commencing until the preceding phase has been completed. Phase I studies usually involve healthy volunteers as participants. These studies investigate primarily, the safety profile of the new compound. Phase II studies recruit patients with the disease that the drug has been designed to treat. These trials are targeted towards assessment of efficacy and safety, as well as towards determination of the appropriate dosage for the new compound. Phase III studies are intended to gather data from greater numbers of patients, to provide substantial evidence of efficacy and safety. Phase III studies are required prior to approval being granted from a regulatory authority, such as the Medicines and Healthcare Products Regulatory Authority (MHRA). Finally, Phase IV trials are undertaken after the drug has been approved for marketing. The aims of Phase IV trials may be further evaluation of efficacy, to investigate other potential uses for the drug, or to provide additional safety data.

Before a clinical research project can start, it must receive approval from the ethics committee and authorization from the NHS trust where the research will be undertaken, via its Research and Development (R&D) Department. In addition, for a clinical trial of an investigational medicinal product, there must be Clinical Trial Authorization from the MHRA. An investigational medicinal product (IMP) is defined in the GCP guidelines as 'a pharmaceutical form of an active substance or placebo being tested or used as a reference in a clinical trial, including products already with a marketing authorization but formulated or packaged in a way different from the authorized form, when used for an unauthorized indication or when used to gain further information about the authorized form'[6]. If a drug is to be investigated for use at a different concentration, or by a different route of administration, it must have a new Clinical Trial Authorization.

Sponsorship

Having developed a research question and a trial design, the next step is to find a sponsor. A sponsor is an individual, company, institution, or organization, which takes responsibility for the initiation, management, and/or financing of that trial.

The decision as to who should act as sponsor to a clinical trial is usually determined by the context of the study. Where the study is commercially funded, for example, a pharmaceutical company developing a new drug, the funder will act as the sponsor. Where funding is being sought from the Medical Research Council or another charity, the funder may be willing to act as sponsor. Where no funding is being sought or the funder is unwilling to act, it is possible to request the NHS Trust and/or the University employing the investigator to act as sponsor.

The sponsor has a responsibility to ensure that the trial design adheres to GCP and all individuals involved in the trial have received GCP training. The sponsor is also responsible for providing notice of amendments to the protocol to the regulating authorities, for example the regional ethics committee, to request the clinical trial authorization (where appropriate), and to report the end of trial data. In clinical trials on an investigational medicinal product, the sponsor is also responsible for pharmacovigilance—to record and report all adverse events related to the investigational medicinal product to the clinical researchers and the MHRA.

Case Scenario: 2

A 73-year-old lady presents with a 6-month history of altered bowel habit, rectal bleeding, and weight loss. Her past medical history includes arterial hypertension and a total hip replacement for osteoarthritis 10 years previously. Following this operation she suffered a deep venous thrombosis and received treatment with warfarin. Her only current medication is a loop diuretic for hypertension. Flexible sigmoidoscopy reveals a mass in the sigmoid colon and biopsies confirm the diagnosis of adenocarcinoma. Subsequent staging investigations show some enlarged mesenteric lymph nodes but no evidence of liver metastases. The surgeon arranges for her to be admitted for anterior resection of the rectum.

The nurse at preoperative assessment mentions that the anaesthetic department is participating in a Phase IIIb clinical trial comparing atracurium to a new muscle relaxant. The patient supports research and asks if she would be eligible to enter the study. The nurse informs her that a member of the trial team will attend and discuss the study with her. The research team reviews the patient and she gives informed consent to participate in the trial. She is assessed as eligible for entry and is enrolled into the study.

The subject receives an investigational medicinal product—the research team is blinded to its identity. Surgery, anaesthesia, and the initial postoperative course are uneventful and the subject is not due to be seen again by the trial team until a week postoperatively. However, on the fourth postoperative day, the subject collapses in the bathroom. The cardiac arrest team is called and finds that she has pulseless electrical activity (PEA). Cardiopulmonary resuscitation is commenced but is abandoned after 30 minutes because no spontaneous cardiac output has been restored: the team decides that to persist would be futile. The coroner is informed and a post mortem examination conducted. The cause of death is found to have been a massive pulmonary embolus arising from a deep venous thrombosis within the femoral vein.

Question: Should the team alert the sponsor to this lady's death?

Comment: Death, by definition, is a serious adverse event and as such requires the investigator to notify the sponsor immediately. If the research team is aware of the death but does not alert the sponsor until its members are in possession of the post mortem report, they are in breach of Good Clinical Practice. If, on the other hand, it was the post mortem report that alerted the trial team to the patient's death and the sponsor was notified within 24 h of the research team becoming aware of the serious adverse event, then Good Clinical Practice guidelines would have been observed.

A second point to consider is the temporal relationship between drug administration and the subject's death. In this scenario, the interval is four days and it would be extremely unlikely for the death to be related to an adverse reaction to such a drug. However, as the time interval between drug administration and death shortens, it becomes increasingly difficult to exclude a relationship between the two events. Where an adverse reaction is suspected, whose nature or severity is not consistent with the product information available in the Investigator's Brochure, a suspected unexpected serious adverse drug reaction must be reported.

Research and development

Once sponsorship arrangements have been dealt with, the next step is to develop a final protocol for the trial. At the same time, the project should be registered with the R&D department at the chief investigator's site. Registration with the R&D department requires submission of a protocol, and copies of the ethics committee application, the consent form, and the patient information leaflet. The R&D department will then organize any required peer review of the project as well as assisting with sponsorship arrangements and project costing, should this not have been arranged already. For all interventional trials, it is necessary for the R&D department to undertake a risk assessment.

For research trials involving administration of an investigational medicinal product, the R&D department will also provide assistance with the application for a EudraCT number and a Clinical Trial Authorization (CTA). The Trial Master File is kept by the principal investigator; it contains documents such as the protocol, ethics committee correspondence, financial arrangements, insurance details, and most importantly, the only source documents by which a patient can be identified.

Obtaining a trial number

Every trial must have a unique trial protocol number in order to obtain a EudraCT number. This is the unique identifier for a trial registered on the European database for clinical trials. The EudraCT number is essential for acquiring a CTA and is a useful identifier for correspondence with ethics committees and the MHRA. In order to ensure a unique trial protocol number for obtaining a EudraCT number, it is possible to enter the details of the trial on the International Standardized Randomized Controlled Trial Number (ISRCTN) Register. Where the research is not a clinical trial, a EudraCT number may not be required. All Medical Research Council-funded clinical trials require an ISRCTN number. The website address is listed at the end of this chapter.

Final approval

Data protection approval is necessary before Trust approval for a clinical trial is issued. It is applied for by completing a questionnaire and by provision of the study documentation to the Data Protection Office at the investigator's site. Approval is not required before submission to an ethics committee but must be confirmed before final Trust approval is granted.

The last step is to submit the final protocol to the ethics committee for review, and to submit the Clinical Trial Authorization application to the MHRA. These steps can occur in parallel. The ethics committee is discussed in more detail in the following paragraphs. Once these bodies have given approval, the R&D department will give the final Trust approval. The trial now has approval to start, and the investigators can begin the process of recruiting and consenting patients.

Trial management and closure

During this period, the investigators have a responsibility to manage and monitor trial patients and to report any untoward events to their sponsor. The sponsor in turn will notify other investigators involved in the trial of any adverse events, as well as the responsible ethics committee and the MHRA. Should these events be of significant concern or serious in nature, the trial may be suspended or terminated early.

Other changes may occur, such as the addition of new sites in a multi-centre clinical trial, and during the course of the study, there may be amendments to the protocol. The site may be subject to audit by the sponsor as a quality control measure and to ensure that the site is GCP-compliant, or to inspection by the MHRA for similar reasons. It is also possible that the regulatory authorities from another country, such as the United States Food and Drug Administration (FDA), may inspect a site prior to granting a licence for a new drug in their own country.

In some countries, such as the United States, it is acceptable for subjects recruited to Phase II and Phase III clinical trials to receive payment for their participation. In the United Kingdom, it is only in Phase I studies, in which the participants are healthy volunteers, that such a payment can be made legally. However, it may be appropriate to reimburse money to Phase II and Phase III study participants for the cost-of-travel expenses for additional journeys to hospital for protocol-related procedures or treatment. There is usually a limit imposed upon the amount that can be reimbursed.

At the end of the trial, recruitment of patients ceases and the data obtained are analysed. The investigator and sponsor have a responsibility to ensure that the data, including positive and negative findings, are published within one year of the end of trial.

Case Scenario: 3

A 37-year-old lady is scheduled to undergo an elective laparoscopic cholecystectomy. She is reviewed at the pre-admission clinic and seen by an anaesthetist who is keen to recruit her to a randomized controlled trial of a new volatile anaesthetic agent. The anaesthetist provides the relevant information and leaves the patient time to consider her decision.

She is admitted to hospital the evening prior to surgery, agrees to enter the trial and gives written informed consent. The anaesthetist then undertakes trial-related procedures including liver function tests (LFTs), which are normal.

Surgery, the following day, is complicated and necessitates conversion from a laparoscopic to an open procedure. In contrast, the anaesthetic is straightforward and causes no concern. As dictated by the trial protocol, the anaesthetist performs repeat blood sampling on several occasions postoperatively and notes that the subject's LFTs are now mildly deranged. The anaesthetist attributes the transient disturbance in liver function to the complicated surgery. The subject remains in hospital for an additional week for observation and is discharged home when her LFTs have returned to normal.

Question: Should these findings be reported to the sponsor and the MHRA?

Comment: The subject's deranged liver function tests may well be attributable to complications from her cholecystectomy but a relationship to the investigational medicinal product, that is, the new volatile anaesthetic agent, cannot be excluded. Whatever the cause of her deranged LFTs, she has experienced an adverse medical event, and it is the duty of the investigator to report this to the study sponsor. In this case, the untoward event prolonged the patient's period of hospitalization and as such would be defined as a serious adverse event. Hence the investigator must report this event to the sponsor within 24 h of becoming aware of it. In turn, the sponsor has a duty to report the event to the MHRA and to other investigators in the trial.

Pregnancy testing

In pre-menopausal female subjects, investigators have additional duties. In the majority of clinical trials of an investigational medicinal product, pregnancy is an undesirable event. In these subjects, the investigator must confirm a negative pregnancy test after obtaining informed consent from the woman and before administering the first dose of the investigational medicine, ideally within 24 h prior to treatment. It is also the responsibility of the investigator to advise appropriate contraceptive precautions to the subject and to highlight the importance of not becoming pregnant whilst she is participating in the trial. The woman must accept that she has the ultimate responsibility in this respect. In certain situations, it may be necessary to advise further contraception in addition to an existing method, for example a barrier method as well as a hormonal method in the context of antibiotic therapy. If the subject does not follow this advice, the investigator and the sponsor are not liable for any resultant pregnancy.

Insurance of subjects

The EU Clinical Trials Directive 2001/20/EC, which sets the legal requirements for clinical research undertaken in the European Union, requires insurance or indemnity covering the liabilities of both the sponsor and the investigator, such as liability for negligence. The Directive does not require no-fault compensation, that is compensation where there is no legal liability. This means that a trial participant who suffers personal injury during clinical research, for example an anaphylactic reaction to another drug not under investigation, may not be entitled to compensation. In the United Kingdom, the EU Directive is implemented by the Medicines for Human Use (Clinical Trials) Regulations 2004. Ethics committees have been given authority by the Regulations to determine whether it is appropriate to seek consent from potential subjects for a clinical trial without no-fault compensation[7].

If a trial participant does suffer personal injury, the circumstances dictate who is responsible for paying compensation[7]. In a situation in which a pharmaceutical company funds a trial, the company usually offers no-fault compensation for personal injury resulting from the clinical research, such as complications arising from the use of an investigational medicinal product or trial-related procedures[7]. Injury may arise as a result of defective medicine, and in this case, the liability lies with the manufacturers[7]. The third scenario in which a subject suffers injury is due to the negligence of the investigator, unrelated to the drug being studied, or as a result of faulty equipment: in this situation, it is the responsibility of the NHS Trust or the University for whom the investigator works[7]. NHS indemnity covers clinical negligence that harms individuals towards whom the NHS has a duty of care and where clinical trials have been conducted with NHS permission. NHS indemnity does not offer no-fault compensation[7]. The responsibility for this indemnity may be shouldered by an individual Trust or may be spread through the Clinical Negligence Scheme for Trusts[1]. The indemnity provided by universities may give cover for negligent harm or a more comprehensive clinical trials insurance that includes both negligence cover and no-fault compensation[7].

The Research Ethics Committee

The role of the research ethics committee (REC) is to protect the dignity, rights, safety, and well-being of potential or actual research participants, a responsibility that is shared with others as part of the Research Governance Framework.[8] It also has to ensure justice, that is the benefits and burdens of research should be distributed fairly among all groups and classes in society. The REC should take into consideration the interest, needs, and safety of the researchers, although the interests of the participants are always paramount.

Committee composition

The committee is an independent body consisting of a maximum of 18 expert and lay people. Each member serves a fixed-term appointment of 5 years and should not serve more than two consecutive appointments.

An expert member is required to have methodological and ethical expertise in clinical and non-clinical research and in qualitative research methods, and to have experience in clinical practice, pharmacy, and statistics relevant to research. The lay members must account for at least a third of the membership of an individual REC and should be independent of the NHS either as employees or in a non-executive role. Their primary personal or professional interest should not be in a research area.

At meetings at which research ethical review is undertaken, a quorum should consist of seven members. This must include the Chair and/or Vice-Chair, one expert with the relevant expertise, one lay member, and one other who is independent of the institution or location where the research is to take place.

There are different types of RECs reviewing research proposals. Some deal only with research involving Phase I healthy volunteer studies or with special population groups such as prisoners. If a clinical trial of an investigational medicinal product is being undertaken at only one site, approval would be sought from the Local Research Ethics Committee (LREC). When an investigational product is being researched at more than one site, the application for ethics approval would be made to a Multi-Centre

Research Ethics Committee (MREC). This has the advantage that if a favourable opinion has been given by an MREC, it covers all sites in the United Kingdom involved in the clinical trial. In addition, there are specific areas of research for which approval must be sought from another body, for example, the Gene Therapy Advisory Committee or the Human Fertilization and Embryo Authority. These are outside the remit of this chapter. The need for ethics approval of research studies into the development of new anaesthetic equipment is still a matter of debate. Recommendations have recently been detailed on how this aspect of anaesthetic research should be taken forward[9].

Research requiring REC approval

Approval from an REC for a research project or clinical trial should be sought when the potential or actual participants are patients or users of the NHS, including past or present treatment, or if individuals are identified as potential research participants because of their status as a relative or carer of a patient or user of the NHS. Approval must also be sought when the research involves access to data, organs, or other bodily material of past and present NHS patients; when it involves the recently dead on NHS premises; or the use of fetal material or IVF in NHS patients. It is also necessary when the research requires use of, or access to, NHS premises and when NHS staff are recruited as research participants by virtue of their professional role.

The need to obtain ethical approval where NHS staff are participants by virtue of their professional role is of particular relevance to research into teaching and training in anaesthesia. There are a significant number of research studies assessing skill performance on manikins, for example comparison of intubation success rates by paramedics with experienced prehospital practitioners using a novel laryngoscope and a standard laryngoscope in a manikin model of difficult intubation[10]. It is important to distinguish between this use of manikins to assess skill performance in a research study and use of manikins to provide a simulated learning environment where the aim is simply to allow individuals to develop skills. The former would need ethics approval, and the latter would not[11].

The key is, if the research is being undertaken on NHS patients or staff on NHS premises, ethics committee approval must be sought.

Case Scenario: 4

The department of anaesthesia in a large teaching hospital is performing an audit to compare the accuracy of calibration of two different vaporizers that are in every day use at the hospital. Because the project is an audit, the team does not submit it for ethics committee approval, nor does it obtain informed consent from the patients. The concentration of volatile anaesthetic agent being delivered to the patient is to be measured using a spectrophotometric device placed within the patient's breathing system and compared to the concentration set at the vaporizer by the anaesthetist. The values for a hundred sequential patients from each vaporizer at steady-state anaesthesia are obtained. The results are analysed and show significant differences in the accuracy of calibration between the two vaporizers. The investigators feel that the results of the audit are so significant that they have a responsibility to share their findings with others. They submit their audit to a peer review anaesthetic journal for publication.

Question: Should the editor publish this article in their journal?

Comment: No matter how flawless the scientific design of the audit, or clinically significant the results, the editor should not publish this work. The audit has involved patient identifiable data and therefore required submission to an ethics committee for approval prior to commencing the study. In addition, as the data are patient-identifiable, informed consent should have been obtained from the patients before they were included in the project. The editor has a duty, laid down in the Declaration of Helsinki, not to publish the article.

Application requirements

The principal investigator should submit the application for ethics committee approval. If the principal investigator is inexperienced, there should be an identified supervisor of adequate quality and experience to countersign the application form and share responsibility for the ethical and scientific conduct of the research.

The full list of documents requiring submission to the ethics committee can be obtained from the responsible REC. It includes:

- A signed and dated application form.
- The protocol of the proposed research.
- A summary or synopsis of the protocol in non-technical language.
- A description of the ethical considerations involved.
- If appropriate, an adequate summary of all safety, pharmacological, pharmaceutical, and toxicological data available on the study product, together with a summary of the clinical experience with the study product to date.
- Applicant's current curriculum vitae.
- Written and other forms of information for potential research participants.
- The informed consent form.
- A description of arrangements for insurance cover for research participants.

Process of review

The primary task of the REC is to conduct an ethical review of the research proposal and supporting documents, with special attention to the nature of any intervention and the safety of participants, the informed consent process, and the suitability and feasibility of the protocol. It should satisfy itself that scientific review has occurred and is of an adequate standard for the nature of the proposal under consideration. It is not the remit of the ethics committee to organize a scientific review. Finally, the committee should consider the relevance of any applicable laws and regulations. Should there be a particular area of concern, the committee may advise that a legal opinion be sought.

The requirements for a favourable opinion to be given by the REC relate to the following:

- Scientific design and conduct of the study.
- Methods of recruitment of research participants.

- Care and protection of research participants.
- Protection of research participant confidentiality.
- Informed consent process.
- Community considerations.

Informed consent

Informed consent is based on the concept that competent individuals have the right to determine what is done, and what is not done, to their body. For the purposes of clinical research, subjects are recruited to trials on the basis not only of meeting the desired criteria for the research in question but also on their capacity to give informed consent. This is in accordance with the principles laid down in the Nuremberg Code and the Declaration of Helsinki. The capacity to consent is determined by the ability of the individual to understand the research in question and how the research applies to his own situation. It also depends on the participant's ability to process this information and make a voluntary decision to enrol in a trial. There is a difference between having the capacity to give informed consent and giving valid consent. The capacity to give informed consent is presumed if an individual is of competent mind with no cognitive impairment. For valid informed consent to be given, the subject must understand the informed consent that he is giving and not simply have the capacity to do so. Described like this, the distinction between the capacity to give informed consent and valid informed consent seems artificial. To put the issue into context, it is estimated that between 20% and 40% of individuals with the capacity to give informed consent have not understood one or more aspects of research participation, such as the risks or the right to withdraw, which are essential to valid consent[12].

Treschan et al.[13] presented patients who believed that they were being asked to participate in a real trial with one of three sham protocols: no risk or pain; risk but no pain; or pain but no risk. They found that understanding was similar between the three groups (67–72%) and that willingness to participate differed significantly, being higher in the' no risk or pain' group. It is interesting that, despite the language in the protocols being extremely blunt and the risks highly exaggerated, 30% of subjects could not identify the degree of pain or risk associated with the sham protocol with they had been presented. The study also found that if understanding was poor or the subject felt pressurized, consent was unlikely to be given.

Research such as Treschan's study[13] shows us that even when we present information using blunt language and in a manner which highlights, or even exaggerates, the risks involved in a trial, a proportion of subjects still have a poor understanding of the risks and hence fail to give valid consent. The literature and research into obtaining valid consent suggest that there is probably no ideal method for obtaining it for clinical research trials[14]. Given the vast number of questions in clinical research and the different types of trial design, as well as differences between subject groups, it is not surprising that there is no one-way-fits-all and foolproof method of obtaining valid consent.

However, there are some elements that are essential for the subject to comprehend. These are the purpose of the research in question and the design of the trial, as well as details of any trial-related procedures. If randomization is involved, the subjects should have an understanding of the concept, that is, that they will receive either a new treatment or an existing treatment or placebo, and that they do not make this choice. The subject needs to understand the potential side-effects of treatment and trial-related procedures and must also appreciate the potential benefits of treatment; even if there is no personal benefit from participation in the trial there may be a gain to the wider population if existing therapy is improved. The subject needs an appropriate length of time to consider the decision and to discuss the trial with family members. Finally, the subject needs to understand that there is no obligation to enter the trial and, if participation is agreed, there is a right to withdraw at any stage without reprisal or compromise of care.

Case Scenario: 5

A 55-year-old lady with no previous medical history presents to the Accident and Emergency department with her first episode of chest pain. She is admitted under the care of the cardiology team. Investigations exclude a myocardial infarction. However, routine observations by the nursing staff reveal that she has an elevated arterial blood pressure on serial examinations. The nursing staff alert the cardiology research nurse who is an investigator on a multi-centre clinical trial comparing an established angiotensin converting enzyme (ACE) inhibitor to a novel ACE inhibitor for the control of hypertension.

The research nurse approaches the patient and discusses the trial at some length with her. The patient appears receptive to the idea of participating in it. The research nurse then proceeds to check the patient's blood pressure to confirm hypertension and to take a blood sample for estimation of urea and electrolytes. Abnormal renal function is an exclusion criterion of the study but the patient's tests are reported as normal. The nurse then obtains informed consent from the patient and enrols her into the trial.

Question: Is this an appropriate way to obtain informed consent?

Comment: Although measurement of both blood pressure and plasma urea and electrolyte concentrations would be considered routine in the management of a newly diagnosed hypertensive patient, they have been undertaken by an individual not directly responsible for her care, and only for the purpose of establishing suitability for a clinical trial. Even though the patient appears willing to enter the trial, she has not formally consented to enter it when the nurse undertakes two trial-related procedures. This is a breach of good clinical practice.

Consent for training

Just as there is a need to obtain consent for clinical research that is additional to a patient's care during anaesthesia, there is also a need to obtain consent for practical procedures undertaken by staff in training during that care. This includes medical students, paramedics, nurses, operating department practitioners, and trainee doctors. This consent should be obtained following a discussion of the procedure with the patient of the proposed benefits and potential risks involved as well as any alternative approach. Consent for any procedure should be sought irrespective of the seniority of the doctor. The magnitude of the benefits and risks, however, depends on the experience of the person performing the procedure.

What is a procedure?

The first issue surrounds the definition of what constitutes a procedure. For example, an epidural or a central venous line insertion can be regarded as a procedure. When considered more closely, however, each procedure is composed of several component parts that could be regarded as procedures in their own right[15]. For example, central venous line insertion comprises aseptic preparation; use of ultrasound to demonstrate anatomy and guide advancement of the needle; puncture of a central vein; and use of a Seldinger technique to facilitate passage of a catheter into the vein. Each of the aspects of the overall 'procedure' has a learning component. The Association of Anaesthetists of Great Britain and Ireland (AAGBI) Working Party on Consent for Anaesthesia (2006) accept that it is 'impossible to seek patients' consent for every aspect of every "procedure" in which there may be a learning component'[16].

It is necessary to assess the benefits and risks of the procedure for which consent is being sought. Some procedures have outcomes that can be clearly defined in terms of success, and with success, the entire benefit of the procedure is achieved, such as tracheal intubation and peripheral venous cannulation. The potential harm and consequences of failure vary dramatically, however. Other procedures are associated with benefits that range in magnitude, for example epidural analgesia and regional nerve blocks, where the degree of benefit varies with the procedure and the experience of the practitioner. In these cases, it is necessary to demonstrate at least some benefit from the procedure, especially when it is performed under supervision[15]. It is difficult to find an example of a risk-free technical procedure: almost all procedures are associated with varying degrees of side-effects or complications. In relation to consent and staff in training, the AAGBI Working Party[16] advocates that:

- The benefits and risks of a procedure to the patient and society are considered.
- As far as possible, the risk of harm is minimized. Strategies to achieve this include practice on manikins and close supervision.
- The benefits of a procedure should be maximized. This may be achieved by close supervision and targeting skills to practitioners likely to use them again in the future.
- Alternative techniques and other methods of learning and maintaining skills should be considered.

The procedural context

The context in which the procedure is being performed is also of importance when obtaining consent. Consider the procedure of awake fibreoptic intubation of the trachea in four different scenarios, which are similar to two described in the AAGBI document[16].

In the first scenario, the intubation is performed by a consultant experienced in endoscopic intubations, as part of his routine technique. In this scenario, the AAGBI states that:

specific consent would not be required since the risks have been minimised and the benefits maximised, and the technique constitutes part of the general procedure of 'orotracheal intubation' (so long as the associated risks remain equivalent to or less than the alternatives)[16].

In the second scenario, the fibreoptic intubation is being performed by a trainee, closely supervised by a consultant experienced in difficult airways, on a patient with a known difficult airway. In this scenario, it would not be necessary to seek specific consent from the patient because, although the procedure is being undertaken by a trainee, the technique should be considered as part of this patient's normal care. It involves a clear benefit to the patient and the risks of harm are minimized by close supervision; they are less than the potential harm associated with alternative techniques for managing the airway.

In the third scenario, a trainee whose only prior experience of fibreoptic intubation has been on manikins, wishes to learn the technique under supervision in an elective situation on a patient who does not have a difficult airway. In this scenario, it should be regarded as mandatory to seek specific consent for the intubation because there is limited, if any, benefit to the patient and a clear potential for harm in terms of anxiety and discomfort.

In the final scenario, an emergency fibreoptic intubation is required out-of-hours for a patient with rapidly progressing stridor secondary to airway burns. In this situation, the intended benefit of securing the airway is life-saving and should be regarded as far outweighing the potential risks of lack of supervision and discomfort. The consequence of failure could be argued to be less serious than having taken no action at all and letting a patient die as a result of loss of the airway. Should consent be refused by the patient (irrespective of the experience of the trainee involved), the trainee could, and should, commence the procedure under common law without waiting for consultant support to arrive from outside the hospital.

Experience

Learning is a constant process, and the experience of the trainee must be taken into account when taking consent. The risk–benefit ratio of a specific procedure in the hands of a senior specialist registrar is likely to be lower than in the hands of a foundation-year-2 doctor. In addition, the impact of the European Working Time Directive on the experience of trainees in practical specialities, such as anaesthesia and surgery, is resulting in less experienced doctors at all grades. This must be accounted for. The AAGBI Working Party advises that:

> consultant anaesthetists should include trainees' experience as part of the assessment of overall risks and benefits, including the need to minimise the former and maximise the latter… [16].

This statement also accepts that, despite efforts to the contrary, complications will still occur. It is important to accept that no matter how undesirable a complication, it still represents a learning experience for the individual or team involved, irrespective of seniority.

Non-medical staff

The final issue to be considered is consent for procedures undertaken by medical students and non-medical staff, such as paramedics, who not only lack the skills of anaesthetists but in addition are not medically qualified. The Department of Health advises that *'Where the procedure will further the patient's care … then assuming the student is appropriately trained in the procedure, the fact that it is carried out by a student does not alter the nature and purpose of the procedure. It is therefore not a legal requirement to tell the patient that the clinician is a student, although it would always be good practice to do so'*[17]. The good practice must be emphasized but the key point is what constitutes 'appropriately trained'? The AAGBI Working Party suggests that the need for specific consent is dependent not only on the competence of the individual but also on the risks involved in the procedure[16]. For example, as the document suggests, specific consent would not be required for a student to hold a facemask as the procedure lies within their competence and the risks are minimal. In contrast, tracheal intubation is a procedure requiring a greater degree of skill and is associated with a greater potential for harm. The AAGBI Working Party suggests that this would require specific consent to be obtained until the student concerned achieved the required level of competence—however that be defined.

Summary

Few anaesthetists obtain substantial experience of clinical research, and their first exposure to it can be daunting. We hope that we have provided some insight into the regulations governing clinical research; that we have explained the necessary steps in planning a research trial; and we have detailed some of the difficulties in obtaining informed consent. Furthermore, we hope that we have highlighted some of the issues surrounding consent for procedures undertaken by trainees.

References

1. http://penelope.uchicago.edu/Thayer/E/Roman/Texts/Celsus/home.html (last accessed 10th December 2008).
2. Scott-Clark, C. and Levy, A. (2001). Survivors of our hell. *The Guardian*, **23 June**.
3. http://www.cdc.gov/nchstp/od/tuskegee
4. The Nuremberg Code. (1949–1953). Trials of War Criminals before the Nuremberg Military Tribunals under Control Council Law No. 10. Nuremberg, October 1946–April 1949. U.S. G.P.O., Washington, D.C.
5. The World Medical Association Declaration of Helsinki. Adopted by the 18th WMA General Assembly, Helsinki, Finland, June 1964. Last amended by the 52nd WMA General Assembly, Edinburgh, Scotland, October 2000.
6. The ICH Guideline for Good Clinical Practice. Use 1996 (revised 2002). International Conference on Harmonisation of Technical Requirements for Registration of Pharmaceuticals for Human. Found at http://www.emea.europa.eu/pdfs/human/ich/013595en.pdf (last accessed 10th December 2008).
7. The Universities UK / Department of Health joint statement on legal responsibilities in clinical trials. October 2004. Statement found at http://www.ct-toolkit.ac.uk/_db/_documents/uniUK+DH_statement.pdf (last accessed 10th December 2008).
8. Governance arrangements for NHS Ethics Committees. Department of Health. August 2001. Document found at http://www.dh.gov.uk/assetRoot/04/05/86/09/04058609.pdf (last accessed 10th December 2008).
9. Wilkes, A.R., Hodzovic, I., and Latto, I.P. (2008). Introducing new anaesthetic equipment into clinical practice. *Anaesthesia*, **63**, 571–5.

10. Woollard, M., Lighton, D., Mannion, W., *et al.* (2008). Airtraq vs standard laryngoscopy by student paramedics and experienced prehospital laryngoscopists managing a model of difficult intubation. *Anaesthesia*, **63**, 26–31.

11. Bogod, D. (2005). Is ethical approval necessary for manikin studies? A reply. *Anaesthesia*, **60**, 94–6.

12. Wendler, D. (2004). Can we ensure that all research subjects give valid consent? *Archives of Internal Medicine*, **164**, 2,201–4.

13. Treschan, T.A., Scheck, T., Kober, A., *et al.* (2003). The influence of protocol pain and risk on patients' willingness to consent for clinical studies: A randomised trial. *Anesthesia and Analgesia*, **96**, 498–506.

14. Edwards, S.J., Lilford, R.J., Thornton, J., and Hewison, J. (1998). Informed consent for clinical trials: in search of the 'best' method. *Social Science and Medicine*, **47**, 1,825–40.

15. Yentis, S.M. (2005). The use of patients for learning and maintaining practical skills. *Journal of the Royal Society of Medicine*, **98**, 299–302.

16. Association of Anaesthetists of Great Britain & Ireland. (2005). *Consent for Anaesthesia*, 2nd edition. Association of Anaesthetists of Great Britain & Ireland, London.

17. Department of Health Reference Guide to Consent for Examination or Treatment. (2001). Document found at http://www.dh.gov.uk/assetRoot/04/01/90/79/04019079.pdf (last accessed 10th December 2008).

Useful web addresses

ICH website	www.ich.org
National Research Ethics Service	www.nres.npsa.nhs.uk
Clinical Trial Toolkit A department of Health/MRC project	www.ct-toolkit.ac.uk
Medicines and Healthcare Products Regulatory Agency	www.mhra.gov.uk
Institute of Clinical Research	www.instituteofclinicalresearch.org
European Database for Clinical Trials	eudract.emea.europa.eu
ISRCTN Register	www.controlled-trials.com
Medicines for Human Use (Clinical Trials) Regulations 2004	www.uk-legislation.hmso.gov.uk/si/si2004/20041031.htm
Clinical Negligence Scheme for Trusts	www.nhsla.com/Claims/Schemes/CNST

Section 3

Risks & benefits

Chapter 10

Mortality associated with anaesthesia

Alan R Aitkenhead

The anaesthetized patient is at risk of complications resulting from the actions, or inaction, of the anaesthetist, from the actions of the surgeon, and from failure or malfunction of anaesthetic equipment. The state of anaesthesia may be considered to be intrinsically unsafe. Patients are subjected to administration of drugs, which have side-effects, particularly on the cardiovascular and respiratory systems. Pharmacological muscle paralysis necessitates the use of artificial ventilation, making the patient dependent on the anaesthetist and his equipment for the fundamental functions of oxygenation and excretion of carbon dioxide. The anaesthetist may deliberately alter physiological functions, for example, by inducing hypotension or ventilating only one lung.

Estimates of mortality

Mortality is a vital estimate of risk associated with anaesthesia, the most important reason being that the definition is clear, in contrast to the more debatable definitions of morbidity. Mortality is also a somewhat crude estimate of risk, because of the relative rarity of this complication[1].

During the three decades up to 1980, a number of investigators in various countries had attempted to estimate the frequency with which death was associated with anaesthesia (Table 10.1)[2–15]. There was a general trend towards reduced mortality attributable primarily to anaesthesia during this period (from about 1:2500 to about 1:5000), but the same principal causes of death continued to be identified: inadequate supervision of trainees, drug overdose, drug mistakes, airway obstruction, aspiration of gastric contents, insufficient monitoring, and lack of postoperative care.

One of the problems that renders comparison between these studies difficult is that different criteria were used to define 'anaesthetic death'. A spectrum of time limits has been used, starting with all deaths occurring before the time of transfer of the patient from the operating theatre or from the recovery room. A limit of deaths occurring within 24–48 h after anaesthesia has reflected coronial requirements in many jurisdictions, with a period of 7–10 days used in other studies. However, some patients who suffer anaesthetic-related complications may not die for weeks, months, or even years after the anaesthetic. These deaths would not be captured in studies using such limits. In addition, some studies of anaesthetic mortality have included patients who suffered hypoxic cerebral damage, with resultant persistent coma.

Table 10.1 Estimates of the incidence of mortality due to anaesthesia between 1954 and 1980

Authors	Year of publication	Number of anaesthetics	Primary cause	Primary and associated cause
Beecher & Todd[2]	1954	599 548	1:2680	1:1560
Dornette & Orth[3]	1956	63 105	1:2427	1:1343
Schapira et al.[4]	1960	22 177	1:1232	1:821
Phillips et al.[5]	1960	—	1:7692	1:2500
Dripps et al.[6]	1961	33 224	1:852	1:415
Clifton & Hotten[7]	1963	295 640	1:6048	1:3955
Memery[8]	1965	114 866	1:3145	1:1082
Gebbie[9]	1966	129 336	—	1:6158
Minuck[10]	1967	121 786	1:6766	1:3291
Harrison[11]	1968	177 928	—	1:3068
Marx et al.[12]	1973	34 145	—	1:1265
Bodlander[13]	1975	211 130	1:14 075	1:1703
Harrison[14]	1978	240 483	—	1:4537
Hovi-Viander[15]	1980	338 934	1:5059	1:1412

More recent studies of mortality are shown in Table 10.2. In 1982, the Association of Anaesthetists of Great Britain and Ireland (AAGBI) published the results of a major study of mortality in five regions in the United Kingdom. An anonymous and confidential system was established to report deaths that occurred within 6 days of surgery. During the study period, an estimated 1 147 362 operations took place[16]. The overall perioperative mortality was 0.53%. Anaesthesia was considered to have been totally responsible for death in less than 1:10 000 operations, but may have contributed to death in 1:1700 operations.

Because of the importance of the findings, and because of the difficulty in separating anaesthetic and surgical factors when reports came only from anaesthetists, the AAGBI initiated the first Confidential Enquiry into Perioperative Deaths (CEPOD) in conjunction with the Association of Surgeons of Great Britain and Ireland. Three regions in the United Kingdom were studied over a 12-month period. The overall perioperative mortality was 0.7%[17]. There were 410 deaths associated with anaesthesia out of a total of 2928 deaths after 555 258 anaesthetics. Factors that were believed to have contributed to death are shown in Table 10.3. However, expert assessors considered that only three deaths resulted solely from anaesthesia, an incidence of 1 in 185 086 anaesthetics.

Studies from other countries have suggested higher rates of death related to anaesthesia than that reported in the CEPOD study. From 1978 to 1982, the French Health Ministry conducted a prospective nationwide survey of major complications during anaesthesia. A representative sample of 198 103 anaesthetics was analysed from

Table 10.2 Estimates of the incidence of mortality due to anaesthesia between 1982 and 2006

Authors	Year of publication	Number of anaesthetics	Primary cause	Primary and associated cause
Lunn & Mushin[16]	1982	1 147 362	1:10 000	1:1700
Tiret et al.[18]	1986	198 103	1:13 207	—
Buck et al.[17]	1987	555 258	1:185 086	1:1354
Holland[19]	1987	—	1:26 000	—
Chopra et al.[20]	1990	113 074	1:16 250	—
Pedersen[21]	1994	200 000	1:2500	—
Tikkanen & Hovi-Viander[22]	1995	325 585	1:66 667	—
Warden & Horan[24]	1996	—	—	1:20 000*
Davis[27]	1999	8 516 436	1:63 085	1:154 844
Arbous et al.[26]	2001	869 483	1:124 212	1:7143
Willis et al.[28]	2002	10 336 200	1:219 919	1:79 509
Kawashima et al.[30]	2003	2 363 038	1:47 619	—
Gibbs[29]	2006	7 759 044	1:56 635	1:184 739

460 institutions selected at random; this represented approximately 8% of the total estimated number of anaesthetics undertaken in France[18]. During anaesthesia, or within 24 h, 268 major anaesthesia-related complications occurred (one in every 739 anaesthetics). There were 67 deaths within 24 h, and 16 patients suffered coma which persisted after 24 h. The incidence of death and persistent coma attributable totally to anaesthesia was 1:7924; death due solely to anaesthesia occurred with an incidence of 1:13 207. In half of all the patients who died or suffered coma, postoperative respiratory depression was responsible.

In New South Wales in Australia, a system was put in place in 1960 to undertake a confidential investigation of deaths related to anaesthesia. Deaths were categorized as anaesthetic, surgical, inevitable, fortuitous, or unassessable. Between 1960 and 1985, the incidence of death attributable to anaesthesia decreased by a factor of five, from 1:5500 to 1:26 000 [19]. However, the pattern of errors by anaesthetists remained largely unchanged during the 25-year period; inadequate preparation of patients, wrong choice of agent or technique, inadvertent overdose, inadequate crisis management, and inadequate resuscitation remained the commonest errors. The proportion of deaths attributable to anaesthesia in which no error could be found in management increased from 2.8% in the period 1960–1969 to 10% in the period 1983–1985. Over the same period, the proportion of specialist anaesthetists involved in deaths attributable to anaesthesia increased from 27% to 62%.

In the Netherlands, a retrospective study of faults, accidents, near accidents, and complications associated with anaesthesia in one institution was conducted between 1978 and 1987[20]. During that period, 97 496 anaesthetics were administered for

Table 10.3 Factors involved in deaths attributable in part to anaesthesia, in decreasing order of frequency[17]

Failure to apply knowledge
Lack of care[a]
Failure of organization
Lack of experience
Lack of knowledge
Drug effect
Failure of equipment
Fatigue

[a] Including failure of a trainee to consult a more senior anaesthetist, grossly inadequate monitoring, inappropriate drug doses, or other clear indication of a poor standard of practice.

Source: From Buck, N., Devlin, H.B., and Lunn, J,N. (1987). Report on the confidential enquiry into perioperative deaths. Nuffield Provincial Hospitals Trust, The Kings Fund Publishing House, London. With permission.

non-cardiac procedures. Cardiac arrest occurred with an incidence of 1:3362 anaesthetics, and mortality from cardiac arrest in these patients had an incidence of 1:5417 anaesthetics. Anaesthesia was considered to have contributed to cardiac arrest in 1:7500 anaesthetics, with a fatal outcome in 1:16 250 anaesthetics. Failure to check, lack of vigilance, and carelessness were the most frequently associated human factors.

In a prospective study conducted in Denmark[21], mortality attributable to anaesthesia occurred with a frequency of 1:2500 (0.04%). The overall perioperative mortality rate was 1.2%, and 0.05% of patients died during anaesthesia. Mortality in patients who developed postoperative cardiovascular complications was 20%.

Mortality associated with anaesthesia and surgery was studied in Finland in 1986 (although not published until 1995) [22]. Death was caused primarily by anaesthesia with an incidence of approximately 1:67 000. This was a substantial improvement on the mortality rate of 1:5000 reported after an earlier study in 1975[15].

Between 1984 and 1990, there were 1503 deaths within 24 h of, or as a result of, anaesthesia in New South Wales. The Special Committee Investigating Deaths Under Anaesthesia in New South Wales attributed 172 deaths (11.4%) to factors under anaesthetists' control. About 10% of the deaths occurred in patients undergoing urgent non-emergency operations, of which 45 (31.3%) were attributed to anaesthetic factors[23,24]. General anaesthesia was used in 31 cases and major regional block (10 spinals and 4 epidurals) in the others. Anaesthetic factors most often identified as contributing to death were inadequate preparation for anaesthesia and surgery, inappropriate choice or application of technique, inadequate postoperative care and overdose. Patients most likely to suffer an anaesthetic-related death were those who were elderly (between 70 and 79 years) and male (almost twice as often as females). The calculated rate of death attributable wholly or in part to anaesthesia was 1 in 20 000 operations. In Canada, the risk factors associated with death within 7 days of anaesthesia were analysed in a study involving 100 000 surgical procedures[25]. There were 71 deaths per 10 000 patients, and differences in anaesthetic practice were of much less importance in contributing to death than were age, physical status, and the type of surgery.

Another study from the Netherlands[26]found that the incidence of mortality in which anaesthesia contributed to death was 1:7143 procedures, but that it was solely responsible for death in only 1:124 000 operations. A number of inadequacies in management of the patients were identified, including poor preoperative assessment, inappropriate anaesthetic technique, inadequate cardiovascular management, poor management of ventilation, and inadequate monitoring. Inadequate communication and lack of supervision were also noted. The highest frequency of anaesthesia-related deaths (45.4%) occurred among ASA 3 patients, whereas mortality rate associated with all operations increased with increasing ASA grade; 39.5% of all deaths occurred in ASA 5 patients, in comparison with only 10.1% of all anaesthesia-related deaths.

All states in Australia have Government-supported Special Committees to collect data about anaesthetic-related deaths. Six successive triennial reports have been collated from all State Committees. The report for 1994–1996[27] concluded that anaesthetic-related deaths occurred with a frequency of approximately 1:63 000 operative or diagnostic procedures; the death rate attributable to anaesthesia alone was considered to be about 1 in 155 000 procedures. The report dealing with the triennium 1997–1999[28] found that the incidence of death had decreased; anaesthesia caused or contributed to death in 1:79 500 procedures, and was the definite cause in approximately 1:220 000. In most deaths, there was more than one causal or contributory factor (mean 2.5). Correctable anaesthetic factors identified most frequently were related to anaesthetic technique, inadequate preoperative assessment, and use of anaesthetic drugs. The authors noted that 73% of deaths involved specialist anaesthetists, but 27% involved non-specialist anaesthetists or trainees working unsupervised. The proportion of ASA 1 or 2 patients among those who died decreased from 42% in 1985–1987 to 10% in 1994–1996, although it increased to 15% in 1997–1999. Death was more frequent among men, and 78% of the patients were over 60 years of age. Almost two-thirds of the deaths occurred in relation to urgent or emergency procedures.

The latest report[29] dealing with the years from 2000 to 2002 used a new coding system to estimate the total number of anaesthetics given. This was lower than previous, probably less accurate methods, resulting in an apparent increase in the incidence of death associated with anaesthesia. The total number of deaths was similar to the numbers in previous triennia, despite a progressive increase in the population. Seventy-six per cent of deaths occurred in patients over the age of 60 years, 46% in patients classified as ASA 4 or 5 and 66% in patients undergoing urgent or emergency surgery. However, the proportion of ASA 1 or 2 patients among those who died increased again to 19%. Most deaths occurred in the operating theatre or an intensive care unit (ICU) or high dependency unit (HDU), but 15% occurred in a general ward, where it was thought that limited monitoring and supervision may have contributed to the adverse outcome. The majority of deaths involved specialist anaesthetists, but 19% involved non-specialist or trainee anaesthetists, and four deaths occurred when anaesthesia was provided by the operator. Death was most likely to occur after orthopaedic or abdominal surgery. In only 31% of deaths associated with anaesthesia was it concluded that it was reasonably certain that death was caused by the anaesthetist or other factors under the control of the anaesthetist, and in 20% of deaths associated with anaesthesia, no correctable factor could be identified, suggesting that in some patients, anaesthetic factors may contribute to death despite optimal anaesthetic management; this probably applied to patients who were significantly medically compromised preoperatively and whose condition could not be improved prior to surgery. Death associated with anaesthesia had an incidence of one death for every 56 000 anaesthetics; for deaths in which it was reasonably certain that anaesthesia was the cause, the incidence was 1:182 000.

A study in Japan[30] investigated mortality between 1994 and 1998. The findings may not be as reliable as those from other studies because data were gathered retrospectively from questionnaires, only 40% of which were returned. Nevertheless, data were gathered relating to 2.3 million operations. The mortality rate attributable to anaesthesia was approximately 1:48 000.

In the United States, an incidence of 1.7 cardiac arrests per 10 000 anaesthetics was reported in 1985[31], although not all were fatal. The study involved 163 240 anaesthetics administered over a 15-year period. Of 449 cardiac arrests, 27 were judged to be attributable solely to anaesthesia, and mortality was 0.9 per 10 000 anaesthetics. Three-quarters of these cardiac arrests were considered to have been preventable. In 1991, the same authors published results relating to 241 934 anaesthetics over a 20-year period from 1969 to 1988[32]. During the second decade, pulse oximetry and capnography were introduced. Cardiac arrest related to anaesthetic causes decreased from 2.1 per 10 000 anaesthetics in the first decade to 1.0 per 10 000 in the second decade. Most of this difference was due to a decrease in cardiac arrests from preventable respiratory causes.

Kawashima et al.[33] also investigated the incidence of cardiac arrest during anaesthesia. They reported that cardiac arrest attributable to anaesthesia (from 1994–1998) occurred with an incidence of 1.0 per 10 000, a figure identical to that reported by Keenan and Boyan[32] from 1979 to 1988. However, mortality following cardiac arrest was 0.13 per 10 000 anaesthetics, much lower than that reported from the United States in the previous decade. The ten most common causes of cardiac arrest attributable to anaesthesia alone are shown in Table 10.4.

A study conducted in one Brazilian tertiary referral hospital over a 9-year period[34] reported 186 cardiac arrests and 118 deaths during surgery or the early postoperative period. Major risk factors were neonates, adults between 51 and 64 years, male gender (2.4 times higher risk than female gender), ASA 3 status or poorer, emergency surgery (11.3 times higher risk), and general anaesthesia (8.3 times higher risk than neuraxial anaesthesia). Anaesthesia was considered to have caused cardiac arrest in only 10% of cases, and death in only 1.5%. Respiratory events were responsible for 55% of anaesthesia-related cardiac arrests, most commonly as a result of loss of the airway or difficulty in tracheal intubation. Pulmonary aspiration and cardiovascular depression were the commonest causes of anaesthesia-related death. The overall

Table 10.4 The ten most common causes of intra-operative cardiac arrest attributable to anaesthesia[33]

Cause	Frequency (%)
Drug overdose or selection error	15.3
Serious arrhythmia	13.9
Myocardial infarction, ischaemia	8.8
Inadequate airway management	7.9
High spinal	7.4
Inadequate vigilance	6.9
Massive haemorrhage managed badly	5.1
Overdose of inhaled anaesthetic	2.8
Suffocation, aspiration	2.8
Dis/misconnection	2.3

Source: From Kawashima, Y., Takahashi, S., Suzuki, M., *et al.* (2003). Anesthesia-related mortality and morbidity over a 5-year period in 2,363,038 patients in Japan. *Acta Anaesthesiologica Scandinavica,* **47**, 809–17.With permission.

mortality associated with anaesthesia and surgery was 1:455; the incidence attributed to anaesthesia alone was 1:8900.

In 2006, a study was published from France, where the number and characteristics of anaesthesia-related deaths were analysed during the year 1999[35]. Over 500 000 death certificates were examined, and deaths that might relate to anaesthesia care or anaesthesia-related complications were studied. Detailed information was obtained about these deaths, and opinions obtained from a committee of experts. The number of anaesthetic procedures during 1999 was estimated to be 7.7 million. It was considered that anaesthesia was primarily responsible for death in 1 in 145 500 anaesthetic procedures, and partly related to anaesthesia in 1 in 21 200 anaesthetics. The mortality rate increased with age and ASA physical status (Table 10.5). Death related totally or partly to anaesthesia was 40 times commoner in patients aged ≥75 years than in those aged 16–39 years, and 137 times higher in patients of ASA status 4 than those with ASA status 1. The risk of death in ASA status 1 patients was 1:250 000. The commonest causes of death were cardiogenic shock, hypovolaemia, respiratory failure caused by drugs, inability to secure access to the airway, and aspiration of vomit. The authors noted that, in comparison with the earlier French study between 1978 and 1982[18], there had been a 10-fold decrease in mortality related to anaesthesia.

It has been suggested recently that depth of anaesthesia and hypotension during anaesthesia may influence mortality rate after surgery[36]. Just over 1000 patients who underwent major non-cardiac surgery were studied. Overall, the mortality rate was 0.7% at 30 days and 5.5% at 1 year. In elderly (≥65 years of age) patients, these rates were 1.8% and 10.3%. The principal causes of death were cancer and cardiovascular

Table 10.5 Incidence of mortality rate totally or partly related to anaesthesia stratified by age and ASA status (derived from Lienhart et al.[35])

	Mortality related to anaesthesia
Age (years)	
0–7	1:166 667
8–15	1:83 333
16–39	1:192 308
40–74	1:19 231
≥75	1:4762
ASA physical status	
1	1:250 000
2	1:20 000
3	1:3704
4	1:1818

Source: From Lienhart, A., Auroy, Y., Péquignot, F., *et al.* (2006). Survey of anesthesia-related mortality in France. *Anesthesiology*, **105**, 1087–97. With permission.

failure; renal failure, liver failure, multiple organ failure, respiratory failure, aspiration, pulmonary embolism, and sepsis also caused a small number of deaths. The relative risk of death was increased particularly by the presence of three or more co-morbidities, ASA status 3 or 4, age ≥65 years, a history of heart disease, previous myocardial infarction or hypertension, a history of hepatic disease, and the duration of surgery. However, it was also found that deep anaesthesia (as defined by a bispectral [BIS] index of less than 45) was associated with an increased risk of death, as was intraoperative hypotension, defined as a systolic blood pressure of <80 mmHg. Both of these risks were time-related, i.e. the longer a patient was deeply anaesthetized or hypotensive, the higher was the risk of death. The authors speculate that the increased risk related to depth of anaesthesia could be associated with alterations to the inflammatory response to surgery and to the postoperative immune response.

This was a relatively small retrospective study, and, as the authors and other commentators have observed[37], prospective studies will be required to establish whether the results of this retrospective study are reliable.

Despite the difficulty in comparing the results of these studies directly, there does appear to have been a considerable reduction in mortality caused primarily by anaesthesia within the last 25 years in countries with high standards of training and well-equipped hospitals. The figures in Table 10.2 should be compared with the mortality rate reported by McKenzie[38]. Death or persistent coma attributable to anaesthesia occurred with a frequency of 1:388 in Zimbabwean teaching hospitals in 1992, and there were avoidable factors in 51% of deaths. Glenshaw and Madzimbamuto[39] reported an avoidable mortality rate from anaesthesia of 1:482 for patients undergoing emergency obstetric procedures in the same country between 1994 and 2001.

The overall incidence of mortality in emergency obstetric patients was 1:293; factors under the control of the anaesthetist accounted for 72% of deaths.

Other sources of information

Closed claims analysis

Because of the high rate of litigation against anaesthetists in some countries, analysis of claims for compensation has been used to examine the pattern of injury which patients may suffer, or believe that they have suffered, as a result of the actions of anaesthetists. There is a risk of bias in analysing claims for compensation, in that the complaints relate predominantly to events that the patient does not expect. Although patients are prepared to accept that surgery may not be entirely successful, or may be associated with a small incidence of complications, they are often unwilling to acknowledge that any consequence which they attribute to anaesthesia, or the anaesthetist, is acceptable.

Between 1996 and 2004, the Danish Patient Insurance Association received 1256 files relating to anaesthesia (4.5% of the total)[40]. The claims included 43 deaths. Analysis indicated that death resulted from anaesthesia in 24 of these. Four were related to airway management, two to ventilation management, four to central venous catheter insertion, four to medication errors, four to infusion pump problems, and four related to regional blocks.

In the United Kingdom, claims involving National Health Service (NHS) hospitals are dealt with by the NHS Litigation Authority through its Clinical Negligence Scheme for Trusts (CNST). Between April 1995 and October 2005, there were 992 claims relating to anaesthetic practice[41]. Of these, 10.5% involved death attributable to anaesthesia, and 6.7% involved brain damage. The risk of death or brain damage was highest in relation to failure of preoperative assessment and errors in procedures in the operating theatre.

Critical incident reporting

Critical incident reporting is a technique, which was developed by psychologists, to evaluate aspects of human behaviour and to study the causes of good and bad performance. An incident is any observable human activity that is sufficiently complete in itself to permit inferences and predictions to be made about the person performing the act. A critical incident is an incident whose purpose or intent is clear to the observer and the consequences of which are sufficiently definite to leave little doubt about its effect. The technique was described first in 1954[42], but had been used extensively by the U.S. Air Force during the Second World War. Trained observers collected large numbers of factual observations which made an important positive or negative contribution to the activity being studied (e.g. the reasons for failure of bombing missions). When these critical incidents were studied, they could be categorized, and steps could be taken to improve success (e.g. in guiding recruitment policy so that pilots with good performance could be predicted), and to reduce failure (e.g. by improving cockpit design).

Critical incident reporting has been adopted widely in anaesthesia over the last two decades. Many anaesthetic departments collect data internally, using the data to identify and correct faults with specific items of equipment, to modify protocols, guidelines and training, and to provide feedback at departmental meetings. One of the largest studies is the Australian Incident Monitoring Study[43], which, in 1993, reported in detail the findings from analysis of the first 2000 incident reports. The findings from the next 2000 incident reports were published in 2005[44]. The commonest incidents reported are shown in Table 10.6, and the most commonly quoted associated factors in Table 10.7. There is a close similarity with the factors which contributed to death in the CEPOD study[17] (Table 10.3).

In the United Kingdom, the National Patient Safety Agency (NPSA) collects information from all hospitals relating to critical incidents. Between January 2004 and February 2006, 12 606 incident reports relating to anaesthesia were filed[45]. Severe harm or death occurred in 2.1% of the reported incidents (2.4% for incidents involving epidural block). However, there is little information about the nature of these incidents.

The Thai Anesthesia Incidents Study[46] was conducted over 12 months starting in February 2003. Over 160 000 patients were studied in 20 hospitals. Any death during surgery or within 24 h after the end of anaesthesia was investigated. The commonest causes of death were exsanguination, traumatic brain injury, sepsis, heart failure,

Table 10.6 Examples of the most commonly quoted critical incidents in the Australian Incident Monitoring Study[43]

Problems with breathing system
Disconnections
Misconnections
Leaks
Problems in administration of drugs
Overdosage
Underdosage
Wrong drug
Problems with intubation and control of airway
Failed intubation
Oesophageal intubation
Endobronchial intubation
Accidental or premature extubation
Aspiration
Failure of equipment
Laryngoscopes
Intravenous infusion devices
Breathing system valves
Monitoring devices

Source: Holland, R. (1993). Symposium – The Australian Incident Monitoring Study. *Anaesthesia and Intensive Care*, **21**, 501. With permission.

Table 10.7 Examples of the commonest factors associated with critical incidents in the Australian Incident Monitoring Study[43]

Inattention/carelessness
Inexperience
Haste
Failure to check equipment
Unfamiliarity with equipment
Poor communication
Restricted visual field or access
Failure of planning
Distraction
Lack of skilled assistance
Lack of supervision
Fatigue and decreased vigilance

Source: From Holland, R. (1993). Symposium – The Australian Incident Monitoring Study. *Anaesthesia and Intensive Care,* **21**, 501. With permission.

and hypoxia. The overall mortality was 1:354. Anaesthesia was considered to have made no contribution to death in 78% of cases. Death was considered to have been directly related to anaesthesia in 6% of deaths (a death rate of 1:5800), and to have been partly related to anaesthesia in a further 14% of deaths (a total death rate of 1:1740 related to anaesthesia). Overall, almost two-thirds of deaths were judged to have been non-preventable. In anaesthesia-related deaths, the commonest problems were drug overdose, uncontrolled haemodynamic status, loss of airway, and early extubation. Other factors identified as contributing to death included lack of ICU beds, inadequate preoperative assessment and preparation, lack of a medically qualified anaesthetist, and inappropriate or unnecessary surgery. More than 90% of the patients who died were classified as ASA 3 or more. Inappropriate decision-making, lack of experience, inadequate knowledge, and inadequate preoperative preparation were the main human failures contributing to death.

Critical incident techniques have an important place in identification of risk and improvement of safety by drawing the attention of anaesthetists to potential errors and by identifying deficiencies in equipment design and function. However, there are potential disadvantages associated with continuous critical incident reporting. Medical staff are much less likely to report a critical incident than non-medical staff, and many reported incidents are trivial. An individual anaesthetist, who is conscientious in reporting critical incidents in a departmental system, or an individual department in a national scheme, may be regarded as a poor performer if there is any breach of anonymity, and this may encourage under-reporting. Similarly, an apathetic individual or department not only causes under-reporting, but may appear (justifiably or not) to be a good performer. Continuous reporting may result in loss of enthusiasm with time, causing progressively increasing under-reporting; limiting reporting to specific areas of anaesthetic practice in rotation might help to maintain enthusiasm. In addition, it is necessary to define the term 'critical incident' carefully; some authors have used Cooper's original definition, but others have used the term to describe events, which may or not be preventable, which may or may not include anaesthetic error or equipment failure, and which may include only incidents which result in an adverse outcome. The term 'real or potential adverse event' has been proposed as a self-explanatory and unambiguous alternative.

Severe brain injury

The incidence of severe brain injury caused by anaesthesia is difficult to ascertain. Severe brain injury is associated usually with either severe hypoxaemia or cerebral ischaemia, and the causes are similar to those which result in death related to anaesthesia. Consequently, it is important to try to learn from studies of severe brain injury and from those which group death and permanent brain injury together.

Severe hypoxaemia in the perioperative period may occur as a result of inadequate ventilation (caused usually by disconnection of the breathing system, oesophageal intubation, ventilatory depression, airway obstruction, or failure or misuse of mechanical ventilation), severe lung disease, delivery of an inappropriately low inspired oxygen concentration, bronchospasm (most commonly caused by asthma, anaphylaxis or aspiration), endobronchial intubation, or haemo- or pneumothorax. Cerebral ischaemia may result from profound hypotension caused by vasodilatation due to adverse effects of drugs or anaphylaxis, severe hypovolaemia, or a greatly reduced cardiac output related to cardiac failure, cardiac arrest, severe bradycardia, or a malignant arrhythmia.

Kawashima et al.[30] found that the incidence of a persistent vegetative state attributable to anaesthesia in surgical patients was approximately 1:170000, more than three times less frequent than death attributable to anaesthesia, but this figure may be misleading because it is possible that some brain-damaged patients were allowed to die and were therefore classified only as deaths related to anaesthesia.

In the mid-1980s, the Committee of Professional Liability of the American Society of Anesthesiologists (ASA) began a structured evaluation of adverse anaesthetic outcomes with the purpose of improving safety by devising strategies to prevent anaesthetic mishaps. Data were extracted from 'closed claims' files of up to 35 insurance organizations, which indemnify doctors (ASA Closed Claims Analysis). Because of the long delays incurred in the legal process, this has generated information about the pattern of injury over 25 years, in addition to data derived from analysing the causes of injury. The most common complications associated with claims in the 1990s are shown in Table 10.8[47]. In 1975, the proportion of total claims for death or brain damage was 56%, and decreased by approximately 1% per year until the year 2000 (the last year available for analysis at the time), when the proportion was 27% of total claims[48]. The two major causes of damage were respiratory and cardiovascular events. Before 1986, respiratory causes of death or permanent brain damage accounted for approximately 50% of claims, and cardiovascular causes for around 27%. By 1992, the proportions of respiratory and cardiovascular causes of damage were both 28%, and remained stable up to the year 2000.

A number of factors are known to influence the risk of serious complications associated with anaesthesia and surgery. Morita et al.[49] reported that the incidences of critical

Table 10.8 Most common complications found on analysis of 1,784 American closed claims related to anaesthetic care in the 1990s[47]

Injury	Frequency (%)
Death	23
Nerve injury	21
Brain damage	9
Burns/skin inflammation	6
Awareness	5
Eye injury	5
Backache	5
Headache	5
Pneumothorax	4
Aspiration pneumonitis	3
Injury to newborn	1.5

Source: From Posner, K.L. (2001). Closed claims project shows safety evolution. *American Patient Safety Newsletter*. With permission.

events, death, and cardiac arrest were greatest at the extremes of age (Figure 10.1), and lowest between the ages of 1 year and 65 years. In the Australian Incident Monitoring Study[50], the incidence of 'harm' that might have resulted from critical incidents was related to the ASA grading of the patient, with ASA 5 patients much more likely to be harmed by an incident than patients in categories 1–4. Chopra *et al.*[20] found that all ASA 4 or ASA 5 patients who suffered perioperative cardiac arrest died, whereas the majority of ASA 1–3 patients survived.

In a study from Denmark, Pedersen[21] investigated the relationship between complications attributable to anaesthesia and both ASA grade and whether the procedure was an emergency or elective procedure; he also studied the influence of these factors on outcome after a complication, and the frequency of preventable errors. He found that complications attributable to anaesthesia were slightly less common during emergency procedures than elective operations, and the number of preventable errors leading to complications was lower in emergency procedures. However, the probability of a negative outcome from an anaesthetic complication was higher in emergency patients. The number of complications attributable to anaesthesia was almost eight times higher in patients in ASA grades 3–5 than in those with ASA grades 1 or 2, and the incidences of a negative outcome and preventable errors were also much higher in patients with a high ASA grade.

Oesophageal intubation is a well-known complication of anaesthesia, and can have devastating consequences if not detected rapidly. The incidence of undetected oesophageal intubation has decreased since the introduction of routine capnography, but it has

Events/10,000 patients

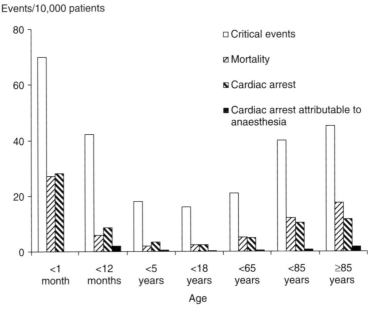

Fig. 10.1 Relationship between age and complications associated with anaesthesia. (adapted from Morita, K., Kawashima, Y., Irita, K., *et al.* (2002). Perioperative mortality and morbidity in the year 2000 in 520 certified training hospitals of Japanese Society of Anesthesiologists: with a special reference to age – report of Japanese Society of Anesthesiologists Committee on Operating Room Safety. *Masui*, **51**, 1285–96. With permission.)

not been eliminated. The Australian Incident Monitoring Study[51] reported that 35 of its first 2000 critical incidents involved oesophageal intubation. In 15 of these incidents, there had been no difficulty reported during intubation. In 18 cases, a trained specialist anaesthetist intubated the trachea; in 15 cases, a trainee was responsible, and in 2 incidents the identity of the individual involved was not known. In the ASA Closed Claims Study[52], analysis of legal claims for damages related to oesophageal intubation revealed that, in more than 80% of claims, the standard of care provided by the anaesthesiologist was considered, on retrospective review, to be substandard. A later study[53] showed that in more than 80% of claims related to oesophageal intubation, the patient had died, and the remainder had suffered brain damage. This information is, of course, rather misleading; provided that oesophageal intubation is detected promptly, no injury is caused and a patient has no grounds for legal action.

The ASA Closed Claims Study also found[47,48] that the standard of care in claims relating to injury caused by inadequate ventilation (again almost always resulting in death or brain injury, but for the same reason) was judged to be inadequate in the large majority of cases. In almost 60% of cases of injury related to difficult intubation, the actions of the anaesthesiologist were judged to have been substandard. In contrast, the standard of care was judged to have been inadequate in approximately 30% of claims that did not involve the respiratory system. As noted earlier, the incidence of claims involving the respiratory system has diminished since the introduction of pulse oximetry and capnography, but hypoxic brain damage and death resulting from failure to ventilate the lungs do still occur and, arguably, are even more culpable if appropriate monitors have not been used, or if the information which they provide has been ignored.

Inability to ventilate the lungs, again with the potential to cause hypoxic brain injury and death, may occur as a result of an obstruction in a tracheal tube, laryngeal mask airway, or the anaesthetic breathing system. The Australian Incident Monitoring Study[54] received reports of obstruction of the tracheal tube caused by kinking, biting, secretions or blood, a surgical gag, and foreign bodies, and there has been a more recent incident in the United Kingdom in which a child died as a result of obstruction of an angle piece by the cap of an intravenous infusion set[55].

In the Australian Anaesthetic Incident Monitoring Study[56], 244 of 2000 critical incidents were related to vomiting or regurgitation associated with anaesthesia, and there were 133 incidents, which involved aspiration. Passive regurgitation occurred three times more commonly than active vomiting. Both regurgitation or vomiting and aspiration occurred approximately twice as commonly in patients undergoing elective surgery in comparison to patients who required emergency treatment. Most incidents occurred during induction of anaesthesia, some took place during maintenance, emergence, and later recovery, and very few occurred in association with the process of extubation. The immediate effect of aspiration was judged to be 'major' in more than half of the incidents, but the final outcome was serious in only about one-third of patients. In the ASA Closed Claims Study[52], approximately half of the patients who sued because of injury associated with aspiration died or suffered brain damage, but this figure is distorted by outcome bias.

Conclusion

Although many claims have been made that the risk associated with anaesthesia has decreased, there is little hard supportive evidence except in relation to serious respiratory complications, where improved monitoring appears to have reduced the incidence substantially over the last three decades. Many assumptions have been based on retrospective analysis of events which 'could have been prevented', but numerous studies have demonstrated that the same pattern of errors, incidents, and accidents continues to occur. Although a small number of studies have suggested that there has been a huge reduction in the incidence of mortality attributable to anaesthesia, other studies suggest that the incidence is not changing significantly, and it remains unacceptably high in some countries. The safety of patients does not depend solely on application of standards of practice, the purchase of new equipment, and the institution of new monitoring techniques. Safety can be increased only by combining the use of modern technology with improvements in education, training, supervision, attitudes, standards of clinical practice, audit, and vigilance.

It is possible that the overall mortality rate associated with anaesthesia in developed countries has reached a plateau or that it may increase as elderly patients with several co-morbidities are offered surgery more readily. The risk of death increases substantially in older and sicker patients, and this must be borne in mind when informing patients of the risk of death.

References

1. Owens, W.D. and Spitznagel, E.L. (1980). Anesthetic side effects and complications: an overview. *International Anesthesiology Clinics*, **18**, 1–9.

2. Beecher, H.K. and Todd, D.P. (1954). A study of the deaths associated with anesthesia and surgery. *Annals of Surgery*, **140**, 2–34.

3. Dornette, W.H.L. and Orth, O.S. (1956). Death in the operating room. *Anesthesia and Analgesia*, **35**, 545–51.

4. Schapira, M., Kepes, E.R., and Hurwitt, E.S. (1960). An analysis of deaths in the operating room and within 24 hours of surgery. *Anesthesia and Analgesia*, **39**, 149–52.

5. Phillips, O.C., Frazier, T.M., Graff, T.D., and DeKornfeld, T.J. (1960). The Baltimore Anesthesia Study Committee. A review of 1,024 postoperative deaths. *Journal of the American Medical Association*, **174**, 2015–20.

6. Dripps, R.D., Lamont, A., and Eckenhoff, J.E. (1961). The role of anesthesia in surgical mortality. *Journal of the American Medical Association*, **178**, 261–6.

7. Clifton, B.S. and Hotten, W.I.T. (1963). Deaths associated with anaesthesia. *British Journal of Anaesthesia*, **35**, 250–9.

8. Memery, H.N. (1965). Anesthesia mortality in private practice. *Journal of the American Medical Association*, **194**, 1185–8.

9. Gebbie, D. (1966). Anaesthesia and death. *Canadian Journal of Anaesthesia*, **13**, 390–6.

10. Minuck, M. (1967). Death in the operating room. *Canadian Journal of Anaesthesia*, **14**, 197–204.

11. Harrison, G.G. (1968). Anaesthetic contributory death—its incidence and causes. I. Incidence *South African Medical Journal*, **42**, 514–8.

12. Marx, G.F., Matteo, C.V., and Otkin, L.R. (1973). Computer analysis of post anesthetic deaths. *Anesthesiology*, **39**, 54–8.

13. Bodlander, F.M.S. (1975). Deaths associated with anaesthesia. *British Journal of Anaesthesia*, **47**, 36–40.

14. Harrison, G.G. (1978). Death attributable to anesthesia: a 10 year survey (1967–1976). *British Journal of Anaesthesia*, **50**, 1041–6.

15. Hovi-Viander, M. (1980). Death associated with anaesthesia in Finland. *British Journal of Anaesthesia*, **52**, 483–9.

16. Lunn, J.N. and Mushin, W.W. (1982). *Mortality associated with anaesthesia*. Nuffield Provincial Hospitals Trust, London.

17. Buck, N., Devlin, H.B., and Lunn, J,N. (1987). *Report on the confidential enquiry into peri-operative deaths*. Nuffield Provincial Hospitals Trust, The Kings Fund Publishing House, London.

18. Tiret, L., Desmonts, J.M., Hatton, F., and Vourc'h, G. (1986). Complications associated with anaesthesia—a prospective survey in France. *Canadian Journal of Anaesthesia*, **33**, 336–44.

19. Holland, R. (1987). Anaesthetic mortality in New South Wales. *British Journal of Anaesthesia*, **59**, 834–41.

20. Chopra, V., Bovill, J.G., and Spierdijk, J. (1990). Accidents, near accidents and complications during anaesthesia: a retrospective analysis of a 10-year period in a teaching hospital. *Anaesthesia*, **45**, 3–6.

21. Pedersen, T. (1994). Complications and death following anaesthesia. A prospective study with special reference to the influence of patient-, anaesthesia-, and surgery-related risk factors. *Danish Medical Bulletin*, **41**, 319–31.

22. Tikkanen, J. and Hovi-Viander, M. (1995). Death associated with anaesthesia and surgery in Finland in 1986 compared to 1975. *Acta Anaesthesiologica Scandinavica*, **39**, 262–7.

23. Horan, B.F., Warden, J.C., and Dwyer, B. (1996). Urgent non-emergency surgery and death attributable to anaesthetic factors. *Anaesthesia and Intensive Care*, **24**, 694–8.

24. Warden, J.C., and Horan, B.F. (1996). Deaths attributed to anaesthesia in New South Wales, 1984–1990. *Anaesthesia and Intensive Care*, **24**, 66–73.

25. Cohen, M.M., Duncan, P.G., and Tate, R.B. (1988). Does anaesthesia contribute to operative mortality? *Journal of the American Medical Association*, **260**, 2859–63.

26. Arbous, M.S., Grobbee, D.E., van Kleef, J.W., *et al.* (2001). Mortality associated with anaesthesia: a qualitative analysis to identify risk factors. *Anaesthesia*, **56**, 1141–53.

27. Davis, N.J. (ed). (1999). *Anaesthesia related mortality in Australia. 1994–1996*. Australian and New Zealand College of Anaesthetists, Melbourne. http://www.anzca.edu.au/resources/books-and-publications/reports/mortality/anaesthesia-related-mortality-in-australia-1994-1996.html (last accessed 22nd December 2008).

28. Willis, R.J. (ed). (2002). *A review of anaesthesia related mortality 1997–1999*. Australian and New Zealand College of Anaesthetists, Melbourne. http://www.anzca.edu.au/resources/books-and-publications/reports/mortality/a-review-of-anaesthesia-related-mortality-1997–1999.html (last accessed 22nd December 2008).

29. Gibbs, N. (ed). (2006, amended 2007). A review of anaesthesia related mortality 2000–2002. Australian and New Zealand College of Anaesthetists, Melbourne. http://www.anzca.edu.au/resources/books-and-publications/reports/mortality/Safety%20of%20Anaesthesia%20in%20Australia.pdf (last accessed 22nd December 2008).

30. Kawashima, Y., Takahashi, S., Suzuki, M., *et al.* (2003). Anesthesia-related mortality and morbidity over a 5-year period in 2,363,038 patients in Japan. *Acta Anaesthesiologica Scandinavica*, **47**, 809–17.

31. Keenan, R.L. and Boyan, C.P. (1985). Cardiac arrest due to anesthesia: a study of incidence and causes. *Journal of the American Medical Association*, **253**, 2373–7.

32. Keenan, R.L. and Boyan, C.P. (1991). Decreasing frequency of anesthetic cardiac arrests. *Journal of Clinical Anesthesia*, **3**, 354–7.

33. Kawashima, Y., Takahashi, S., Suzuki, M., *et al.* (2003). Anesthesia-related mortality and morbidity over a 5-year period in 2,363,038 patients in Japan. *Acta Anaesthesiologica Scandinavica*, **47**, 809–17.

34. Braz, L.G., Módolo, N.S.P., do Nascimento, P., *et al.* (2006). Perioperative cardiac arrest: a study of 53 718 anaesthetics over 9 yr from a Brazilian teaching hospital. *British Journal of Anaesthesia*, **96**, 569–75.

35. Lienhart, A., Auroy, Y., Péquignot, F., *et al.* (2006). Survey of anesthesia-related mortality in France. *Anesthesiology*, **105**, 1087–97.

36. Monk, T.G., Saini, V., Weldon, and B.C., Sigl, J.C. (2005). Anesthetic management and one-year mortality after noncardiac surgery. *Anesthesia and Analgesia*, **100**, 4–10.

37. Cohen, N.H. (2005). Anesthetic depth is not (yet) a predictor of mortality! *Anesthesia and Analgesia*, **100**, 1–3.

38. McKenzie, A.G. (1996). Mortality associated with anaesthesia at Zimbabwean teaching hospitals. *South African Medical Journal*, **86**, 338–42.

39. Glenshaw, M. and Madzimbamuto, F.D. (2005). Anaesthesia associated mortality in a district hospital in Zimbabwe: 1994 to 2001. *Central African Journal of Medicine*, **51**, 39–44.

40. Hove, L.D., Steinmetz, J., Christoffersen, Møller, A., Nielsen, J., and Schmidt, H. (2007). Analysis of deaths related to anesthesia in the period 1996-2004 from closed claims registered by the Danish Patient Insurance Association. *Anesthesiology*, **106**, 675–80.

41. National Patient Safety Agency, personal communication.

42. Flanagan, J.C. (1954). The critical incident technique. *Psychological Bulletin*, **51**, 327–58.

43. Holland, R. (1993). Symposium – The Australian Incident Monitoring Study. *Anaesthesia and Intensive Care*, **21**, 501.

44. Runciman, W.B. and Merry, A.F. (2005). Crises in clinical care: an approach to management. *Quality and Safety in Health Care*, **14**, 156–63.

45. Catchpole, K., Bell, M.D.D, and Johnson, S. (2008). Safety in anaesthesia: a study of 12 606 reported incidents from the UK National Reporting and Learning System. *Anaesthesia*, **63**, 340–346.

46. Charuluxananan, S., Chinachoti, T., Pulnitiporn, A., Klanarong, S., Rodanant, O., and Tanudsintum, S. (2005). The Thai incidents study (THAI study) of perioperative death: analysis of risk factors. *Journal of the Medical Association of Thailand*, **88 (Suppl. 7)**, S30–S40.

47. Posner, K.L. (2001). Closed claims project shows safety evolution. *American Patient Safety Newsletter*.

48. Cheney, F.W., Posner, K.L., Lee, L.A., Caplan, R.A., and Domino, K.B. (2006). Trends in anesthesia-related death and brain damage: a closed claims analysis. *Anesthesiology*, **105**, 1081–6.

49. Morita, K., Kawashima, Y., Irita, K., Iwao, Y., Seo, N., and Tsuzaki, K. (2002). Perioperative mortality and morbidity in the year 2000 in 520 certified training hospitals of Japanese Society of Anesthesiologists: with a special reference to age – report of Japanese Society of Anesthesiologists Committee on Operating Room Safety. *Masui*, **51**, 1285–96.

50. Webb, R.K., Currie, M., Morgan, C.A., *et al.* (1993). The Australian Incident Monitoring Study: an analysis of 2000 incident reports. *Anaesthesia and Intensive Care*, **21**, 520–8.

51. Holland, R., Webb, R.K., and Runciman, W.B. (1993). The Australian Incident Monitoring Study. Oesophageal intubation: an analysis of 2000 incident reports. *Anaesthesia and Intensive Care*, **21**, 608–10.

52. Caplan, R.A., Posner, K.L., Ward, R.J., and Cheney, F.W. (1990). Adverse respiratory events in anesthesia: a closed claims analysis. *Anesthesiology*, **72**, 828–33.

53. Cheney, F.W., Posner, K.L., and Caplan, R.A. (1991). Adverse respiratory events infrequently leading to malpractice suits: a closed claims analysis. *Anesthesiology*, **75**, 932–9.

54. Szekely, S.M., Webb, R.K., Williamson, J.A., and Russell, W.J. (1993). The Australian Incident Monitoring Study. Problems related to the endotracheal tube: an analysis of 2000 incident reports. *Anaesthesia and Intensive Care*, **21**, 611–6.

55. *Hospital 'neglect' led to boy's death in routine surgery.* The Times, 20 May 2003, p. 9.

56. Kluger, M.T. and Short, T,G. (1999). Aspiration during anaesthesia: a review of 133 cases from the Australian Anaesthetic Incident Monitoring Study (AIMS). *Anaesthesia*, **54**, 19–26.

Chapter 11

Awareness during anaesthesia

Alan R Aitkenhead

Awareness during anaesthesia has been recognized as a clinical entity for many years, and had an incidence of 1–2% in the United Kingdom during the 1960s and 1970s[1-3], when most anaesthetics comprised nitrous oxide and an opioid analgesic, but no volatile anaesthetic agent. Despite this high incidence, there was only a very modest number of law suits annually, partly because the culture of medical litigation was very different to the present day, partly because some patients were led to believe that awareness was an inevitable complication of anaesthesia, and partly because many patients were disbelieved when they reported awareness and became convinced that their experience must have been imagined.

A dramatic change occurred in 1985. In that year, a patient who had experienced severe and prolonged pain during Caesarean section, with profound psychological sequelae, sued her anaesthetist, and was awarded damages in excess of £13 000[4] amidst a blaze of publicity generated by her solicitor, who knew that a number of other patients treated by the same anaesthetist were also seeking compensation. The publicity resulted in an enormous increase in litigation by patients who claimed that they had been aware during anaesthesia. Some of the alleged experiences had occurred up to 20 years earlier, but many of these claims were allowed to proceed despite the normal limitation period. The large majority of claims were sustainable. Claims for awareness during anaesthesia suddenly escalated.

A cause of some alarm is that claims against anaesthetists which relate to awareness during anaesthesia continue, despite the fact that the surge of historical claims which followed the Ackers case was short-lived, and despite the fact that the deliberate use of predictably inadequate anaesthetic techniques involving the use of nitrous oxide, which was not supplemented by volatile or intravenous anaesthetic agents stopped in the mid-1980s. In the United Kingdom, claims involving National Health Service (NHS) hospitals are dealt with by the NHS Litigation Authority through its Clinical Negligence Scheme for Trusts (CNST). Between April 1995 and October 2005, there were 51 reports of anaesthetic awareness, with 34 injuries described as psychological, 9 described as unnecessary pain, and 10 as 'anaesthetic'[5]. The cost of claims totalled £1 574 507, with a mean of £30 873.

The reason for the persistence of claims for awareness during anaesthesia may be that delivery systems for anaesthetic gas mixtures have become more complex, with an increased potential for misuse. However, in some cases it is apparent that, despite the availability of monitoring apparatus, which can confirm that predictably adequate concentrations of inhaled anaesthetics are being delivered to the patient's lungs, some anaesthetists fail to detect inadequate delivery. This may be because of leaks from the breathing system or dilution of anaesthetic gases by oxygen or air used to drive mechanical ventilators, or failure to deliver the anticipated concentration of volatile anaesthetic agent from a vaporizer, either because it has emptied or because it is not connected correctly to its seating on the back bar of the anaesthetic machine.

It should not be forgotten that the principal reason for attempting to minimize the incidence of awareness should be humanitarian, not fear of litigation. Myles *et al.*[6] undertook a study of patient satisfaction after anaesthesia. The overall level of satisfaction was high (96.8%). Factors that were significantly associated with dissatisfaction were moderate or severe postoperative pain (odds ratio 3.94), severe nausea and vomiting (odds ratio 4.09), and 'any other postoperative complications' (odds ratio 2.04). In patients who experienced awareness during anaesthesia, the odds ratio for dissatisfaction was 54.9, many orders of magnitude above any other complications. Awareness during anaesthesia is a major complication, which causes severe distress at the time of injury, and often results in prolonged psychological injury.

Awareness during anaesthesia has been defined[2] as the 'ability to recall, with or without prompting, events which occurred during the period at which it was thought the patient was fully unconscious'. Subsequently, there has been considerable debate concerning the definition of the word 'unconscious' in relation to anaesthesia, and several demonstrations that patients may be able to recall, at least subconsciously, information perceived by some areas of the brain during otherwise adequate anaesthesia. Nevertheless, Brice's definition remains useful because it refers to the variety of awareness, which is of most clinical relevance, and because it draws attention to the difficulties faced by the anaesthetist in determining the level of consciousness in the anaesthetized patient.

What is anaesthesia?

Prys-Roberts[7] considered that anaesthesia is an all-or-none phenomenon, and thus suggested that there can be no degrees or depths of anaesthesia. This is technically correct if the term anaesthesia is taken to mean lack of conscious recall of events or noxious stimuli, but is unhelpful in attempting to understand the functional mechanism of action of anaesthetic and analgesic agents. Much has been written about the meaning of 'consciousness' during anaesthesia[8–12], and it is likely that no satisfactory solution to this philosophical argument will be found. The practising anaesthetist, who is, quite reasonably, content to equate clinical awareness with conscious recall of intra-operative events, seeks a more pragmatic approach which is consistent with the clinical signs that accompany anaesthesia and with the pattern of recall of patients who complain spontaneously of awareness.

White[13] has described a continuum of anaesthesia (Figure 11.1). Increasing 'depth of anaesthesia' results in a progression from full consciousness through a phase of intoxication to a 'level' at which conscious perception of pain is decreased. There follows a loss of conscious memory of the various sensory modalities; pain is the first modality to be affected, followed by tactile sensation, and subsequently by auditory, visual, and other senses. At this stage, the patient may still respond to stimuli, including the spoken word, but retains no conscious memory of the event. Further movement down the continuum results in loss of responsiveness to command, and then to loss of the motor and autonomic responses to noxious stimuli.

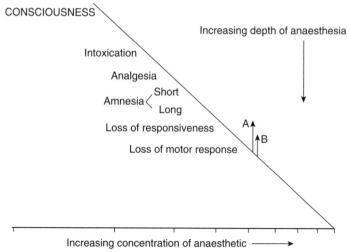

Fig. 11.1 Diagrammatic representation of the continuum of anaesthesia, adapted from White, with permission. Arrow A represents diagrammatically the response to a surgical stimulus, which tends to produce an effect opposite to that of the anaesthetic agent; arrow B represents the influence of opioids on the response to surgical stimulation. See text for details.(Adapted from White, D.C. (1987). Anaesthesia: a privation of the senses. An historical introduction and some definitions. In *Consciousness awareness and pain in general anaesthesia* (eds. M. Rosen and J.N. Lunn), pp. 1–9. Butterworths, London. With permission.)

It may be considered, simplistically, that increasing brain concentrations of anaesthetic agents result in movement down the continuum. However, clinical evidence suggests that noxious stimulation causes an increased 'level of consciousness', resulting in some 'upward' movement from the continuum (Figure 11.1, arrow A). Although opioids may produce an anaesthetic state in very large doses, they appear to act in more conventional analgesic doses by reducing the 'upward' movement in response to a noxious stimulus, from a point on the continuum determined by the concentration of anaesthetic agent in the brain (Figure 11.1, arrow B); this effect is presumably a reflection of the action of opioids in reducing the transmission of noxious stimuli along the pain pathways to the brain. Thus, the 'level of consciousness' is determined by the balance between the cerebral concentration of anaesthetic agent (determined by the anaesthetist) and the degree of cerebral arousal induced by surgical stimuli (which varies during the procedure, and which may be modified by analgesic drugs). This concept is also of importance in considering methods of detecting 'depth of anaesthesia'.

What is awareness?

Jones and Konieczko[14] have suggested that the effect of progressively increasing concentrations of anaesthetic drugs on the brain can be represented crudely by four stages:

Stage I. Conscious awareness without amnesia

Stage II. Conscious awareness with amnesia

Stage III. Subconscious awareness with amnesia

Stage IV. No awareness

The majority of studies undertaken to investigate the incidence of awareness have depended on spontaneous recall upon questioning during the postoperative period (Stage I). This approach has been criticized[15] on the basis that it relies not only on the patient's awareness of events, but also on his ability to remember them. A much higher incidence of awareness may be found using more sensitive tests of memory function, such as prompting under hypnosis, and recognition testing (Stage III) or by using the isolated forearm technique to identify intra-operative response to command, but without conscious recall (Stage II). However, it remains unclear whether awareness without recall is of clinical importance. In contrast, recall of intra-operative events is distressing to the patient and may result in psychological sequelae, which include insomnia, anxiety, irritability, repetitive nightmares, and depression; a preoccupation with death may develop and there may be a morbid fear of hospitals, doctors and, in particular, of the need for future surgery. This 'post-traumatic stress syndrome' may persist for months or years, although it may be ameliorated or cured if the patient is able to discuss the memories openly, and is assured that the memories are genuine. While those who pursue litigation represent only a proportion of patients who remember intra-operative events, the fact that, to date, patients have sought recourse through the courts in respect only of 'conscious awareness without amnesia' suggests that this is the category of awareness that is of greatest clinical importance. It is also the category referred to by most anaesthetists who use the term 'awareness'.

A distinction must be made between spontaneous recall of intra-operative events and dreams, illusions or hallucinations occurring during unconsciousness. An illusion has been defined by Garfield et al.[16] as 'a misinterpretation of a real sensory experience', and a hallucination as 'a false sensory perception in the absence of a sensory experience'. Wilson et al.[17] defined a dream as 'a train of thoughts or images passing through the mind, which the patient believes occurred between the induction of anaesthesia and the first moment of consciousness after the completion of the anaesthetic procedure'. Usually, spontaneous recall can be differentiated from dreams, illusions, or hallucinations by the presence of verifiable conversation or events that occurred during operation. It is important also to differentiate between recall of experiences during anaesthesia and memories of events that occurred in the postoperative period.

Incidence of awareness

Spontaneous recall

Studies of the ability of the patient to recall spontaneously, events that occurred during anaesthesia and surgery, are reliable only if there has been a structured interview, consisting of questions such as:

What is the last thing you remember before going to sleep for your operation?

What is the first thing you remember on waking up after your operation?

Do you remember anything in between?

The incidence of spontaneous recall after non-obstetric procedures in such studies was up to 1.67% in the 1960s and 1970s[1-3,17], when paralysed patients were given only nitrous oxide and an opioid analgesic (Table 11.1); up to 26% of patients reported dreams. More recent studies of patients who have received either nitrous oxide and a volatile anaesthetic agent or total intravenous anaesthesia (TIVA) indicate that the incidence of spontaneous recall is now much lower[6,18-25]; the majority of these studies suggest that the incidence is 1–3 patients per 1000 anaesthetics. It should be noted that most of these patients did not experience pain or distress during their episode of awareness. The incidence of 'severe' awareness is much lower; it has been estimated that about 10% of patients with spontaneous recall remember pain[26].

The incidence of recall may be slightly higher during anaesthesia for obstetric operations (see following paragraphs). In the author's experience of analysing allegations of awareness in more than 140 cases, the large majority of episodes of awareness occur in non-obstetric procedures (Table 11.2), but this probably reflects the fact that most anaesthetics are administered outside the obstetric unit.

Table 11.1 Incidences of awareness during non-obstetric anaesthesia reported between 1970 and 2008

First author (year of publication)	n	Incidence (%)	Gender (F/M)	Notes
Hutchinson (1960)[1]	656	1.22	8/0	N$_2$O/relaxant
Brice (1970)[2]	120	1.67	1/1	N$_2$O/relaxant
McKenna (1973)[3]	200	1.50	0/3	N$_2$O/relaxant
Wilson (1975)[17]	490	0.82	4/0	
Liu (1991)[18]	1000	0.20	1/1	
Sandin (1993)[19]	1727	0.29	5/0	TIVA
Nordström (1997)[20]	1000	0.29	2/0	
Ranta (1998)[21]	2612	0.38	8/2	Another 0.3% might have been aware
Sandin (2000)[22]	11785	0.16	12/7	
Myles (2000)[6]	10811	0.11	Unknown	
Wennervirta (2002)[23]	3843	0.10	4/0	Another 0.18% might have been aware
Sebel (2004)[24]	19575	0.13	16/9	Another 0.24% might have been aware
Avidan (2008)[25]	1941	0.21	1/3	Another 0.31% might have been aware
Errando (2008)[59]	4001	1.0	10/7	TIVA appeared to offer greater risk than inhalational anaesthesia

TIVA= total intravenous anaesthesia.

Table 11.2 Distribution of allegations of awareness by specialty in 142 claims analysed by the author; the events occurred between 1979 and 2007

Speciality	Percentage of claims (%)
Gynaecology	28
General surgery	25
Obstetrics	24
Orthopaedics	7
ENT	6
Dental	4
Cardiac	3
Neurosurgery	1
Others	2

Hearing is the most common sensation recalled, and is the last sense to disappear on losing consciousness. A more distressing complaint is recall of the sensation of pain during surgery. Some patients are aware of being paralysed, and of being unable to indicate to the anaesthetist that they are awake; these patients may not experience pain, but are usually distressed.

Causes of awareness with recall

Spontaneous recall of intra-operative events is, by definition, due to delivery of inadequate concentrations of anaesthetic agents to the brain for the needs of the individual patient. The commonest causes in the cases which the author has analysed are shown in Figure 11.2.

Failure to check apparatus In the author's experience, this is the commonest single cause of awareness with recall. Apparatus must be checked before and during

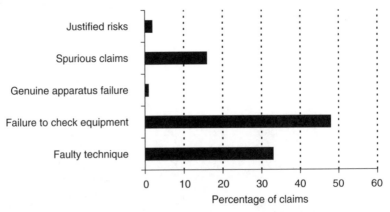

Fig. 11.2 Causes of awareness in 142 cases analysed by the author. The events occurred between 1979 and 2007.

every anaesthetic. Common causes of recall include failure to ensure that the anaesthetic gases are delivered to a mechanical ventilator of a type that does not depend upon the supply of fresh gas for its power; loose connections in the ventilator tubing or breathing system, which result in loss of fresh gas and rebreathing or entrainment of air; failure to connect the vaporizer into the fresh gas supply at all or at least securely, or to lock the vaporizer on to a Selectatec block; failure to ensure that the vaporizer contains the anaesthetic agent; and failure to notice that a nitrous oxide cylinder has become empty. The emergency oxygen flush may be switched on accidentally, diluting the concentration of anaesthetic gases. An infusion of intravenous agent may become disconnected, leak or 'tissue' or the syringe in the infusion pump may become empty. A number of these events may occur during anaesthesia, even though a pre-anaesthetic check has been undertaken. There may also be misinterpretation of signs of light anaesthesia if ECG monitors and automated blood pressure devices are not checked regularly. Recall may occur if an inaccurate inspired oxygen monitor or pulse oximeter causes the anaesthetist to increase the inspired concentration of oxygen inappropriately.

Faulty anaesthetic technique A faulty technique is one which could reasonably be predicted to result in recall of intra-operative events, or in which drug doses are not adjusted when clinical signs of inadequate anaesthesia become apparent. In general, the likelihood of recall is related inversely to the dose or concentration of anaesthetic drug administered (Figure 11.1). However, high concentrations of most anaesthetic agents result in an increased incidence and severity of side-effects, and delayed recovery. Consequently, it became common in the United Kingdom in the 1960s and 1970s for anaesthetists to use paralysing doses of a muscle relaxant to prevent movement during surgery (in contrast to the smaller doses used in North America), and to administer nitrous oxide alone, or with an opioid analgesic, to maintain anaesthesia. Awareness with unpleasant recall occurs almost exclusively in patients who have received a muscle relaxant.

Inhalational anaesthetics The alveolar concentration of inhaled anaesthetic agents required to produce loss of consciousness (i.e. hypnosis) is approximately 0.6 MAC (often termed the MAC_{awake})[27]. However, this is in the absence of surgical stimulation; a higher proportion of MAC is required to ensure amnesia during surgery. In addition, there is individual variability in response; MAC and MAC_{awake} are average values, and the distribution of values among individuals conforms approximately to a normal distribution curve. Thus some patients require significantly higher alveolar concentrations of inhaled anaesthetics than others to ensure loss of consciousness.

Any technique that results in an alveolar concentration of inhaled anaesthetic, which equates to 0.6–0.7 MAC will predictably result in awareness with recall in an unacceptably high proportion of patients. The use of unsupplemented nitrous oxide in concentrations of 67–70% provides about 0.65 MAC, and is unsatisfactory. Utting[28] reported definite or probable recall in 2.2% of 500 patients anaesthetized with unsupplemented nitrous oxide 70% in oxygen. The addition of opioids may reduce the incidence of recall, but only slightly. Rosen[29] demonstrated that auditory perception occurred in some patients breathing 60–75% nitrous oxide, despite an opioid premedication. Brown and Catton[30] reported an incidence of recall of 5.3% in patients premedicated with pethidine or promethazine, and moderately hyperventilated using nitrous oxide 60% in oxygen.

The alveolar concentration of an inhalational agent is normally lower than the delivered concentration and 'overpressure' with volatile agents may be required initially to achieve the desired effect. Uptake is more rapid for agents with a low blood/gas solubility coefficient, and this may be of particular relevance to recall during tracheal intubation or at the start of surgery.

The concentration of an inhalational agent delivered to a patient may be considerably less than the concentration set on the flowmeters or vaporizer if a circle system with vaporizer outside the circle (VOC) is used, especially with low fresh gas flow rates.

Intravenous anaesthetics Anaesthetic drugs administered intravenously are less predictable than inhalational agents. Distribution volumes vary widely between individual patients. Whereas distribution volume has some influence on the rate of uptake of inhalational drugs, its effect is relatively small because increased distribution is to a large extent compensated for by increased uptake from the lungs, and the total dose of anaesthetic administered is increased. In contrast, the total dose of an intravenous drug is selected by the anaesthetist, and the blood and brain concentrations are determined, at least in the short term, by redistribution to tissues, which receive high blood flow. Recall may occur during tracheal intubation if a muscle relaxant has been given before clear signs of loss of consciousness have become apparent, or if inhalational anaesthetics are not given between induction and tracheal intubation; this risk is highest if a non-depolarizing relaxant has been used. In general, higher doses of intravenous anaesthetics are required to ensure lack of recall in unpremedicated outpatients in comparison to premedicated inpatients. A potential problem with total intravenous anaesthesia (TIVA) is that, unlike inhaled anaesthetics, the concentration of drug in the blood cannot be measured during anaesthesia; continuous measurement of end-tidal concentrations of inhaled anaesthetics allow early detection of unexpected failure of delivery of drug to the patient. However, there is little evidence that the incidence of awareness is significantly larger in patients receiving total intravenous anaesthesia than in those anaesthetized using halogenated volatile agents (Table 11.1).

Supplements of non-anaesthetic drugs Lorazepam and diazepam have been used to contribute amnesia to an anaesthetic technique. They do not appear to offer reliable retrograde amnesia, as recall and unpleasant dreams still occurred when either of these drugs was administered following delivery of the baby at Caesarean section using nitrous oxide anaesthesia[31]. Their capacity to induce anterograde amnesia has also been questioned. Indeed, diazepam has been shown to improve the memory of anxious individuals[32], and in normal individuals only certain aspects of memory are depressed[33]. Lorazepam appears to impair alertness and attention rather than memory *per se*[34].

Caesarean section In the 1970s and early 1980s, there was a high incidence of awareness during anaesthesia for Caesarean section conducted under general anaesthesia, due to a reluctance to use inhalational agents in adequate concentrations, because of fears of inducing depression of the fetus and of increased haemorrhage from the uterus. There is no evidence that these fears are justified. General anaesthetics cross the placenta and depress the neonate, and the effects are most apparent at the 1-min

Apgar score. One authority described the 1-min score as an indicator for the need for resuscitation, and the 5-min score as a marker of resuscitative success[35]. Without underlying asphyxia, the 1-min score has no sinister prognosis, as the effects of general anaesthetics are reversible. However, when general anaesthesia is used, an individual who is trained in neonatal resuscitation must be present.

Moir[36] found an incidence of recall of 4% during Caesarean section in patients receiving 70% nitrous oxide, but no recall in patients anaesthetized with 50% nitrous oxide supplemented by halothane 0.5%. However, the incidence of recall using this technique was 0.21% when the number of patients studied was extended to 1400[37], and 'under 1%' after 3000 patients had been interviewed[38]. This was reinforced by investigations using the isolated forearm technique[39]; following a standard dose of thiopentone 250 mg, a suxamethonium infusion, halothane 0.5% in 50% nitrous oxide, and an abdominal incision made immediately after tracheal intubation, the majority of 30 women indicated that they were experiencing pain in the first minute, although none had spontaneous recall.

A review of more than 3000 Caesarean sections described a series of steps that greatly reduced the incidence of awareness[40]. In summary, they included giving thiopentone 5–7 mg kg^{-1} instead of the recommended 3–4 mg kg^{-1}, and using nitrous oxide 50% with isoflurane set at 1% prior to delivery, and nitrous oxide 67% with isoflurane 0.5%, together with administration of an intravenous opioid, after delivery. The incidence of awareness was reduced from 1.3% to 0.4%.

A current recommendation is that anaesthesia should be induced using thiopentone 5–7 mg kg^{-1}, and ventilation and the inhaled gas mixture should be adjusted to deliver target oxygen saturation and end-tidal carbon dioxide values. The vaporizer settings should be continually adjusted to give a target end-tidal concentration. This entails turning the vaporizer to a high setting initially, to ensure that the target is met at the start of the operation. It is recommended that maternal oxygen saturation is maintained at more than 94% with administration of up to 70% nitrous oxide, that the end-tidal carbon dioxide concentration should be maintained between 3.5 and 4 kPa, and that the end-tidal vapour concentration should be maintained at the equivalent of 1 MAC up to delivery[41]. Although propofol is often used for induction of general anaesthesia for Caesarean section, there is still widespread use of thiopentone[42].

Awareness during Caesarean section continues to occur. A low incidence is possibly inevitable because of the very short induction-to-incision time and the diminishing experience of the use of general anaesthesia for Caesarean section. There is an argument in favour of warning patients scheduled to undergo Caesarean section under general anaesthesia of the possibility that awareness may occur (see following paragraphs).

Difficult intubation It is often desirable to discontinue the administration of nitrous oxide in order to maintain adequate oxygenation, if tracheal intubation is difficult. This may lead to awareness with recall, unless anaesthesia is maintained while attempts are made to intubate the trachea, either by administration of adequate concentrations of a volatile agent in oxygen between attempts, or by further doses of an intravenous anaesthetic agent.

Premature discontinuation of anaesthesia A desire to produce unnecessarily rapid recovery of consciousness after surgery may lead the anaesthetist to discontinue administration of a volatile anaesthetic agent or intravenous infusion of anaesthetic drug several minutes before the end of the operation, or to switch off the nitrous oxide before reversal of the effects of neuromuscular blockers.

Failure to understand apparatus Air is entrained by some mechanical ventilators if the supply of anaesthetic gases from the anaesthetic machine is less than the total minute volume delivered by the ventilator. Oxygen or air may dilute anaesthetic gases if tubing with an inadequate volume is used to connect a ventilator to a Bain system. Failure to understand the principles of the circle system may result in delivery of inadequate concentrations of anaesthetic gases.

Genuine apparatus failure In some circumstances, failure of apparatus could not reasonably have been predicted or detected by the anaesthetist. Flexible hoses connecting the supply of anaesthetic gases to the vaporizer may become perforated, resulting in a reduction in fresh gas flow rate. There may be a loss of fresh gas because of leaks in the back bar of the anaesthetic machine or a damaged flowmeter. Vaporizers may very occasionally deliver grossly inaccurate concentrations of volatile agent. Infusion pumps may malfunction without sounding an alarm. Ventilators may operate incorrectly despite appropriate external connections.

Spurious claims Occasionally, patients complain of recall without foundation. Others may claim recall of intra-operative events, which are found on detailed questioning, to be memories of the early postoperative period, or a dream.

Justified risks In a very small number of cases, the patient is so seriously ill that there is a genuine risk to life if normally adequate doses or concentrations of anaesthetic drug are administered. The commonest cause is profound hypotension caused by hypovolaemia when only surgery can effect a cure. Another example is recall of paralysis before the effects of suxamethonium have worn off, following failed tracheal intubation in an emergency situation, when the anaesthetist decides to allow the patient to awaken and delivers 100% oxygen.

Monitoring depth of anaesthesia

It is clear that the probability of recall is related to depth of anaesthesia. The major problem lies in detecting depth of anaesthesia accurately, and quantifying the relationship. A number of methods of monitoring depth of anaesthesia have been described.

Clinical monitoring

During balanced anaesthesia involving the use of paralysing doses of muscle relaxants, the clinical signs, which are sought, are predominantly those associated with stimulation of the autonomic nervous system. These may be affected by intercurrent disease, or by the action of drugs.

Pupil size

In general, the pupil size tends to decrease with increasing depth of anaesthesia, although the degree of constriction varies with different anaesthetic drugs, and the pupil may dilate during very deep anaesthesia. The response to light may be present during inadequate anaesthesia. Opioids constrict the pupil, and anticholinergics dilate it. Intense constriction or dilation of the pupil may limit the ability to detect a light response.

Cardiovascular changes

Arterial pressure tends to decrease as anaesthesia deepens, except with ketamine. Heart rate tends to decrease with increasing depth of anaesthesia. However, other drugs, e.g. muscle relaxants, may influence cardiovascular parameters without altering the conscious level. In addition, haemorrhage, drug reactions, and body fluid abnormalities may affect the interpretation of arterial pressure and heart rate, as also drugs acting directly on the cardiovascular system, e.g. ß-blockers, which may be administered by the anaesthetist or which the patient may have received preoperatively. Peripheral vasoconstriction may be associated with light anaesthesia, but is influenced also by body temperature and volaemic status.

Sweating and lacrimation

These signs may be found during light anaesthesia, but may be present when anaesthesia is adequate. Lacrimation is a more sensitive index of light anaesthesia than sweating. Both may be reduced if anticholinergic drugs have been administered.

Limitations

Clinical monitoring has always been, and remains, by far the commonest method of attempting to gauge the depth of anaesthesia. There is no evidence that any instrument is more reliable during routine anaesthesia. Clinical signs may be difficult to interpret in the presence of other drugs that act on the cardiovascular system, and if hypovolaemia is present. Clinical signs of light anaesthesia are relatively common, and usually are not associated with recall of intra-operative events. Conversely, awareness with recall may occur in the absence of clinical evidence of inadequate anaesthesia. However, in the author's experience, recall of intra-operative pain or distress is almost invariably associated with clinical evidence of light anaesthesia if no confounding factors are present and if accurate recordings are available. Consequently, evidence of increased sympathoadrenal activity should be regarded as an indication to increase depth of anaesthesia immediately, by administration of further doses or higher concentrations of anaesthetic agents. It may be appropriate to supplement, but not to substitute, the anaesthetic agent with an opioid analgesic and/or a muscle relaxant.

Monitoring anaesthetic drug delivery

Because many episodes of awareness occur because of inadvertent failure of delivery of the intended anaesthetic drug concentrations, or delivery of predictably inadequate doses, there is a cogent argument in favour of routine monitoring of drug delivery where that is possible. Currently, it is not possible to measure blood concentrations of intravenous anaesthetics, but it is possible to measure inspired and end-tidal concentrations of inhaled anaesthetics breath by breath. This allows the anaesthetist to receive an early warning of failure of delivery, and to ensure that a predictably adequate concentration is being delivered at all times. It is known[43] that a concentration of 70% nitrous oxide (just under 0.7 MAC) is associated with a risk of awareness of around 2%, and it has been recommended that, other than in exceptional circumstances, a minimum end-tidal concentration of 0.8 MAC should be used in an attempt to prevent awareness[33].

Instrumental monitoring

A number of instruments, based on analysis of the electroencephalogram (EEG) trace have been developed in an attempt to monitor depth of anaesthesia. Currently, only three of these devices have been evaluated extensively.

Evoked potentials (EPs)

Auditory, visual, or peripheral nerve (somatosensory) stimulation produces characteristic changes in the EEG. These changes are of very low amplitude and high frequency, and are obscured in other electrical activity in an EEG trace. However, by using repeated stimuli and computerized averaging techniques, it is possible to eliminate other EEG activity, and obtain a display of the electrical changes produced as the impulse generated by the stimulus progresses up the brain stem and into the cortex.

Thornton et al.[44] (1984) found dose-related increases in latency and decreases in amplitude of some waves in the brain stem auditory EP in patients anaesthetized with nitrous oxide and enflurane or halothane; however, intravenous anaesthetic agents had no effect on the brain stem EP[45]. The later (more peripheral) waves of the cortical auditory EP are abolished by volatile anaesthetic agents. However, the earliest cortical waves remain relatively intact even during administration of inhalational anaesthetic agents in excess of MAC, suggesting that auditory stimuli may reach the inner areas of the cerebral cortex even during surgical anaesthesia; this may be related to the phenomenon of unconscious perception of auditory stimuli. The administration of inhalational anaesthetic agents is associated with a decrease in amplitude and an increase in latency of the waveform. Similar changes accompany the administration of intravenous anaesthetic drugs. Of particular significance is the fact that the changes in the waveform are reversed in part by surgical stimulation, suggesting that EPs may indicate true depth of anaesthesia, and are not acting only as bioassays of anaesthetic drug concentration in the brain.

Somatosensory EPs also show changes in latency and amplitude in response to the administration of anaesthetic and opioid drugs. However, the mid-latency auditory EP offers greater promise as a clinically useful index of depth of anaesthesia. A number of devices have been produced, which derive an index from the pattern of the early cortical EP waveform, and many studies have demonstrated a relationship between these indices, depth of anaesthesia, and return of consciousness[46–48]. However, the apparatus used to generate EPs is expensive and complex, and is sensitive to interference from other equipment, particularly diathermy, and from other components of the EEG[49].

Entropy

Entropy is a term derived from thermodynamics, where it describes the state of a gas or fluid system and the distribution probability of molecules. In a highly ordered system, such as a solid, every molecule has a pre-set place and there are fewer possibilities of motion and distribution of molecules than in a disordered system such as a fluid. EEG signals reflect the underlying state of brain activity. In general terms, a patient who is awake has an irregular EEG pattern, which becomes more orderly and regular if an individual falls asleep or is anaesthetized.

The concept of entropy has been applied to EEG analysis to provide an index of conscious level[50]. Spectral analysis of the EEG is performed by fast Fourier transformation, and a value for what is termed state entropy (SE) is calculated from the entropy analysis of the resulting frequency pattern. EEG recordings over the forehead also detect EMG activity from muscles, which may also provide some information about the state of responsiveness of an individual. A second entropy value, response entropy (RE), is derived from analysis of the spectrum representing both EEG and EMG activity; SE and RE should be the same if there is no EMG activity.

Clinical studies have demonstrated relationships between SE and hypnotic effects of drugs except for ketamine and nitrous oxide. RE probably reflects response to noxious stimulus, and may prove to be a better index of depth of anaesthesia. The techniques require further evaluation.

Bispectral index

Bispectral (BIS[TM]) analysis is a statistical technique that analyses interfrequency phase relationships in the EEG, and computes these with the presence or absence of burst suppression, frequency domain, and EMG in a complex, weighted multivariate model, which has been 'calibrated' against a database of recordings, matched to varying states of consciousness[51]. The analysis derives a dimensionless number (the BIS index) with a value between 0 and 100. Awake, unpremedicated patients have been reported to have BIS values of 93 or more. Loss of recall occurs in about 90% of individuals at BIS values of 75–80. Values of ≤60 have been associated with a low probability of recall and a high probability of unresponsiveness during surgery under general anaesthesia[52].

Hundreds of peer-reviewed papers, describing the use of BIS have been published in the last 20 years or so. The BIS monitor has been approved by the American Food and Drug Administration (FDA) as a device, which can be used to reduce the incidence of intra-operative awareness during general anaesthesia. However, although it is clear that there is a relationship between the BIS index and depth of anaesthesia, evidence that it reduces the incidence of awareness in routine use is currently slim. The only study to demonstrate a statistically significant reduction in the incidence of awareness during routine anaesthesia is a prospective cohort trial of 4945 patients, who were compared with a historical control group of 7826 patients; the incidence of awareness in the historical control group was 0.18%, compared with 0.04% in those monitored with BIS[53].

In the widely publicized 'B-Aware' trial, 2463 high-risk patients (e.g. cardiac surgery, Caesarean section, trauma, previous awareness) were anaesthetized either without BIS guidance, or with the BIS index maintained as far as possible between 40 and 60. The incidence of awareness in the control group was 0.91%, compared to an incidence of 0.17% in the BIS-guided group, a difference of 82%[54].

However, in a randomized prospective study in which depth of anaesthesia was guided either by BIS monitoring (target 40–60) or end-tidal anaesthetic gas monitoring (target 0.7–1.3 MAC), but in which the data from both types of monitoring were available to those who analysed the results, two patients out of around 970 in each group were judged to have been definitely aware; four patients in the BIS-guided group were judged to have been possibly aware, compared with one in the end-tidal gas guided group[25]. Of note, the BIS value was 60 or less in three of the four patients with definite awareness, and in six of the nine patients with definite or possible awareness. The end-tidal anaesthetic gas concentration was more than 0.7 MAC in only one of the patients with definite awareness and in only two of the patients with definite or possible awareness. This suggests that controlling the end-tidal concentration may be a better means of minimizing the risk of awareness than monitoring BIS, particularly if a lower threshold of 0.8 MAC is employed, as recommended by Ghoneim[43].

Currently, in common with the American Society of Anesthesiologists[55] and the Australian and New Zealand College of Anaesthetists[56], the Association of Anaesthetists of Great Britain and Ireland does not recommend the routine use of electronic monitors of depth of anaesthesia[57], although it is the author's view that they may be useful in high-risk patients, when total intravenous anaesthesia is employed or when an infusion of remifentanil is used in conjunction with a vapour concentration equating to less than 0.8 MAC.

Monitoring of inspired and end-tidal anaesthetic gas concentrations is regarded as mandatory when inhaled anaesthetic agents are employed[57].

What should the patient be told?[58]

It is important that any patient who has experienced recall of intra-operative events should be identified. Ideally, this would be accomplished by regular postoperative visits by all anaesthetists. However, this is not always achieved in practice, and it is important that ward nurses and non-anaesthetic medical staff are educated about the subject in order that any complaint is dealt with appropriately. If informed of a patient who complains of recall, the anaesthetist should interview the patient in the presence of a witness and listen carefully to the complaint. If it is clear that intra-operative recall has occurred, the anaesthetist should acknowledge the fact that he/she believes the account of events. The anaesthetist should apologize to the patient and explain that recall can occur without fault during anaesthesia in which muscle relaxants are employed, because of the desire to avoid high and potentially toxic concentrations of anaesthetic drugs, and because of difficulty in interpreting clinical signs. The patient should be reassured and informed that a note will be made in the hospital record so that other anaesthetists will know of the problem if anaesthesia and surgery are required in future. A full account of the interview should be recorded in the clinical notes. Junior anaesthetists should inform a consultant, who should be present when the patient is counselled. The surgeon and the patient's general practitioner should be informed. The patient should be told to report any psychological symptoms, should be given a contact name within the Department of Anaesthesia, and should be referred for psychiatric or psychological assessment and treatment if symptoms ensue.

It may be advisable to warn all 'high-risk' patients (e.g. the seriously ill, and patients undergoing Caesarean section under general anaesthesia, if low concentrations of anaesthetic agents are to be used) of the possibility of recall during anaesthesia.

Many patients are already anxious about the possibility of awareness because of media publicity. In addition, the psychological stress resulting from awareness with recall may be reduced if a warning has been given. However, this should not be used as an excuse to omit the measures outlined above to reduce to a minimum the occurrence of this extremely distressing experience.

References

1. Hutchinson, R. (1960). Awareness during surgery. *British Journal of Anaesthesia*, **33**, 463–9.

2. Brice, D.D., Hetherington, R.R., and Utting, J.E. (1970). A simple study of awareness and dreaming during anaesthesia. *British Journal of Anaesthesia*, **42**, 535–41.

3. McKenna, J. and Wilton, T.N.P. (1973). Awareness during endotracheal intubation. *Anaesthesia*, **28**, 599–602.

4. *Ackers v Wigan Health Authority. Med L R* (1991) **2**, 232–3.

5. Catchpole, K., Bell, D., Johnson, S., and Boult, M. (2006). Reviewing the evidence of patient safety incidents in anaesthetics. *Internal Report*. The National Patient Safety Agency, London.

6. Myles, P.S., Williams, D.L., Hendrata, M., Anderson, H., and Weeks, A.M. (2000). Patient satisfaction after anaesthesia and surgery: results of a prospective study of 10 811 patients. *British Journal of Anaesthesia*, **84**, 6–10.

7. Prys-Roberts, C. (1987). Anaesthesia: a practical or impractical construct? *British Journal of Anaesthesia*, **59**, 1341–5.

8. Pinsker, M.C. (1986). Anesthesia: a pragmatic construct. *Anesthesia and Analgesia*, **65**, 819–20.

9. Vickers, M.D. (1987). Detecting consciousness by clinical means. In *Consciousness awareness and pain in general anaesthesia* (eds. M. Rosen and J.N. Lunn), pp. 12–7, Butterworths, London.

10. Kissin, I. and Gelman, S. (1987). Three components of anesthesia: one more reason to accept the concept. *Anesthesia and Analgesia*, **66**, 98.

11. Russell, I.F. (1989). Conscious awareness during general anaesthesia: relevance of autonomic signs and isolated arm movements as guides to depth of anaesthesia. In: Jones JG (ed.). Depth of anaesthesia. *Baillière's Clinical Anaesthesiology: International Practice and Research*, **3**, 511–32.

12. Rupreht, J. and Valkenburg, M. (1990). The anaesthetic state: evolution of a concept. In *Memory and awareness in anaesthesia* (eds. B. Bonke, W. Fitch, and K. Millar), pp. 70–5. Swetz and Zeitlinger, Amsterdam.

13. White, D.C. (1987). Anaesthesia: a privation of the senses. An historical introduction and some definitions. In *Consciousness awareness and pain in general anaesthesia* (eds. M. Rosen and J.N. Lunn), pp. 1–9. Butterworths, London.

14. Jones, J.G. and Konieczko, K. (1986). Hearing and memory in anaesthetised patients. *British Medical Journal*, **292**, 1291–3.

15. Millar, K. and Watkinson, N. (1983). Recognition of words presented during general anaesthesia. *Ergonomics*, **26**, 585–94.

16. Garfield, J.M, Garfield, F.B., Stone, J.G., and Hopkins, D. (1972). A comparison of psychologic responses to ketamine and thiopental-nitrous oxide-halothane anesthesia. *Anesthesiology*, **36**, 329–38.

17. Wilson, S., Vaughan, R., and Stephen, C. (1975). Awareness, dreams and hallucinations associated with general anaesthesia. *Anesthesia and Analgesia*, **54**, 609–19.

18. Liu, W.H., Thorp, T.A., Graham, S.G., and Aitkenhead, A.R. (1991). Incidence of awareness with recall during general anaesthesia. *Anaesthesia*, **46**, 435–7.

19. Sandin, R. and Nordström, O. (1993). Awareness during total iv anaesthesia. *British Journal of Anaesthesia*, **71**, 782–7.

20. Nordström, O., Engstrom, A., Persson, S., and Sandin, R. (1997). Incidence of awareness in total iv anaesthesia based on propofol, alfentanil and neuromuscular blockade. *Acta Anaesthesiologica Scandnavica*, **41**, 978–84.

21. Ranta, S.O-V., Laurila, R., Saario, J., Ali-Melkkilä, T., and Hynynen, M. (1998). Awareness with recall during general anesthesia: incidence and risk factors. *Anesthesia Analgesia*, **86**, 1084–9.

22. Sandin, R., Enlund, G., Samuelsson, P., and Lennmarken, C. (2000). Awareness during anesthesia: a prospective case study. *Lancet*, **355**, 707–11.

23. Wennervirta, J., Ranta, S.O-V., and Hynynen, M. (2002). Awareness and recall in outpatient anesthesia. *Anesthesia and Analgesia*, **95**, 72–7.

24. Sebel, P.S., Bowdle, T.A., Ghoneim, M.M., *et al.* (2004). The incidence of awareness during anesthesia: a multicenter United States study. *Anesthesia and Analgesia*, **99**, 833–9.

25. Avidan, M.S., Zhang, L., Burnside, B.A., *et al.* (2008). Anesthesia awareness and the bispectral index. *New England Journal of Medicine*, **358**, 1097–108.

26. Crawford, J.S. (1984). *Principles and Practice of Obstetric Anaesthesia*, p 297, 5th edition. Blackwell Scientific Publications, Oxford.

27. Stoelting, R.K., Longnecker, D.E., and Eger, E.I. (1970). Minimum alveolar concentrations in man on awakening from methoxyflurane, halothane, ether and fluroxene anesthesia: MAC awake. *Anesthesiology*, **33**, 5–9.

28. Utting, J.E. (1987). Awareness: clinical aspects. In *Consciousness, awareness and pain in general anaesthesia* (eds. M. Rosen and J.N. Lunn JN), pp. 171–9. Butterworths, London.

29. Rosen, J. (1959). Hearing tests during anaesthesia with nitrous oxide and relaxants. *Acta Anaesthesiologica Scandnavica*, **3**, 1–8.

30. Browne, R.A. and Catton, D.V. (1973). Awareness during anaesthesia: a comparison of anaesthesia with nitrous oxide-oxygen and nitrous oxide-oxygen with Innovar. *Canadian Anaesthesia Society Journal*, **20**, 763–8.

31. Barr, A.M., Moxon, A., Woollam, C.H., and Fryer, M.E. (1977). Effect of diazepam and lorazepam on awareness during anaesthesia for Caesarean section. *Anaesthesia*, **32**, 873–8.

32. Desai, N., Taylor-Davies, A., and Barnett, D.B. (1983). The effects of diazepam and oxprenolol on short term memory in individuals of high and low state anxiety. *British Journal of Clinical Pharmacology*, **15**, 197–202.

33. Jones, D.M., Jones, M.E.L., Lewis, M.J., and Spriggs, T.L.B. (1979). Drugs and human memory: effects of low doses of nitrazepam and hyoscine on retention. *British Journal of Clinical Pharmacology*, **7**, 479–83.

34. File, S.E. and Lister, R.G. (1982). Do lorazepam-induced deficits in learning result from impaired rehearsal, reduced motivation or increased sedation? *British Journal of Clinical Pharmacology*, **14**, 545–50.

35. Rolbin, S.H., Cohen, M.M., Levinton, C.M., Kelly, E.N., and Farine, D. (1994). The premature infant: anesthesia for Cesarean delivery. *Anesthesia and Analgesia*, **78**, 912–7.

36. Moir, D.D. (1970). Anaesthesia for Caesarean section. *British Journal of Anaesthesia*, **42**, 136–42.

37. Moir, D.D. (1976). *Obstetric anaesthesia and analgesia*, p. 145. Baillière Tindall London.

38. Moir, D.D and Thorburn, J. (1986). *Obstetric anaesthesia and analgesia*, p. 193, 3rd edition. Baillière Tindall, London.

39. King, H., Ashley, S., Braithwaite, D., Decayette, J., and Wooten, D. (1993). Adequacy of general anesthesia for Cesarean section. *Anesthesia and Analgesia*, **77**, 84–8.

40. Lyons, G. and Macdonald, R. (1991). Awareness during Caesarean section. *Anaesthesia*, **46**, 62–4.

41. Lyons, G. and Akerman, N. (2005). Problems with general anaesthesia for Caesarean section. *Minerva Anestesiologica*, **71**, 27–38.

42. Paech, M.J. (2002). Complications of obstetric anesthesia and analgesia. In *Handbook of Obstetric Anesthesia* (eds. C.M. Palmer, R. d´Angelo, and M.J. Paech), pp. 227–30. Bios Scientific, Oxford.

43. Ghoneim, M.M. (2000). Awareness during anesthesia. *Anesthesiology*, **92**, 597–602.

44. Thornton, C., Heneghan, C.P.H., James, M.F.M., and Jones, J.G. (1984). Effects of halothane or enflurane with controlled ventilation on auditory evoked potentials. *British Journal of Anaesthesia*, **56**, 315–23.

45. Thornton, C. and Newton, D.E.F. (1989). The auditory evoked response: a measure of depth of anaesthesia. *Baillière's Clinical Anaesthesiology: International Practice and Research*, **3**, 559–85.

46. Mantzaridis, H. and Kenny, G.N.C. (1997). Auditory evoked potential index: a quantitative measure of changes in auditory evoked potentials during general anaesthesia. *Anaesthesia*, **52**, 1030–6.

47. Weber, F., Seidl, M., and Bein, T. (2005). Impact of the AEP-Monitor/2-derived composite auditory-evoked potential index on propofol consumption and emergence times during total intravenous anaesthesia with propofol and remifentanil in children. *Acta Anaesthesiologica Scandinavica*, **49**, 277–83.

48. Plourde, G. (2006). Auditory evoked potentials. *Best Practice and Research Clinical Anaesthesiology*, **20**, 129–39.

49. Wenningmann, I., Paprotny, S., Strassmann, S., *et al.* (2006). Correlation of the A-line™ ARX index with acoustically evoked potential amplitude. *British Journal of Anaesthesia*, **97**, 666–75.

50. Bein, B. Entropy. (2006). *Best Practice and Research Clinical Anaesthesiology*, **20**, 101–9.

51. Johansen, J.W. and Sebel, P.S. (2000). Development and clinical applications of electroencephalographic bispectrum monitoring. *Anesthesiology*, **93**, 1336–44.

52. Johansen, J.W. (2006). Update on Bispectral Index monitoring. *Best Practice and Research Clinical Anaesthesiology*, **20**, 81–99.

53. Ekman, A., Lindholm, M.L., Lennmarken, C., and Sandin, R. (2004). Reduction in the incidence of awareness using BIS monitoring. *Acta Anaesthesiologica Scandinavica*, **48**, 20–6.

54. Myles, P.S., Leslie, K., McNeil, J., Forbes, A., and Chan, M.T.V. (2004) for the B-Aware trial group. *Lancet*, **363**, 1757–63.

55. American Society of Anesthesiologists' Task Force on Intraoperative Awareness. Practice advisory for intraoperative awareness and brain function monitoring: a report by the American Society of Anesthesiologists' task force on intraoperative awareness. (2006). *Anesthesiology*, **104**, 847–64.

56. Australian and New Zealand College of Anaesthetists ABN 82 055 042 852 Recommendations on monitoring during anaesthesia – 2006 http://www.anzca.edu.au/resources/professional-documents/professional-standards/ps18.html (last Accessed 1st December 2008).

57. Association of Anaesthetists of Great Britain and Ireland. (2007). *Recommendations for Standards of Monitoring during Anaesthesia and Recovery*, 4th edition. London.

58. Aitkenhead, A.R. (1990). Awareness during anaesthesia: what should the patient be told? *Anaesthesia*, **45**, 351–2.

59. Errando, C.L., Sigl, J.C., Robles, M., *et al.* (2008). Awareness with recall during general anaesthesia: a prospective observational evaluation of 4001 patients. *British Journal of Anaesthesia*, **101**(2), 178–85.

Chapter 12

Respiratory risk

Iain K Moppett

This chapter discusses respiratory complications associated with anaesthesia during the intraoperative and postoperative periods. Factors that influence these risks will be discussed, as well as anaesthetic approaches that may have benefit in reducing risks of complications. Complications will be divided into intraoperative and postoperative, though there is clearly some overlap.

Intraoperative complications

Adverse respiratory events during anaesthesia include breath-holding, coughing, laryngospasm, bronchospasm, and difficulties with airway management.

Failed intubation

The incidence of failed tracheal intubation is influenced by many factors: the environment, the patient, the urgency, and the training of the practitioner, to name the most common. It is therefore difficult to describe a 'real' figure. However, in the out-of-hospital environment, anaesthesia-trained physicians reported multiple intubation attempts in 4% and failed intubation in 2% of attempted intubations[1]. Intensive care patients have a relatively high rate of difficult intubation (8%)[2]. The rate of failed intubation is approximately 1 in 250[3,4] to 1 in 500[5] in the general obstetric population. The incidence of failed intubation in the general population has been reported at around 0.7–4% of patients[6–8]. Difficult laryngoscopy occurs in around 5–10% of patients[6,7,9]. A number of sub-groups of patients (e.g. those with craniofacial abnormalities, temporomandibular joint disease, fused cervical spine, etc.) are predictable as being potentially difficult to intubate, but for the general population, anaesthetists can use bedside predictive tests. Unfortunately, none of these is particularly sensitive or specific for difficult intubation[10].

Difficult mask ventilation

There has been only limited research related to the frequency of difficult mask ventilation (DMV). The incidence of DMV clearly depends upon the experience and training of the anaesthetist and the definition used. The most recent study[11] suggests that Grade 3/4 DMV occurs in around 1.5% of anaesthetics. Grade 3 is defined as difficult (inadequate to maintain oxygenation or requiring two providers). Grade 4 DMV is impossible mask ventilation (absence of end-tidal carbon dioxide measurement and lack of perceptible chest wall movement during positive pressure ventilation attempts, despite airway adjuvants and additional personnel). Risk factors include Mallampati Grade IV, male gender, higher Cormack and Lehane grade[12], poor mandibular protrusion, history of snoring and a full beard[11]. Only the beard is really amenable to pre-anaesthetic intervention.

12.1 Predictors of difficult mask ventilation

Grade 3 mask ventilation

Body mass index ≥ 30 kg.m^{-2}

Beard

Mallampati III or IV

Age ≥ 57 years

Jaw protrusion—severely limited

Snoring

Grade 3 or 4 mask ventilation and difficult intubation

Jaw protrusion—limited or severely limited

Thick/obese neck anatomy

Sleep apnoea

Snoring

Body mass index ≥ 30 kg.m^{-2}

Malpositioning of tracheal tubes

The incidence of unintended endobronchial intubation is unknown because the majority are probably diagnosed and remedied shortly after intubation. One study of out-of-hospital intubation found endobronchial intubation in 7% and tube tip position within 2 cm of the carina in 13% of chest radiographs reviewed retrospectively[13]. A prospective study with on-site evaluation of tube position following non-physician intubation found undiagnosed endobronchial intubation in 11% and oesophageal intubation in 7% (of whom 70% died). Emergency intubation in hospital is associated with a 15% rate of malpositioning; in three-quarters of cases, the tip of the tube lay too close to the carina[14]. Approximately 8% and 4% of intensive care intubations were initially oesophageal or endobronchial, respectively, in one study[2]. Older studies put the incidences somewhat higher, but a modern emphasis on the importance of maintaining oxygenation and limiting time spent attempting laryngoscopy may have contributed to the lower rates in more recent reports[15]. Repeated attempts (≤ 2 attempts vs. >2) at emergency laryngoscopy are associated with higher rates of complications: hypoxaemia (12% vs. 70%), regurgitation of gastric contents (2% vs. 22%), aspiration of gastric contents (0.8% vs. 13%), bradycardia (2% vs. 21%), and cardiac arrest (0.7% vs. 11%)[15].

Movement (flexion or rotation) of the head and neck[16] and creation of pneumoperitoneum may result in delayed endobronchial intubation[17,18].

Aspiration of gastric contents

The loss of protective airway reflexes combined with changes in oesophageal sphincter tone may predispose patients undergoing general anaesthesia or sedation to aspiration of gastric contents. A proportion of patients who aspirate may then develop significant complications including death.

The classic description by Mendelson of pulmonary aspiration in pregnant patients undergoing face mask anaesthesia[19] found 66 cases of aspiration in 44 000 anaesthetics. Among the 40 women who aspirated liquids, there were no deaths; two of five patients who aspirated solids died. Two reports from Scandinavia involving over 270 000 anaesthetics found an incidence of aspiration of 0.7–4.7 per 10 000 general anaesthetics in 1986[20] and 2.9 per 10 000 in 1996[21]. US studies found similar rates in adults (3.1 per 10 000)[22] and children (3.8 per 10 000)[22] although a separate paediatric study found considerably higher rates in children (10.2 per 10 000)[23]. Emergency intubation in hospital has been associated with a 4% incidence of new pulmonary infiltrates on chest X-ray, despite the use of cricoid pressure[2]. Although pregnant patients are generally held to be at higher risk for physiological and anatomical reasons, one Israeli study found a similar level of risk in obstetric patients undergoing general anaesthesia without tracheal intubation (5.3 per 10 000), although the study was relatively small (1850 women) and did not include women undergoing caesarean section. The incidence of pulmonary aspiration in patients managed with the laryngeal mask airway (LMA) (2 per 10 000)[24] appears to be similar to that in patients managed with a tracheal tube, although it should be borne in mind that the patients and surgical procedures associated with these methods of airway management are usually different. There have been reports of death following aspiration of gastric contents associated with use of the LMA[25]. Patients who have suffered pulmonary aspiration have approximately a 5% risk of death[22]. Patients who are managed with an LMA may be at a lower risk than this because they should be patients with less risk of solid/particulate aspiration, though there is no direct evidence for this. There is theoretical evidence suggesting that the LMA used in association with positive pressure ventilation may predispose to a greater risk of aspiration; however Verghese and colleagues found no increased risk in an observational study[26].

Airway reactivity

The incidence of adverse events due to reactive airways is influenced by anaesthetic technique, drugs, and patient factors. The 'real-life' rate for these events is therefore unknown, but various studies have identified factors associated with higher adverse incident rates at induction and emergence, and intraoperatively.

Upper-respiratory-tract infection

Ongoing upper respiratory tract infection (URTI) is a risk factor for predominantly minor adverse respiratory events during anaesthesia in children[27–29] and possibly in adults. Around 40% of children with a current URTI suffer an adverse respiratory event during anaesthesia[30]. Increased airway reactivity probably persists for around 6 weeks after the acute symptoms have subsided[31]. Young age (<1 year) and tracheal intubation increase the risk of adverse events[29]. Although there has been a case report of death following laryngospasm, associated with a common cold[32], there is no good evidence that systemically well children with URTI are more at risk of serious respiratory adverse events than children without.

Various strategies have been investigated to reduce the incidence of adverse events. Neither preoperative bronchodilator therapy[33] nor peri-induction glycopyrrolate[30] have been shown to reduce the rate of adverse events.

Smoking

Current active or passive smoking increases the incidence of adverse respiratory events compared to that in non-smokers (43% vs. 24%)[34]. Effective strategies to reduce this risk include: nebulized 4% lidocaine [35] (32% vs. 13% adverse event rate); using sevoflurane rather than isoflurane for maintenance[36] (10% vs. 45% adverse event rate); and avoidance of desflurane for induction, although desflurane maintenance appears not to increase risk[37] despite its lack of bronchodilator effect[38].

Anaesthetic drugs

Potentially, any drug can cause anaphylaxis and consequent airway obstruction. Predictable adverse respiratory effects are encountered in association with the use of several commonly used anaesthetic drugs. Desflurane is an upper- and lower-airway irritant and is not a bronchodilator *in vivo*[39]; this effect can be ameliorated by the concomitant use of opioids[40]. Thiopentone is a less potent suppressant of airway reflexes than propofol[41]. Atracurium and mivacurium have been associated with bronchospasm more frequently than vecuronium or rocuronium[42].

Postoperative

Major morbidity

Major respiratory morbidity following surgery and anaesthesia is relatively uncommon, although it may be related to nearly a quarter of early postoperative deaths, increases postoperative length of stay, and may predict long-term postoperative mortality in the elderly[43]. Postoperative pulmonary complications (POPC) are strongly associated with mortality: the relative risk of death associated with POPC in the general surgical population is 10–20[44–46], and notably similar risk has been identified after thoracic surgery (relative risk of death with POPC 15)[47]. A prospective American study of over 1000 elective, non-thoracic surgical patients found significant POPC in 2.7%, with an increase in average length of hospital stay from 4.5 to 28 days[46]. The rate of POPC is similar to the rate of cardiac events in patients with hip fracture[48] (2.6. vs. 2.0%) and non-daycase, non-cardiac elective surgery[49] (1.8% vs. 2.2%). For daycase patients, the rates are much lower, with only 5 out of over 45 000 patients (0.01%) developing respiratory failure in an American daycase series[50].

Numerous studies of varying size and quality have attempted to quantify the risk associated with various patient (history and investigation) and procedural factors.

The definition of POPC varies among the studies, with many small studies using either indirect measures of respiratory function (e.g. change in spirometry) or clinically insignificant changes in oximetry as markers of respiratory morbidity. Postoperative pneumonia has been investigated most frequently, partly because it is easier to define (see Box 12.2) and also because it is associated with a high mortality. Unsurprisingly, different studies have found different strengths of association between risk factor and outcome. The American College of Physicians has recently carried out an extensive systematic review of this topic[51]. The consistent risk factors for POPC are discussed in the following paragraphs (Table 12.1).

12.2 "Definition of postoperative pneumonia used in studies"

Patient met one of the following two criteria postoperatively:

1. Rales or dullness to percussion on physical examination of chest AND any of the following:

    New onset of purulent sputum or change in character of sputum

    Isolation of organism from blood culture

    Isolation of pathogen from specimen obtained by transtracheal aspirate, bronchial brushing, or biopsy

2. Chest radiography showing new or progressive infiltrate, consolidation, cavitation, or pleural effusion AND any of the following:

    New onset of purulent sputum or change in character of sputum

    Isolation of organism from blood culture

    Isolation of pathogen from specimen obtained by transtracheal aspirate, bronchial brushing, or biopsy

    Isolation of virus or detection of viral antigen in respiratory secretions

    Diagnostic single antibody titre (IgM) or fourfold increase in paired serum samples (IgG) for pathogen

    Histopathological evidence of pneumonia

Patient factors

Age Age over 50 years is an independent risk factor for POPC, with odds ratios increasing for each decade over 50 years from 1.5 (50–59 years) to 5.6 ($\geq$ 80 years)[51]. This effect is independent of the effect of other co-morbidities and procedural factors.

General health The most commonly used assessment of general health is the ASA physical status score. Various studies have found increased risk of POPC with ASA grade greater than 2 or 3[51]. Similarly, the Charlson co-morbidity index, which provides a weighted composite of co-morbidities, is associated with the incidence of POPC[52]. Functional dependence (inability to perform activities of daily living) or partial dependence (assistance required for some activities of daily living), which may

Table 12.1 Risk factors for postoperative pulmonary complications

Risk factor	Odds ratio
Advanced age	2.1 (>60 years); 3.04 (>70 years)
ASA status	2.6 (≥II); 4.87 (≥III)
Heart failure	2.9
Functional dependence	1.6 (partial); 2.5 (full)
Cigarettes	1.3
Medical comorbidities	1.5
Impaired consciousness	1.4
Surgical site	
Aortic	6.9
Thoracic	4.3
Abdominal	3.0
Neurosurgery	2.5
Head and neck	2.2
Vascular	2.1
Emergency surgery	2.2
General anaesthesia	1.8
Tests	
Abnormal chest X-ray	4.8
Serum albumin <35 g.L^{-1}	2.5
Blood urea >7.5 mmol.L^{-1}	1.4

be markers of co-morbidity and functional reserve, are associated with increased risk of POPC (odds ratio 2.5 and 1.6, respectively).

Chronic obstructive pulmonary disease Chronic obstructive pulmonary disease (COPD) is the most commonly reported risk factor for POPC, although not the strongest, with a combined odds ratio of 1.8. However, this may be an underestimate because most of the studies dichotomized the population into COPD or not. Severe COPD may well carry a significantly higher risk of POPC, although at present the magnitude of this risk is not clear.

Cardiac history Both the Goldman cardiac risk index[52] and a history of congestive cardiac failure[51] (odds ratio 2.9) are risk factors for POPC. One study of patients over 80 years of age[53] found preoperative arrhythmia to be a risk factor for POPC.

Cigarette use Current cigarette use is associated with a higher risk of POPC (combined odds ratio 1.26). Some caution is needed in interpreting this figure because study defini-tions of current smoking vary: some use any tobacco use within the last 12 months[45], whereas others used smoking within 2 weeks of surgery[46]. Furthermore, smoking cessation or reduction within 6–8 weeks of surgery may be associated with a higher risk of POPC, although this is not consistent across studies, and may apply only to patients undergoing thoracic surgery[54]. Whether this paradoxical rise in POPC risk is due to physiological changes or selection bias is not clear.

Obesity Although obesity undoubtedly reduces lung volumes, only one of several studies assessing its effect on POPC found obesity to be an independent risk factor. Even in univariate studies, the risk of POPC was similar for obese and non-obese subjects. Within the obese population, there is no evidence to suggest that marked obesity is associated with higher risk[51]. Of course, given that none of these studies is randomized, the confounding effect of changes in perioperative care cannot be excluded. Obstructive sleep apnoea has had little direct investigation, but the limited results available suggest that it may be a risk factor for POPC, with a higher rate of unplanned intensive care unit transfers, prolonged length of stay, and (non-significant) increased rates of hypoxaemia, hypercapnia, and re-intubation in patients following lower limb arthroplasty[55].

Conscious level Acutely impaired consciousness is associated with a higher incidence of POPC (odds ratio 1.39)[51]. The evidence for this comes only from the Veterans Affairs National Surgical Quality Improvement Program (NSQIP), which because of its catchment population, only has 3% of female subjects[45]. Chronic neurological disease such as previous cerebrovascular accident (odds ratio 1.47)[45] and impaired cognition (odds ratio 5.93 but non-significant)[56] may also be associated with POPC.

Procedural factors

Surgical site Open abdominal aortic surgery carries the highest risk of POPC (odds ratio 6.9; around 25% of patients experience POPC). Thoracic, abdominal, neurosurgical, and head and neck surgery carry significant but lower risks. Endovascular aortic aneurysm repair is associated with a lower risk of POPC than open repair (odds ratio 0.14)[57]. Gynaecological and urological procedures are associated with a lower risk of POPC.

Duration of surgery Prolonged duration of surgery is a risk factor for POPC (odds ratio 2.3), although the definition of 'prolonged' varies from 2.5 to 4 h. This is a somewhat crude measure of surgical duration, especially because it does not take into account whether operations were longer than expected for individual procedures.

Emergency surgery Unsurprisingly, patients undergoing emergency surgery have a higher risk of POPC even when multivariate analysis is performed (odds ratio 2.2)[51].

Nasogastric tubes Nasogastric tubes (NGT) are a risk factor for POPC in multivariate analysis, and meta-analysis of selective versus routine NGT placement found routine placement to be a risk factor for POPC despite decreased rates of nausea and abdominal distension[58].

General anaesthesia General anaesthesia is relatively consistent as a risk factor for POPC. Smetana and colleagues found an overall odds ratio of 1.8[51]. Clearly, for many operations, it is difficult to distinguish between the patient and procedural factors leading to the choice of general anaesthesia from the effect of general anaesthesia itself. The impact of adjuvant techniques such as intra- and postoperative epidural analgesia or postoperative opioids on POPC is discussed separately in the following paragraphs.

Neuromuscular blockade The use of neuromuscular blockade to facilitate tracheal intubation and provide safe operating conditions is generally held to be beneficial. It is associated with a reduced incidence of postoperative sore throat. Tracheal intubation with a cuffed tube is held to be the gold standard for protection against aspiration, and thoracic or abdominal surgery may be technically too difficult without paralysis. However, the use of neuromuscular blocking agents is possibly associated with POPC. Residual paralysis (train-of-four<0.9) has been found in 88% of patients at extubation[59] and 32–35% of patients in the recovery area[59,60]. Inadequate return of neuromuscular function is associated with impaired airway protective reflexes, upper airway obstruction, decreased ability to mount a hypoxic ventilatory response, and postoperative hypoxaemia[59].

Preoperative tests

Chest radiography Abnormal chest radiographs are associated with POPC[52,61], with a pooled odds ratio of 4.8[51]. The importance of this is diminished by the finding that only rarely does an abnormal chest radiograph influence clinical decision-making[62,63] because most are associated with an abnormal history or examination.

Spirometry As with chest radiography, abnormal preoperative spirometry is associated with higher rates of POPC[63]. Univariate studies have found that mean forced vital capacity (FVC) and forced expiratory volume in 1 second (FEV_1) are lower in patients with POPC than without, but with no clear cut-off for predicting POPC. Multivariate studies have found FEV_1:FVC ratio <50%[64], FEV_1< 61% of predicted[65], FEV_1< 79% of predicted [65] and value of FEV_1 % predicted (as a continuous variable)[66] to be independent markers of POPC risk. However, other clinical associations (age, co-morbidity, respiratory examination, mucus hypersecretion) were generally more significant markers of risk for POPC[51].

In selected sub-groups, spirometry may be of more value. Patients who undergo lung resection are at particular risk of respiratory failure and ventilator-dependence. Numerous studies have investigated the association between preoperative spirometry and postoperative complications following surgery, with FVC > 1.5 L[67], predicted FVC < 80% (odds ratio 5.9)[68] and FEV_1 < 2.0 L (odds ratio 2.74)[47] being predictors of poor outcome. However, as with the general surgical population, spirometry may not be independent of other factors such as ASA status ≥ 3 (odds ratio 2.1)[47].

Renal function High blood urea (>7.5 mmol l^{-1}) (odds ratio 1.4)[45] and creatinine (>133 μmol.L^{-1}) (odds ratio 1.4)[69] concentrations are associated with increased risk of POPC.

Serum albumin Serum albumin concentration <36 g.L^{-1} is associated with POPC. Univariate analysis gives POPC rates of 28% vs. 7% for patients with serum albumin concentration <36 g.L^{-1}. Multivariate analysis in the NSQIP study found the association less strong, with an adjusted odds ratio of 2.53[44].

Other blood tests Various other blood tests have been found to be predictive of POPC in sub-groups, such as serum troponin concentration after surgery for subarachnoid haemorrhage[70] and lactate dehydrogenase in patients who have undergone thoracic surgery[68]. Whether they add much extra information to the patient and procedural factors is doubtful.

Pneumonia

Pneumonia is the third commonest postoperative infection and is associated with a mortality of around 20–40%[45]. Definitions of postoperative pneumonia (POP) vary, but most studies use the Centers for Disease Control approach (Box 12.2). The largest prospective study of postoperative pneumonia comes from the NSQIP programme[45]. Risk factors for POP were broadly similar to those for POPC as a whole. Using a multivariate logistic regression approach, the authors produced odds ratios and a pneumonia risk index to predict the rates of POP, with a good correlation between predicted and actual rates. Their data exclude patients with preoperative pneumonia, those who developed pneumonia after postoperative respiratory failure, patients who underwent cardiac and transplant surgery and very low mortality procedures. Only 5% of patients were female. Their predictors and risk scoring index are detailed in Table 12.2 and Table 12.3.

Lung surgery is a particular risk factor for POP, with an incidence of up to 40%. One well-conducted prospective study[71] found that 25% of patients developed POP after lung surgery, with an associated 19% mortality. In this highly selected group of patients, male sex, moderate COPD, and lobectomy/pneumonectomy were all strong predictors of POP (odds ratio all > 4)[71].

Respiratory failure

Definitions of postoperative respiratory failure (PRF) vary, but the term is commonly applied to patients who require mechanical ventilation for more than 48 h after surgery or who require re-intubation and artificial ventilation after extubation[44]. On this basis, 5–20% of patients who have undergone thoraco-abdominal aortic aneurysm repair may develop PRF, with around 40% mortality for those with PRF and 6% for those without[72]. Approximately 20% of patients required ventilation for more than 24 h in one small series of abdominal vascular surgical patients[73].

A large prospective case series ($n=180\,000$) from the NSQIP program has been used to develop and validate a multifactorial risk index for the development of PRF. The overall incidence of PRF was 3.4% in this all-male cohort, which was a separate cohort from the pneumonia study. There were significant exclusions including: comatose, ventilator-dependent, and 'do not resuscitate' patients; 'very low risk' surgery/procedures (endoscopy, line insertion, dressings changes); and transplantation.

Table 12.2 Risk factors and 'risk index' scores for postoperative pneumonia

Predictor	Odds ratio	Risk index score
Type of surgery		
Abdominal aortic aneurysm	4.3	15
Thoracic	3.9	14
Upper abdominal	2.7	10
Neck	2.3	8
Neurosurgery	2.1	8
Vascular	1.3	3
Emergency surgery	1.3	3
Transfusion > 4 units	1.3	3
Urea		
<2.9 mmol.L^{-1}	1.5	4
7.9–10.7 mmol.L^{-1}	1.2	2
>10.7 mmol.L^{-1}	1.4	3
Partially/fully dependent functional status	1.8/2.8	6/10
History of CVA	1.5	4
Impaired consciousness	1.5	4
History of COPD	1.7	5
Smoking within 1 year	1.3	3
Steroids for chronic condition	1.3	3
Alcohol >2 drinks per day in last 2 weeks	1.2	2
Weight loss >10% over 6 months	1.9	7
Age (years)		
≥80	5.6	17
70–79	3.6	13
60–69	2.4	9
50–59	1.5	4

Source: Arozullah, A.M., Khuri, S.F., Henderson, W.G., *et al.* (2001). Development and validation of a multifactorial risk index for predicting postoperative pneumonia after major noncardiac surgery. *Annals of Internal Medicine*, **20**,135(10), 847–57. With permission.

Note: Total Risk index scores can be summated to give an aggregate risk score, which when inputted in a regression equation, gives an estimate of risk of postoperative pneumonia (See Table 12.3).

Overall mortality in the PRF group was 27% and 1% in patients without PRF. The simplified model from their data is shown in Table 12.4 and Table 12.5. The risk factors for PRF are essentially the same as for POPC. Obesity was not found to be a risk factor. It can be noted that all the of the factors identified are 'fixed' and not readily amenable to intervention by the anaesthetist or surgeon[44].

Table 12.3 Stratification of scores using the pneumonia risk index

Class	Risk index score total	Predicted risk of postoperative respiratory failure (%)
1	≤15	0.24
2	16–25	1.2
3	26–40	4.0
4	41–55	9.4
5	>55	15.3

Source: From Arozullah, A.M., Khuri, S.F., Henderson, W.G., et al. (2001). Development and validation of a multifactorial risk index for predicting postoperative pneumonia after major noncardiac surgery. Annals of Internal Medicine, **20**,135(10), 847–57. With permission.

Major respiratory tract injury

Direct gross injury to the oesophagus, trachea, or respiratory tree following airway management is rare, consisting mainly of pneumothorax, oesophageal perforation, or tracheal or bronchial rupture. There are no data reporting the incidence of pneumothorax after elective tracheal intubation. One study reported an incidence of

Table 12.4 Risk factors and 'risk index' scores for postoperative respiratory failure

Predictor	Odds ratio	Risk index score
Type of surgery		
Abdominal aortic aneurysm	14.3	27
Thoracic	8.1	21
Neurosurgery, upper abdominal or peripheral vascular	4.2	14
Neck	3.1	11
Emergency surgery	3.1	11
Albumin (<30 g.L^{-1})	2.5	9
Urea (>10.7 mmol.L^{-1})	2.2	8
Partially or fully dependent functional status	1.9	7
History of COPD	1.8	6
Age (years)		
≥70	1.9	6
60–69	1.5	4

Source: From Arozullah, A.M., Daley, J., Henderson, W.G., et al. (2000). Multifactorial risk index for predicting postoperative respiratory failure in men after major noncardiac surgery. The National Veterans Administration Surgical Quality Improvement Program. Annals of Surgery, **232**(2), 242–53. With permission.

Note: Total Risk index scores can be summated to give an aggregate risk score, which when inputted in a regression equation gives an estimate of risk of postoperative respiratory failure (see Table 12.5).

Table 12.5 Stratification of scores using the respiratory failure risk index

Class	Risk index score total	Predicted risk of postoperative respiratory failure (%)
1	≤10	0.5
2	11–19	2.2
3	20–27	5.0
4	28–40	11.6
5	>40	30.5

Source: From Arozullah, A.M., Daley, J., Henderson, W.G., *et al.* (2000). Multifactorial risk index for predicting postoperative respiratory failure in men after major noncardiac surgery. The National Veterans Administration Surgical Quality Improvement Program. *Annals of Surgery*, **232**(2), 242–53. With permission.

pneumothorax of 1% after emergency intubation[2]. The published literature for tracheobronchial injuries consists largely of case reports and small case series[74]. Airway injuries accounted for 6% of claims in the American Closed Claims study[74]. Among patients in the closed-claims database, tracheal intubation was difficult in 39% of those who suffered airway injury compared to 9% in other claimants. Tracheal intubation was difficult in 68% of patients who suffered pharyngeal perforation and 62% of those whose oesophagus was perforated. Logistic regression analysis of this cohort gave an odds ratio of 4.5 for difficult intubation and oesphagopharyngeal injury compared to other airway injuries.

The incidence of tracheobronchial rupture following tracheal intubation is unknown. Two French centres reported 20 cases over 23 years, and speculated that overinflation of the tracheal cuff, movement of the tube or coughing were the predominant causes[75,76].

Amelioration of respiratory risk

Following the identification of the risk factors for developing complications, various strategies have been investigated to reduce the risks. These have been reviewed recently in detail by the American College of Physicians[77].

Smoking

The data are conflicting regarding the effect of short-term cessation of smoking. One small prospective randomized study found a lower incidence of complications overall in the cessation group, but the study was underpowered to find a change in the rate of pulmonary complications[78].

Neuraxial blockade

Cohort studies identify general anaesthesia as a risk factor for POPC and POP[44,45,51]. However, this may be influenced by various biases in clinical care. The results of randomized trials are less clear. One meta-analysis of over 9500 patients[79] found that general anaesthesia alone was associated with worse respiratory outcomes than neuraxial anaesthesia (with or without general anaesthesia). However, most of the studies were old and relatively small, whilst sub-group analysis found benefit in only orthopaedic patients. In the same year, a smaller (2000 subjects) meta-analysis of hip fracture studies[80] found no difference in POP rates (5%) in patients undergoing general or neuraxial anaesthesia. There have been some large randomized trials comparing general anaesthesia alone and general anaesthesia with epidural block. One study of 168 patients undergoing open abdominal aortic aneurysm repair compared intraoperative and postoperative epidural anaesthesia/analgesia with general anaesthesia alone and intravenous analgesia in a well-standardized 4-group design. In this high-risk group, there were no significant differences in POPC. Time to extubation was shorter in the epidural patient-controlled analgesia(PCA) group[81].

The MASTER trial investigated epidural anaesthesia with general anaesthesia versus general anaesthesia alone in nearly 900 patients at high risk of cardiorespiratory complications[82,83]. Analysis of the trial overall[83] and of data from a pre-specified sub-group of 'respiratory high risk' patients[82], showed that there was no difference in outcome between control and treatment groups. The incidence of respiratory failure was higher in the control group (45% vs 29%; odds ratio 0.5) However, the trial authors suggest that this is largely an artefact of the definition of respiratory failure used, because mild hypercapnia/hypoxia are common in patients treated with intravenous opioids. The incidence of prolonged artificial ventilation was the same in the epidural and control groups. Another large study of 1021 subjects who underwent abdominal surgery compared general anaesthesia and postoperative opioid (Group 1) with light general anaesthesia, intraoperative epidural block and postoperative epidural morphine (Group 2). There was a non-significant trend towards lower POPC in Group 2; sub-group analysis found a significantly lower rate of respiratory failure in Group 2 patients who had undergone abdominal aortic aneurysm[84].

Neuromuscular blocking agents

Quantitative monitoring of neuromuscular function is believed to be the most reliable method to reduce the incidence of postoperative partial blockade although even this is not a panacea[59,85] and some argue that good clinical practice and the use of simple train-of-four monitoring may be adequate[86].

Laparoscopic versus open surgery

Although laparoscopic abdominal surgery avoids a large surgical incision and reduces the physiological stress response, the evidence that laparoscopic procedures reduce POPC is lacking. Postoperative atelectasis was reduced following laparoscopic compared to open cholecystectomy in two small studies[77], although the incidences of clinically significant POPC were not reported. For colectomy, the available data suggest that the risk of POPC may be reduced by laparoscopic surgery although statistical significance was found only for surrogate spirometric markers[87].

Nasogastric tubes

Meta-analysis of trials of selective versus routine nasogastric decompression after abdominal surgery is reported as showing a strong trend towards benefit from selective (i.e. with a clear indication) rather than non-selective use of a nasogastric tube.

Ventilatory pattern

Although large tidal volumes are associated with worse outcome in intensive care patients with acute lunge injury or acute respiratory distress syndrome (ARDS), and even short periods of positive pressure ventilation cause biological changes similar to those seen in ARDS[88], there is little evidence that intraoperative ventilatory patterns influence subsequent development of POPC for most patients. This may be for several reasons: the variation in ventilation pattern between individuals and institutions is small, most patients have positive pressure ventilation for a relatively short period, and the risk of ventilator-induced injury is small in patients with healthy lungs. One study has found an association between intraoperative tidal volume and POPC in patients undergoing pneumonectomy[89]. Alveolar recruitment strategies have been shown to reduce atelectasis and improve arterial oxygenation in both low-risk[90] and high-risk groups[91] for a short period of time. This has not translated into clinically significant reductions in POPC.

Postoperative lung expansion

A number of researchers have investigated the use of different lung-expansion therapies to reduce POPC in the postoperative period. Although the studies have flaws, the consensus is that some form of lung-expansion technique (physiotherapy, incentive spirometry, deep-breathing excercises, continuous positive airway pressure) is better than nothing, but that there is little to choose between the techniques[77].

Postoperative analgesia

Effective postoperative analgesia is associated with a reduction in POPC. If studies using comparably efficacious mechanisms for postoperative analgesia (patient-controlled intravenous or epidural analgesia) are assessed, there is probably no difference in POPC between epidural and intravenous groups[92]. The more recent large randomized studies of intra- and postoperative epidural analgesia did not find consistent improvements in significant POPC[82–84], although abdominal vascular surgery may be the exception to this [84,92]. Postoperative patient-controlled intravenous analgesia (PCA) may be associated with less POPC than morphine given intramuscularly or by continuous intravenous infusion[93]. Although the addition of paracetamol to morphine PCA reduces morphine consumption, there is no evidence to suggest that it reduces POPC[94].

Table 12.6 Strategies to reduce postoperative pulmonary morbidity

Strategy	Evidence
Postoperative lung expansion	Supportive
Intra-operative alveolar recruitment	Short-term benefits in arterial oxygenation only
Short-acting, monitored neuromuscular blockade	Definite benefits of using NMB, reasonable evidence for good clinical practice reducing POPC
Laparoscopic approach	Only indirect evidence of benefit
Smoking cessation	Long-term beneficial but conflicting evidence for perioperative cessation

Minor postoperative respiratory morbidity

A number of investigators have studied the associations between airway management technique, duration of anaesthesia, and minor morbidities (Table 12.6). The data from these studies are somewhat inconsistent, probably because of differences in study design.

Face mask anaesthesia is associated with the lowest incidence of postoperative sore throat (around 8%). Laryngeal mask anaesthesia generally has a higher incidence of sore throat. The incidence varies between studies from 0[95] to 40%[96]. Some investigators have found that the risk of sore throat is higher in women[97,98], but others have found no gender-related difference[96]. High-pressure inflation of the LMA cuff is associated with a higher incidence of postoperative sore throat in some[95] but not all studies[99]. Lubrication with 2% lidocaine gel does not appear to reduce the risk of sore throat[100]. Filling the tracheal tube cuff with alkalinized lidocaine reduces early postoperative sore throat, compared to an air-filled cuff with both nitrous oxide and air-based anaesthesia[101]. Tracheal tube size correlates with postoperative sore throat[102]. Postoperative hoarseness (44% vs. 17%) and vocal cord injuries (44% vs. 17%) are more common with double lumen tubes than bronchial blockers, although the incidences of sore throat and bronchial injury are similar for both techniques[103].

References

1. Timmermann, A., Eich, C., Russo, S.G., *et al.* (2006). Prehospital airway management: a prospective evaluation of anaesthesia trained emergency physicians. *Resuscitation*, **70**(2), 179–85.

2. Schwartz, D.E., Matthay, M.A., and Cohen, N.H. (1995). Death and other complications of emergency airway management in critically ill adults. A prospective investigation of 297 tracheal intubations. *Anesthesiology*, **82**(2), 367–76.

3. Barnardo, P.D. and Jenkins, J.G. (2000). Failed tracheal intubation in obstetrics: a 6-year review in a UK region. *Anaesthesia*, **55**(7), 690–4.

4. Hawthorne, L., Wilson, R., Lyons, G., and Dresner, M. (1996). Failed intubation revisited: 17-yr experience in a teaching maternity unit, *British Journal of Anaesthesia*, **76**(5), 680–4.

5. Saravanakumar, K. and Cooper, G.M. (2005). Failed intubation in obstetrics: has the incidence changed recently? *British Journal of Anaesthesia*, **94**(5), 690.

6. Butler, P.J. and Dhara, S.S., (1992). Prediction of difficult laryngoscopy: an assessment of the thyromental distance and Mallampati predictive tests. *Anaesthesia and Intensive Care*, **20**(2), 139–42.

7. Ezri, T., Weisenberg, M., Khazin, V., *et al.* (2003). Difficult laryngoscopy: incidence and predictors in patients undergoing coronary artery bypass surgery versus general surgery patients. *Journal of Cardiothoracic and Vascular Anesthesia*, **17**(3), 321–4.

8. Koay, C.K. (1998). Difficult tracheal intubation–analysis and management in 37 cases. *Singapore Medical Journal*, **39**(3), 112–4.

9. Wilson, M.E., Spiegelhalter, D., Robertson, J.A., and Lesser, P. (1988). Predicting difficult intubation. *British Journal of Anaesthesia*, **61**(2), 211–6.

10. Lee, A., Fan, L.T., Gin, T., Karmakar, M.K., Ngan and Kee, W.D. (2006). A systematic review (meta-analysis) of the accuracy of the Mallampati tests to predict the difficult airway. *Anesthesia and Analgesia*, **102**(6), 1867–78.

11 Kheterpal, S., Han, R., Tremper, K.K., *et al.* (2006). Incidence and predictors of difficult and impossible mask ventilation. *Anesthesiology*, **105**(5), 885–91.

12. Yildiz, T.S., Solak, M., and Toker, K. (2005). The incidence and risk factors of difficult mask ventilation. *Journal of Anesthesia*, **19**(1), 7–11.

13. Bissinger, U., Lenz, G., and Kuhn, W. (1989). Unrecognized endobronchial intubation of emergency patients. *Annals of Emergency Medicine*, **18**(8), 853–5.

14. Schwartz, D.E., Lieberman, J.A., and Cohen, N.H. (1994). Women are at greater risk than men for malpositioning of the endotracheal tube after emergent intubation. *Critical Care Medicine*, **22**(7), 1127–31.

15. Mort, T.C. (2004). Emergency tracheal intubation: complications associated with repeated laryngoscopic attempts. *Anesthesia and Analgesia*, **99**(2), 607–13.

16. Hartrey, R. and Kestin, I.G. (1995). Movement of oral and nasal tracheal tubes as a result of changes in head and neck position. *Anaesthesia*, **50**(8), 682–7.

17. Lobato, E.B., Paige, G.B., Brown, M.M., Bennett, B., and Davis, J.D. (1998). Pneumoperitoneum as a risk factor for endobronchial intubation during laparoscopic gynecologic surgery. *Anesthesia and Analgesia*, **86**(2), 301–3.

18. Inada, T., Uesugi, F., Kawachi, S., and Takubo, K. (1996). Changes in tracheal tube position during laparoscopic cholecystectomy. *Anaesthesia*, **51**(9), 823–6.

19. Mendelson, C.L. (1945). The aspiration of stomach contents into the lungs during obstetric anesthesia. *American Journal of Obstetrics and Gynecology*, **52**, 191–204.

20. Olsson, G.L., Hallen, B., and Hambraeus-Jonzon, K. (1986). Aspiration during anaesthesia: a computer-aided study of 185 358 anaesthetics. *Acta Anaesthesiologica Scandinavica*, **30**(1), 84–92.

21. Mellin-Olsen, J., Fasting, S., Gisvold, S.E., Mellin-Olsen, J., Fasting, S., and Gisvold, S.E. (1996). Routine preoperative gastric emptying is seldom indicated. A study of 85 594 anaesthetics with special focus on aspiration pneumonia. *Acta Anaesthesiologica Scandinavica*, **40**(10), 1184–8.

22. Warner, M.A., Warner, M.E., and Weber, J.G. (1993). Clinical significance of pulmonary aspiration during the perioperative period. *Anesthesiology*, **78**(1), 56–62.

23. Borland,.L.M., Sereika, S.M., Woelfel, S.K., *et al.* (1998). Pulmonary aspiration in pediatric patients during general anesthesia: incidence and outcome. *Journal of Clinical Anesthesia*, **10**(2), 95–102.

24. Brimacombe, J.R. and Berry, A. (1995). The incidence of aspiration associated with the laryngeal mask airway: a meta-analysis of published literature. *Journal of Clinical Anesthesia*, **7**(4), 297–305.

25. Keller, C., Brimacombe, J., Bittersohl, J., *et al.* (2004). Aspiration and the laryngeal mask airway: three cases and a review of the literature. *British Journal of Anaesthesia*, **93**(4), 579–82.

26. Verghese, C. and Brimacombe, J.R. (1996). Survey of laryngeal mask airway usage in 11 910 patients: safety and efficacy for conventional and nonconventional usage. *Anesthesia and Analgesia*, **82**(1), 129–33.

27. Rolf, N. and Cote, C.J. (1992). Frequency and severity of desaturation events during general anesthesia in children with and without upper respiratory infections. *Journal of Clinical Anesthesia*, **4**(3), 200–3.

28. DeSoto, H., Patel, R.I., Soliman, I.E., and Hannallah, R.S. (1988). Changes in oxygen saturation following general anesthesia in children with upper respiratory infection signs and symptoms undergoing otolaryngological procedures. *Anesthesiology*, **68**(2), 276–9.

29. Cohen, M.M. and Cameron, C.B. (1991). Should you cancel the operation when a child has an upper respiratory tract infection? *Anesthesia and Analgesia*, **72**(3), 282–8.

30. Tait, A.R., Burke, C., Voepel-Lewis, T., Chiravuri, D., Wagner, D., and Malviya, S. (2007). Glycopyrrolate does not reduce the incidence of perioperative adverse events in children with upper respiratory tract infections. *Anesthesia and Analgesia*, **104**(2), 265–70.

31. Aquilina, A.T., Hall, W.J., Douglas, R.G., Jr., and Utell, M.J. (1980). Airway reactivity in subjects with viral upper respiratory tract infections: the effects of exercise and cold air. *American Review Respiratory Diseases*, **122**(1), 3–10.

32. Konarzewski, W.H., Ravindran N., Findlow, D., and Timmis, P.K. (1992). Anaesthetic death of a child with a cold. *Anaesthesia*, **47**(7), 624.

33. Elwood, T., Morris, W., Martin, L.D., *et al.* (2003). Bronchodilator premedication does not decrease respiratory adverse events in pediatric general anaesthesia. *Canadian Journal of Anaesthesia*, **50**(3), 277–84.

34. Dennis, A., Curran, J., Sherriff, J., and Kinnear, W. (1994). Effects of passive and active smoking on induction of anaesthesia. *British Journal of Anaesthesia*, **73**(4), 450–2.

35. Caranza, R., Raphael, J.H., Nandwani, N., and Langton, J.A. (1997). Effect of nebulised lignocaine on the quality of induction of anaesthesia in cigarette smokers. *Anaesthesia*, **52**(9), 849–52.

36. Wild, M.R., Gornall, C.B., Griffiths, D.E., and Curran, J. (2004). Maintenance of anaesthesia with sevoflurane or isoflurane effects on adverse airway events in smokers. *Anaesthesia*, **59**(9), 891–3.

37. McKay, R.E., Bostrom, A., Balea, M.C., and McKay, W.R. (2006). Airway responses during desflurane versus sevoflurane administration via a laryngeal mask airway in smokers. *Anesthesia and Analgesia*, **103**(5), 1147–54.

38. Goff, M.J., Arain, S.R., Ficke, D.J., Uhrich, T.D., and Ebert, T.J. (2000). Absence of bronchodilation during desflurane anesthesia: a comparison to sevoflurane and thiopental. *Anesthesiology*, **93**(2), 404–8.

39. Klock, P.A., Jr., Czeslick, E.G., Klafta, J.M., Ovassapian, A., and Moss, J. (2001). The effect of sevoflurane and desflurane on upper airway reactivity. *Anesthesiology*, **94**(6), 963–7.

40. Kong, C.F., Chew, S.T., and Ip-Yam, P.C. (2000). Intravenous opioids reduce airway irritation during induction of anaesthesia with desflurane in adults. *British Journal of Anaesthesia*, **85**(3), 364–7.

41. Driver, I., Wilson, C., Wiltshire, S., Mills, P., and Howard-Griffin, R. (1997). Co-induction and laryngeal mask insertion. A comparison of thiopentone versus propofol. *Anaesthesia*, **52**(7), 698–700.

42. Bishop, M.J., O'Donnell, J.T., and Salemi, J.R. (2003). Mivacurium and bronchospasm. *Anesthesia and Analgesia*, **97**(2), 484–5.

43. Manku, K., Bacchetti, P. and Leung, J.M. (2003). Prognostic significance of postoperative in-hospital complications in elderly patients. I. Long-term survival. *Anesthesia and Analgesia*, **96**(2), 583–9.

44. Arozullah, A.M., Daley, J., Henderson, W.G., and Khuri, S.F. (2000). Multifactorial risk index for predicting postoperative respiratory failure in men after major noncardiac surgery. The National Veterans Administration Surgical Quality Improvement Program. *Annals of Surgery*, **232**(2), 242–53.

45. Arozullah, A.M., Khuri, S.F., Henderson, W.G., and Daley, J. (2001). Development and validation of a multifactorial risk index for predicting postoperative pneumonia after major noncardiac surgery. *Annals of Internal Medicine*, **135**(10), 847–57.

46. McAlister, F.A., Bertsch, K., Man, J., *et al.* (2005). Incidence of and risk factors for pulmonary complications after nonthoracic surgery. *American Journal of Respiratory and Critical Care Medicine*, **171**(5), 514–7.

47. Stephan, F., Boucheseiche, S., Hollande, J., *et al.* (2000). Pulmonary complications following lung resection: a comprehensive analysis of incidence and possible risk factors. *Chest*, **118**(5), 1263–70.

48. Lawrence, V.A., Hilsenbeck, S.G., Noveck, H., *et al.* (2002). Medical complications and outcomes after hip fracture repair. *Archives of Internal Medicine*, **162**(18), 2053–7.

49. Thomas, E.J., Goldman, L., Mangione, C.M., *et al.* (1997). Body mass index as a correlate of postoperative complications and resource utilization. *American Journal of Medicine*, **102**(3), 277–83.

50. Warner, M.A., Shields, S.E., and Chute, C.G. (1993). Major morbidity and mortality within 1 month of ambulatory surgery and anesthesia. *Journal of the American Medical Association*, **270**(12), 1437–41.

51. Smetana, G.W., Lawrence, V.A., and Cornell, J.E. (2006). Preoperative pulmonary risk stratification for noncardiothoracic surgery: systematic review for the American College of Physicians. *Annals of Internal Medicine*, **144**(8), 581–95.

52. Lawrence, V.A., Dhanda, R., Hilsenbeck, S.G., and Page, C.P. (1996). Risk of pulmonary complications after elective abdominal surgery. *Chest*, **110**(3), 744–50.

53. Liu, L.L. and Leung, J.M. (2000). Predicting adverse postoperative outcomes in patients aged 80 years or older. *Journal of the American Geriatric Society*, **48**(4), 405–12.

54. Theadom, A. and Cropley, M. (2006). Effects of preoperative smoking cessation on the incidence and risk of intraoperative and postoperative complications in adult smokers: a systematic review. *Tobacco control*, **15**(5), 352–8.

55. Gupta, R.M., Parvizi, J., Hanssen, A.D., *et al.* (2001). Postoperative complications in patients with obstructive sleep apnea syndrome undergoing hip or knee replacement: a case-control study. *Mayo Clinic Proceedings*, **76**(9), 897–905.

56. Brooks-Brunn, J.A. (1997). Predictors of postoperative pulmonary complications following abdominal surgery. *Chest*, **111**(3), 564–71.

57. Elkouri, S., Gloviczki, P., McKusick, M.A., *et al.* (2004). Perioperative complications and early outcome after endovascular and open surgical repair of abdominal aortic aneurysms. *Journal of Vascular Surgery*, **39**(3), 497–505.

58. Cheatham, M.L., Chapman, W.C., Key, S.P., *et al.* (1995). A meta-analysis of selective versus routine nasogastric decompression after elective laparotomy. *Annals of Surgery*, **221**(5), 469–76, discussion 476–8.

59. Murphy, G.S., Szokol, J.W., Marymont, J.H., *et al.* (2005). Residual paralysis at the time of tracheal extubation. *Anesthesia and Analgesia*, **100**(6), 1840–5.

60. Debaene, B., Plaud, B., Dilly, M.P., *et al.* (2003). Residual paralysis in the PACU after a single intubating dose of nondepolarizing muscle relaxant with an intermediate duration of action. *Anesthesiology*, **98**(5), 1042–8.

61. Bluman, L.G., Mosca, L., Newman, N., and Simon, D.G. (1998). Preoperative smoking habits and postoperative pulmonary complications. *Chest*, **113**(4), 883–9.

62. Archer, C., Levy, A.R., and McGregor, M. (1993). Value of routine preoperative chest x-rays: a meta-analysis. *Canadian Journal of Anaesthesia*, **40**(11), 1022–7.

63. Smetana, G.W. and Macpherson, D.S. (2003). The case against routine preoperative laboratory testing. *Medical Clinics of North America*, **87**(1), 7–40.

64. Wong, D.H., Weber, E.C., Schell, M.J., *et al.* (1995). Factors associated with postoperative pulmonary complications in patients with severe chronic obstructive pulmonary disease. *Anesthesia and Analgesia*, **80**(2), 276–84.

65. Fuso, L., Cisternino, L., Di Napoli, A., *et al.* (2000). Role of spirometric and arterial gas data in predicting pulmonary complications after abdominal surgery. *Respiratory Medicine*, **94**(12), 1171–6.

66. Barisione, G., Rovida, S., Gazzaniga, G.M., and Fontana, L. (1997). Upper abdominal surgery: does a lung function test exist to predict early severe postoperative respiratory complications? *European Respiratory Journal*, **10**(6), 1301–8.

67. British Thoracic Society, Society of Cardiothoracic Surgeons of Great Britain and Ireland Working Party (2001). BTS guidelines: guidelines on the selection of patients with lung cancer for surgery. *Thorax*, **56**(2), 89–108.

68. Uramoto, H., Nakanishi, R., Fujino, Y., *et al.* (2001). Prediction of pulmonary complications after a lobectomy in patients with non-small cell lung cancer. *Thorax*, **56**(1), 59–61.

69. O'Brien, M.M., Gonzales, R., Shroyer, A.L., *et al.* (2002). Modest serum creatinine elevation affects adverse outcome after general surgery. *Kidney International*, **62**(2), 585–92.

70. Schuiling, W.J., Dennesen, P.J.W., Tans, J.T.J., Kingma, L.M., Algra, A., and Rinkel, G.J.E. (2005). Troponin I in predicting cardiac or pulmonary complications and outcome in subarachnoid haemorrhage. *Journal of Neurology, Neurosurgery, and Psychiatry*, **76**(11), 1565–9.

71. Schussler, O., Alifano, M., Dermine, H., *et al.* (2006). Postoperative pneumonia after major lung resection. *American Journal of Respiratory and Critical Care Medicine*, **173**(10), 1161–9.

72. Money, S.R., Rice, K., Crockett, D., *et al.* (1994). Risk of respiratory failure after repair of thoracoabdominal aortic aneurysms. *American Journal of Surgery*, **168**(2), 152–5.

73. Jayr, C., Matthay, M.A., Goldstone, J., Gold, W.M., and Wiener-Kronish, J.P. (1993). Preoperative and intraoperative factors associated with prolonged mechanical ventilation. A study in patients following major abdominal vascular surgery. *Chest*, **103**(4), 1231–6.

74. Domino, K.B., Posner, K.L., Caplan, R.A., and Cheney, F.W. (1999). Airway injury during anesthesia: a closed claims analysis. *Anesthesiology*, **91**(6), 1703–11.

75. Marty-Ane, C.H., Picard, E., Jonquet, O., and Mary, H. (1995). Membranous tracheal rupture after endotracheal intubation. *Annals of Thoracic Surgery*, **60**(5), 1367–71.

76. Massard, G., Rouge, C., Dabbagh, A., *et al.* (1996). Tracheobronchial lacerations after intubation and tracheostomy. *Annals of Thoracic Surgery*, **61**(5), 1483–7.

77. Lawrence, V.A., Cornell, J.E., Smetana, G.W., *et al.* (2006). Strategies to reduce postoperative pulmonary complications after noncardiothoracic surgery: systematic review for the American College of Physicians. *Annals of Internal Medicine*, **144**(8), 596–608.

78. Moller, A.M., Villebro, N., Pedersen, T., *et al.* (2002). Effect of preoperative smoking intervention on postoperative complications: a randomised clinical trial. *Lancet*, **359**(9301), 114–7.

79. Rodgers, A., Walker, N., Schug, S., *et al.* (2000). Reduction of postoperative mortality and morbidity with epidural or spinal anaesthesia: results from overview of randomised trials. *British Medical Journal*, **321**(7275), 1493.

80. Urwin, S.C., Parker, M.J., and Griffiths, R. (2000). General versus regional anaesthesia for hip fracture surgery: a meta-analysis of randomized trials.[erratum appears in British Journal of Anaesthesia 2002 88(4):619]. *British Journal of Anaesthesia*, **84**(4), 450–5.

81. Norris, E.J., Beattie, C., Perler, B.A., *et al.* (2001). Double-masked randomized trial comparing alternate combinations of intraoperative anesthesia and postoperative analgesia in abdominal aortic surgery. *Anesthesiology*, **95**(5), 1054–67.

82. Peyton, P.J., Myles, P.S., Silbert, B.S., Rigg, J.A., Jamrozik, K., and Parsons, R. (2003). Perioperative epidural analgesia and outcome after major abdominal surgery in high-risk patients. *Anesthesia and Analgesia*, **96**(2), 548–54.

83. Rigg, J.R., Jamrozik, K., Myles, P.S., *et al.* (2002). Epidural anaesthesia and analgesia and outcome of major surgery: a randomised trial. *Lancet*, **359**(9314), 1276–82.

84. Park, W.Y., Thompson, J.S., and Lee, K.K. (2001). Effect of epidural anesthesia and analgesia on perioperative outcome: a randomized, controlled Veterans Affairs cooperative study. *Annals of Surgery*, **234**(4), 560–9, discussion 569–71.

85. Mortensen, C.R., Berg, H., el-Mahdy, A., Viby-Mogensen, J., and Mortensen, C.R. (1995). Perioperative monitoring of neuromuscular transmission using acceleromyography prevents residual neuromuscular block following pancuronium. *Acta Anaesthesiologica Scandinavica*, **39**(6), 797–801.

86. Kopman, A.F., Zank, L.M., Ng, J., Neuman, G.G. (2004). Antagonism of cisatracurium and rocuronium block at a tactile train-of-four count of 2: should quantitative assessment of neuromuscular function be mandatory? *Anesthesia and Analgesia*, **98**(1), 102–6.

87. Abraham, N.S., Young, J.M., and Solomon, M.J. (2004). Meta-analysis of short-term outcomes after laparoscopic resection for colorectal cancer. *British Journal of Surgery*, **91**(9), 1111–24.

88. Dos Santos, C.C. and Slutsky, A.S. (2000). Cellular responses to mechanical stress: Invited Review: Mechanisms of ventilator-induced lung injury: a perspective. *Journal of Applied Physiology*, **89**(4), 1645–55.

89. Fernandez-Perez, E.R., Keegan, M.T., Brown, D.R., Hubmayr, R.D., and Gajic, O. (2006). Intraoperative tidal volume as a risk factor for respiratory failure after pneumonectomy. *Anesthesiology*, **105**(1), 14–8.

90. Tusman, G., Bohm, S.H., Vazquez de Anda, G.F., do Campo, J.L., and Lachmann, B. (1999). 'Alveolar recruitment strategy' improves arterial oxygenation during general anaesthesia. *British Journal of Anaesthesia*, **82**(1), 8–13.

91. Claxton, B.A., Morgan, P., McKeague, H., Mulpur, A., and Berridge, J. (2003). Alveolar recruitment strategy improves arterial oxygenation after cardiopulmonary bypass. *Anaesthesia*, **58**(2), 111–6.

92. Liu, S.S. and Wu, C.L. (2007). Effect of postoperative analgesia on major postoperative complications: A systematic update of the evidence. *Anesthesia and Analgesia*, **104**(3), 689–702.

93. Walder, B., Schafer, M., Henzi, I., and Tramer, M.R. (2001). Efficacy and safety of patient-controlled opioid analgesia for acute postoperative pain. A quantitative systematic review. *Acta Anaesthesiologica Scandinavica*, **45**(7), 795–804.

94. Remy, C., Marret, E., and Bonnet, F. (2005). Effects of acetaminophen on morphine side-effects and consumption after major surgery: meta-analysis of randomized controlled trials. British Journal of Anaesthesia, **94**(4), 505–13.

95. Burgard, G., Mollhoff, T., and Prien, T. (1996). The effect of laryngeal mask cuff pressure on postoperative sore throat incidence. *Journal of Clinical Anesthesia*, **8**(3), 198–201.

96. Brimacombe, J., Holyoake, L., Keller, C., *et al.* (2000). Pharyngolaryngeal, neck, and jaw discomfort after anesthesia with the face mask and laryngeal mask airway at high and low cuff volumes in males and females. *Anesthesiology*, **93**(1), 26–31.

97. Rieger, A., Brunne, B., Hass, I., *et al.* (1997). Laryngo-pharyngeal complaints following laryngeal mask airway and endotracheal intubation. *Journal of Clinical Anesthesia,* **9**(1), 42–7.

98. Nott, M.R., Noble, P.D., and Parmar, M. (1998). Reducing the incidence of sore throat with the laryngeal mask airway. *European Journal of Anaesthesiology,* **15**(2), 153–7.

99. Rieger, A., Brunne, B., and Striebel, H.W. (1997). Intracuff pressures do not predict laryngopharyngeal discomfort after use of the laryngeal mask airway. *Anesthesiology,* **87**(1), 63–7.

100. Keller, C., Sparr, H.J., and Brimacombe, J.R.(1997). Laryngeal mask lubrication. A comparative study of saline versus 2% lignocaine gel with cuff pressure control. *Anaesthesia,* **52**(6), 592–7.

101. Estebe, J-P., Gentili, M., Le Corre, P., Dollo, G., Chevanne, F., and Ecoffey, C. (2005). Alkalinization of intracuff lidocaine: efficacy and safety. *Anesthesia and Analgesia,* **101**(5), 1536–41.

102. Stout, D.M., Bishop, M.J., Dwersteg, J.F., and Cullen, F.C. (1987). Correlation of endotracheal tube size with sore throat and hoarseness following general anaesthesia. *Anesthesiology,* **67**, 419–21.

103. Knoll, H., Ziegeler, S., Schreiber, J-U., *et al.* (2006). Airway injuries after one-lung ventilation: a comparison between double-lumen tube and endobronchial blocker. *Anesthesiology,* **105**, 471–7.

Chapter 13

Cardiovascular risk

Henry J Skinner

Cardiovascular risk, perhaps more than any other risk associated with anaesthesia, has been studied in great detail. Cardiovascular complications account for approximately a third of postoperative complications and up to half of perioperative deaths. Surgery causes tissue trauma, fluid shifts, and tachycardia, and elicits a stress response, which results in an increase in cardiac workload. Adverse cardiac events commonly are produced by an unfavourable myocardial oxygen supply–demand ratio or inability to carry the increased burden. However, the aetiology may be complex and multifactorial, and it can be difficult to establish the role of anaesthesia in this. Most general anaesthetic drugs reduce left ventricle (LV) contractility, impair diastolic function, and dilate arteries and veins[1]. Vasodilatation may be important in patients with fixed coronary flow obstruction as flow becomes pressure-dependent. Induction of anaesthesia reduces sympathetic tone. A proportion of patients with impaired cardiac function (especially the elderly) depend on sympathetic activity to maintain adequate perfusion pressure[2]. On the other hand, volatile agents reduce cardiac workload and may protect the heart against ischaemic insults[3]. The notion that anaesthesia is simply a vehicle to facilitate surgery with its incumbent risks is thus incorrect.

The purpose of quantifying cardiovascular risk is threefold. Firstly, it is important to inform the patient how much risk a proposed procedure carries. For example, if a 65-year-old lady, who is otherwise fit and well, is scheduled for a hip replacement to relieve hip pain and get her back on her feet, a <1% risk of a serious perioperative cardiac complication seems acceptable. On the other hand, if she was 80 years old and had suffered a myocardial infarction (MI) six months ago with subsequent heart failure (HF) and renal impairment, the risk of significant cardiac morbidity is in the order of 10% or more. She may decide to live with the pain rather than take this degree of risk; it remains her decision but she must be adequately informed. Patients want to know the risk associated with the entire procedure rather than its various components, and it is the responsibility of the surgical team, of which the anaesthetist is an integral part, to impart this information in clear and simple terms. Surgeons usually discuss surgical risks, but the input from the anaesthetist becomes paramount as co-morbidity and degree of incapacity increase. The second aim of risk stratification is to identify the subset of higher-risk patients in whom it may be possible to reduce the risk. For example, the physician could treat uncompensated HF, commence beta-blockers, or consider further cardiological assessment. Finally, patients at increased risk may warrant a modification of anaesthesia technique such as invasive vascular pressure monitoring, or regional anaesthesia. Based on evidence that intensive care significantly reduces mortality rates in nonsurgical patients with myocardial infarction[4], intensive postoperative monitoring and treatment have been recommended for patients having surgery who are at high risk for cardiac complications[5]. There are excellent reviews and updates on assessing and reducing cardiac risk[5,6].

What are the risks?

Death

Current data suggest an overall mortality rate of approximately 1 in 500 anaesthetics within the first two postoperative days[7], half of that within 24 h of anaesthesia[8]. Up to half of all perioperative deaths are related to cardiac events. In Lagasse's large prospective study in 2002, anaesthesia was a contributing factor to death in 1.4 in 10 000 anaesthetics, just over 50% associated with cardiovascular management[7]. Others suggest the contribution of anaesthesia care *per se* is nearer to 1 in 100 000[9,10]. Most studies of anaesthetic death cover the time from induction to leaving recovery or the first 24 h. Important complications like HF or MI often only present two or three days after surgery and it is difficult to know what role intraoperative factors like hypotension or fluid overload may have had. Cardiac death usually refers to death in the setting of MI, ventricular arrhythmias, cardiogenic shock, or if death was sudden and unexplained. MI caused death in two-thirds of patients with HF, and arrhythmias accounted for the rest[11]. Unexpected perioperative cardiac death in otherwise healthy individuals is fortunately exceedingly rare and usually associated with a previously undiagnosed structural abnormality. Tabib in 2000 reported a retrospective analysis of 1700 forensic autopsies following unexpected sudden cardiac death[12]. Fifty cases could have been related to surgery and/or anaesthesia. Structural cardiac lesions were found in 94%, the most common being arrhythmogenic right ventricular cardiomyopathy, coronary artery disease (CAD), cardiomyopathy, and abnormalities of the His bundle.

Cardiac arrest

Cardiac arrests are often the final common pathway of a variety of factors, anaesthetic care (or lack of) being one of them. The reported incidence of perioperative cardiac arrests has varied during the past several decades, ranging between about 4 and 20 in 10 000 anaesthetics[9]. Sprung and colleagues peer-reviewed 223 cases of perioperative cardiac arrest that occurred before discharge from the recovery room after non-cardiac surgery. After bleeding (44%), the dominant causes were judged to be cardiac in origin (21%). This included MI, heart blocks and dysrhythmias, placement of pacemaker wires, and medication-related asystole. Just over 10% of arrests were judged to be attributable primarily to anaesthesia (0.5 in 10 000); thus, most perioperative cardiac arrests were not directly related to anaesthesia. Again, the relationship between anaesthetic care and arrests further into the postoperative period has not been established. Patients who have a cardiac arrest after non-cardiac surgery have a hospital mortality rate of 65% and nonfatal perioperative cardiac arrest is a risk factor for cardiac death during the 5 years following surgery[13].

Perioperative myocardial ischaemia and infarct

Perioperative MI may follow plaque rupture with coronary thrombosis as seen in the non-operative setting. On the other hand, prolonged ischaemia secondary to limited myocardial oxygen supply and increased oxygen demand can cause MI[14], and is typical in patients with severe but stable CAD. Post-mortem examinations suggest that the incidence of both types is roughly equal[15,16]. Myocardial ischaemia and MI represents a continuum. Priebe found a 20–63% reported incidence of perioperative myocardial ischaemia in patients at risk[17]. Mangano's group observed myocardial ischaemia most commonly on the second and third day after surgery[18]. The same investigators saw postoperative ischaemia was associated with a sharp risk increase, 2.8-fold for serious cardiac events and 9-fold for subsequent acute coronary syndrome[19].

Table 13.1 Incidence of perioperative cardiac morbidity and mortality

Risk	Incidence	Comment	Reference
Cardiac arrest	0.04–0.4%		[9,34]
MI	0.03–0.7%	Low risk/ambulatory surgery	[96,25,24]
	1.4–1.9%	Major surgery	[34,45,28]
	3.1%	Question of cardiac risk	[46]
	4.7%	IHD or >70 years of age	[70]
	2.7–5.6%	IHD	[62,28,23]
	0.8%	Prior coronary bypass surgery	[62]
	2.3–6.5%	Vascular surgery	[44,105,106] [107,108]
Serious cardiac event*	>1.6%	Men >40 years of age, major surgery	[28]
	0.4%	Subset of lower risk patients	[28]
	2.1%	>50 years of age, major surgery	[34]
	3.2%	Suspected heart disease	[29]
	3.9%	Mostly patients at risk	[11]
	2.6%	>40 years of age, not minor surgery	[35]
	>4%	Major surgery with IHD	[62]
	4.6%	Question of cardiac risk	[46]
	5.1–8.0%	Vascular surgery	[44,54]
Cardiac death	0.3–1.9%	Major surgery	[34,28,45]
Serious arrhythmia	1.2%	Ventricular tachycardia	[45]
	6.1%	Sustained supraventricular tachycardia	[38]
HF	1–3.6%	Major surgery	[34,45]
	6.3%	IHD	[19]

Note: Cardiac death and nonfatal MI; includes arrest [28,29,34,35], pulmonary oedema [34,44,46], VT [35,45].

Perioperative MI after non-cardiac surgery was most prevalent on postoperative days 2 and 3 [20,21] but sooner in other studies[22,23]. We are clearer about the incidence of perioperative MI (Table 13.1). In the absence of IHD, the chance of a MI was low even after major surgery (0.5%)[24]. Because the large majority of perioperative MI is believed to be asymptomatic, unaccompanied by a Q-wave, and not associated with ventricular failure[22,25], there is an increased reliance on markers of myocardial damage. Until recently there has not been a widely accepted cut-off for the diagnosis of MI[26] and this accounts in part for the wide range in the reported incidence[27]. Cardiac troponin is highly specific and sensitive for myocardial injury and is the preferred marker. The cut-off value for troponin (or creatine kinase-MB) should be >99th percentile of the reference control group. Elevated markers in the right time context, accompanied by either ischaemic symptoms or ECG changes, confirms the diagnosis[26]. In 1993, Ashton[28] found (Table 13.2) that factors independently associated with perioperative MI included age>75 years old, preoperative HF, CAD, and a planned vascular operation. Perioperative MI carried a high hospital mortality of 15%–25% [22, 28,29], and nonfatal perioperative MI is an independent risk factor for cardiovascular death and nonfatal MI during the 6 months following surgery (OR 18; 95% CI 6–57)[30]. There are no data that definitively extrapolate results of randomized trials for the treatment of the acute coronary syndromes or acute MI to the perioperative setting.

Heart failure

Cowie (1999) showed that 0.13% of adults in the London area were diagnosed with HF each year and the incidence approached 1% in those over 75 years of age[31]. The main known causes of HF are IHD and hypertension (HT). As the surgical population gets older and sicker, it is anticipated that more patients with HF will undergo surgery. LV dysfunction begins with some insult to the myocardium, and this may be precipitated by increased perioperative metabolic demand. Surgery activates the renin–angiotensin system and elevates cortisol as well as epinephrine levels[32] and failure ensues then if the heart cannot meet the systemic demands. HF may worsen immediately after surgery because of the insult of surgery, ischaemia, and rapid fluid shifts, or a few days later when third-spaced fluid is reabsorbed. Almost half of HF occurred after the third postoperative day in Mangano's study[19]. About 70% of cases of HF are related to LV systolic dysfunction and 30% are due to diastolic dysfunction[33]. Impaired LV contractility causes systolic dysfunction. LV dysfunction is not equivalent to HF but describes possible structural or functional reasons for the development of HF. Impaired LV relaxation and reduced compliance are the hallmarks of diastolic dysfunction. These patients are at risk for marked elevation in LV filling pressures in the presence of volume overload, but also for hypotension if they are underfilled. Diagnosing HF postoperatively can be difficult as there are other causes of dyspnoea, bilateral rales, and pulmonary infiltrates on chest films, such as increased capillary permeability due to sepsis, transfusion-related lung injury, and atelectasis to name a few. The availability of assays for natriuretic peptides may improve diagnosis. Overall, the incidence of perioperative HF is around 1%[34] but may be up to 6.3% in patients at risk of or with ischaemic heart disease (IHD)[19], and even higher, if there are persistent

Table 13.2 Influence of risk factors on adverse cardiac outcome

Risk factor	Odds ratio % (95% CI)	Reference	Endpoint
>75 years of age	4.8 (1.2–19.4)	[28]	MI
>70 years of age	1.6 (0.9–3.0)	[54] [70]	Serious cardiac risk
>65 years of age	2.3 (1.4–3.6)	[109]	Serious risk
CAD	10.4 (2.3–47.7)	[28]	MI
	2.6 (1.6–4.3)	[109]	Serious risk
	2.4 (1.3–4.2)	[34]	Serious cardiac risk
MI ever	3.2	[57]	Death
MI< 6 months	4.5 (1.9–2.9)	[29]	Serious cardiac risk
MI >6 months	2.2 (1.4–3.5)		
Valvular heart disease	2.1 (1.1–3.9)	[22]	MI after major vascular surgery
Severe aortic stenosis	5.2 (1.6–17.0)	[68]	Serious risk
Hypertension	1.9	[57]	Death
	3.8 (1.1–13)	[72]	Death
Renal failure			
Cr >150 μmol L^{-1}	3.6	[57]	Death
Cr >177 μmol L^{-1}	3.0 (1.4–6.8)	[34]	Serious cardiac risk
Cr clearance <0.83 mL.s^{-1}	6.8 (2.8–16)	[72]	Death
Smoking	2.0	[73]	Serious complication
Postoperative ischaemia	2.0–4.9	[110]	Serious cardiac risk
	2.8 (1.6–4.9)	[19]	Serious cardiac risk
Postoperative MI	20	[30]	Long-term cardiac complication
Poor exercise tolerance	2	[73]	Serious complication
	< 5	[73]	Myocardial ischaemia
	9.7 (2.5–37)	[72]	Death
Heart failure	1.9 (1.2–3.0)	[29]	Serious cardiac risk
	2.2 (1.9–2.5)	[53]	30-day mortality
	2.7-3.6	[54,55]	Serious cardiac risk
	3.3 (1.0–11.4)	[28]	MI
	3.4 (2–5.7)	[34]	Serious cardiac risk
	13.6 (3.6–58.6)	[22]	Cardiac death
	14.8 (2.5–87)	[56]	Cardiac death after emergency surgery
Cerebrovascular disease	3.2 (1.8–6.0)	[34]	Serious cardiac risk
Diabetes on insulin	3.0 (1.3–7.1)	[34]	Serious cardiac risk

Table 13.2 (continued) Influence of risk factors on adverse cardiac outcome

Risk factor	Odds ratio % (95% CI)	Reference	Endpoint
Non-sinus rhythm	1.7 (0.9–3.2)	[29]	Serious cardiac risk
Emergency surgery	2.6 (1.2–5.6)	[29]	Serious cardiac risk
Vascular surgery	3.7 (1.2–2.4)	[28]	MI
Neuraxial blockade	0.7 (0.5–1.0)	[100]	MI

Note: Serious cardiac risk implies cardiac death or nonfatal MI [54, 55] and includes arrest [28,29, 34, 35,110], pulmonary oedema [34,44,46,110], VT [35,45], heart block [34,110]

Serious risk is 30-day all-cause mortality or significant cardiac morbidity.

Serious complications are cardiac, pulmonary, neurological, or infective complications.

Cr = creatinine.

signs of congestive HF at the time of surgery[35]. Mangano and colleagues[19] found a history of dysrhythmias, diabetes, duration of anaesthesia, vascular surgery, and high-dose opioids were all associated with postoperative heart failure. Charlson and colleagues[36] found that the risk for postoperative HF was limited to patients with preoperative symptomatic cardiac disease, especially in patients with diabetes. Hernandez felt inability to continue taking oral anti-failure treatment postoperatively may also be a factor[37].

Serious dysrhythmias and complete heart block

There is increased sympathetic activity perioperatively. Arrhythmias in this context are common and mostly benign, but some may cause decompensation in patients with critical aortic stenosis or CAD. In a study of over 4000 patients ≥ 50 years of age in sinus rhythm who had major, routine, non-cardiac procedures, supraventricular tachycardia occurred in 7.6%[38]. A quarter occurred during surgery and three-quarters after surgery. Independent correlates were significant valvular disease (OR 2.1), history of supraventricular tachycardia (OR 3.4), asthma (OR 2.0), congestive heart failure (OR 1.7), premature atrial complexes (OR 2.1), and intrathoracic procedures (OR 9.2). Development of supraventricular tachycardia was associated with increased risk for perioperative acute cardiac events and increase in length of stay[38], but this is not a consistent finding. Perioperative dysrhythmias were not a predictor of adverse outcome in patients with structural heart disease undergoing non-cardiac surgery[39]. For example, 15% of patients had ventricular tachycardia after thoracic surgery but none was sustained or associated with poor outcome[40]. O'Kelly *et al.* in 1992 found significant ventricular arrhythmias in 44% of patients at risk or with CAD[41]. A third occurred during, and the rest after-surgery. Not surprisingly, preoperative ventricular arrhythmias predicted later recurrence. In Foster's study, 3.3% of patients after major surgery had dysrhythmias warranting drug interventions[24]. Patients with underlying structural heart disease were at greatest risk for developing either supraventricular or ventricular arrhythmias during the induction of anaesthesia secondary to hypotension, autonomic imbalance, or airway manipulation[42]. Anaesthesia also interferes with vagal control of heart rate. New conduction defects usually result from enhanced vagal tone or medication that suppress AV nodal conduction or AV nodal ischaemia[43]. The incidence of complete heart block was 0.1% in Lee's study[34].

Serious cardiac risk

Serious cardiac risks are often pooled together. It is easier to compare events with a higher incidence and it can simplify discussion of risk. Serious cardiac events represent a bad outcome in itself or may be a precursor to poor outcome. Events are often inter-related; for example, a patient may develop acute HF following a perioperative MI, which may be further complicated by ventricular tachycardia or worse. Many investiga-tors considered a serious cardiac events as an endpoint in itself[11,29,34,35,44]. These events usually constitute cardiac death, MI, pulmonary oedema, cardiac arrest, and sustained ventricular tachycardia, but may also include unstable angina[19,29], new or worsened HF[29] and complete heart block[34]. Serious cardiac events occur with incidences of 2.1% in unselected major surgery and 8% in high-risk surgery (Table 13.1).

How is cardiac risk estimated?

A complex interaction exists between individual risk factors. HT, for example, causes IHD, HF, and renal impairment, themselves independent risk factors. Logistic regres-sion verifies which factors, independent of others, alter outcome. Even if it has been difficult to show that HT worsens outcome independently, it seems likely that HT is at least indirectly related to increased cardiac risk. The likelihood of a cardiac complica-tion depends on the patient's co-morbidity, functional capacity, and type of surgery. Risk indices have been designed to collate individual risk factors into a probability of an adverse outcome. Indices[34,35,45] estimate risk through a combination of patient and surgical factors. In their original study, Goldman and colleagues (1977) enrolled 1001 patients ≥40 years of age, undergoing major non-cardiac surgery[45]. They used multivariate analysis to identify nine risk factors and attributed a score to each. The sum total placed the patient into one of four risk categories. For example, if a 70-year-old patient with a raised jugular venous pulse in atrial fibrillation, undergoing elective bowel resection, had a total score ≥26; mortality in this highest risk category was 56%. If the same patient had his operation when he was a year younger, his lesser score would put him in the second highest category where the mortality was much lower. This illustrates that risk categories are somewhat artificial, and caution should be exer-cised when predicting outcomes. Detsky and colleagues felt Goldman's index did not reflect adequately the influence of severity of CAD and modified the index[46]. They and others[29] adjusted the patient's individual risk score for the hospital's average cardiac complication rate for the proposed surgical procedure. This increased the predictive ability but made it slightly more complex to use. However, few high-quality studies have established contemporary complication rates for non-cardiac surgery, and it is unknown whether complication rates at one institution are applicable to others. Kumar et al. in 2001 found five clinical variables were independently associated with adverse cardiac outcomes after non-cardiac surgery: MI within the last 6 months, a remote infarction, emergency surgery, history of congestive HF, and non-sinus rhythm. Lee and colleagues (1999)[34] proposed a revised cardiac risk index (RCRI).

The index was derived in 2893 patients over 50 years of age, scheduled for major surgery, and then verified in a large cohort. Through logistic regression they identified six independent risk factors: high-risk surgery, IHD, congestive HF, cerebrovascular disease, diabetes on insulin, and preoperative serum creatinine >177 µmol L^{-1}. The risk ratios for these factors were similar, therefore risk was reflected by the number of risk factors present. Rates of major cardiac complication with 0, 1, 2, or ≥ 3 of these factors were 0.5%, 1.3%, 4%, and 9%, respectively, in the derivation cohort and similar in the validation cohort. The RCRI outperformed Goldman's and Detsky's indices (area under the receiver operating characteristic curve)[34] and features strongly in the American College of Cardiology/American Heart Association (ACC/AHA) markers of clinical risk[47]. Interestingly, in the RCRI, age, aortic stenosis, and arrhythmia were not independent predictors. This could have reflected patient selection and increased attention to these issues. The authors felt these factors might be important predictors in patients undergoing emergent operations. A problem with all risk indices is poorer

Table 13.3 Active cardiac conditions for which the patient should undergo evaluation and treatment before non-cardiac surgery (Class I, level of evidence: B)

Condition	Examples
Unstable coronary syndromes	Unstable or severe angina (CCS class III or IV)†
	Recent MI‡
Decompensated HF (NYHA functional class IV; worsening or new-onset HF)	
Significant arrhythmias	High-grade atrioventricular block
	Mobitz II atrioventricular block
	Third-degree atrioventricular heart block
	Symptomatic ventricular heart block
	Supraventricular arrhythmias (including atrial fibrillation) with uncontrolled ventricular rate (HR greater than 100 bpm at rest)
	Symptomatic bradycardia
	Newly recognized ventricular tachycardia
Severe valvular disease	Severe aortic stenosis (mean pressure gradient greater than 40 mm Hg, aortic valve area less than 1.0 cm^2, or symptomatic)
	Symptomatic mitral stenosis (progressive dyspnoea on exertion, presyncope, or HF)

CCS indicates Canadian Cardiovascular Society; HF, heart failure; HR, heart rate; MI, myocardial infarction; NYHA, New York Heart Association.

†May include "stable" angina in patients who are unusually sedentary.

‡The American College of Cardiology National Database Library defines recent MI as more than 7 days but less than or equal to 1 month (within 30 days)

Source: From Fleisher, L.A., *et al.* (2007). ACC/AHA 2007 Guidelines on Perioperative Cardiovascular Evaluation and Care for Noncardiac Surgery. *Circulation,* **116**, e418–e499.

performance when used in populations other than in which it was derived. Scoring systems may be specific, but they are not sensitive-with a low predictive accuracy[11,48]. Given the overall low incidence of complications (risk), there are more false positives than true positives, but risk indices remain clinically and epidemiologically useful.

The ACC/AHA algorithm for cardiac risk assessment

The ACC/AHA has recently updated their practice guidelines for perioperative cardio-vascular evaluation and care for non-cardiac surgery[47]. They identified active cardiac conditions which are major predictors of risk and for which the patient should undergo evaluation and treatment before non-cardiac surgery (Table 13.3). The algorithm then takes into account risk of surgery (Table 13.4), whether the patient is able to perform 4 metabolic equivalents (light work around the house like dusting or wash dishes or climb a flight of stairs) without symptoms, and the number of clinical risk factors present (IHD, history of HF, diabetes mellitus, renal insufficiency, and cerebrovascular disease), to help guide which patients ought to undergo further evaluation (provided it will change management) and which patients should proceed to surgery with or without perioperative beta-blockade (Figure 13.1). The previous algorithm was not derived from a prospective study and despite validation[49], there remain questions regarding its predictive ability[11].

What factors determine cardiac risk?

Risk factors are patient, surgery, or anaesthesia related.

Patient factors

Renal failure Cardiovascular complications are common in patients with renal failure, and cardiac death is the main cause of death in the nonsurgical setting. The metabolic

Table 13.4 Cardiac risk* stratification for non-cardiac surgical procedures

Risk stratification	Procedure examples
Vascular (reported cardiac risk often more than 5%)	Aortic and other major vascular surgery
	Peripheral vascular surgery
Intermediate (reported cardiac risk generally 1% to 5%)	Intraperitoneal and intrathoracic surgery
	Carotid endarterectomy
	Head and neck surgery
	Orthopaedic surgery
	Prostate surgery
Low† (reported cardiac risk generally less than 1%)	Endoscopic procedure
	Superficial procedure
	Cataract surgery
	Breast surgery
	Ambulatory surgery

*Combined incidence of cardiac death and nonfatal myocardial infarction.

†These procedures do not generally require further preoperative cardiac testing.

Source: From Fleisher, L.A., et al. (2007). ACC/AHA 2007 Guidelines on Perioperative Cardiovascular Evaluation and Care for Noncardiac Surgery. Circulation, **116**, e418–e499.

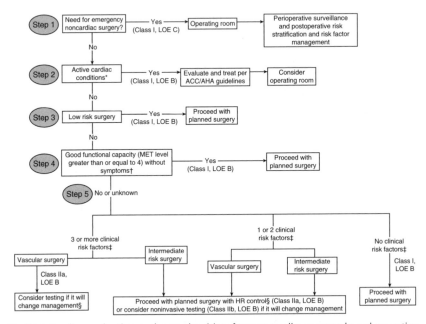

Fig 13.1 Cardiac evaluation and care algorithm for non-cardiac surgery based on active clinical conditions, known cardiovascular disease, or cardiac risk factors for patients 50 years of age or greater. *See Table 2 for active clinical conditions. †See table 3 for estimated MET level equivalent. ‡Clinical risk factors include ischaemic heart disease, compensated or prior HF, diabetes mellitus, renal insufficiency, and cerebrovascular disease, § Consider perioperative beta-blockade (see Table 11) for populations in which this has been shown to reduce cardiac morbidity/mortality. ACC/ACH indicates American College of Cardiology/American Heart Association, HR, heart rate; LOE, level of evidence; and MET, metabolic equivalent.

Source: From Fleisher, L.A., et al. (2007). ACC/AHA 2007 Guidelines on Perioperative Cardiovascular Evaluation and Care for Noncardiac Surgery. *Circulation*, **116**, e418–e499.

milieu in renal failure has a direct relationship with the pathogenesis of atherosclerosis, acute coronary syndromes, HF, and arrhythmias. It is likely that in uraemic patients myocardial ischaemia is more poorly tolerated even in the absence of classical atherosclerosis[50]. This can be explained by structural and metabolic abnormalities of the myocardium, and in part, by alterations of the extracardiac vasculature. Impaired renal function has been shown to be associated with increased cardiac mortality after major[34] and vascular surgery[51] and features as an independent predictor in several cardiac risk indices[34,45,46].

Heart failure Hernandez reviewed the assessment of the HF patient for non-cardiac surgery[37]. Most patients presenting for the first time with HF are already in their seventies, and the prognosis is poor. A third die within one year, and nearly one in two patients are dead by two years[52]. Not surprisingly, patients in HF do less well after surgery. They may not be able to cope with fluid shifts associated with major surgery.

In a large retrospective study, Hernandez reported nearly twice the 30-day mortality rate after major surgery in HF patients compared to controls (11.6% vs. 6.2%), and a readmission rate of 20%[53]. In Goldman's index, signs of HF carried the greatest weight[45]. HF was also recognized as a risk factor in other risk indices[34,35,46]. In one study in particular[35], patients with persistent pulmonary congestion at the time of surgery had a serious cardiac event rate >10%. Preoperative HF predicted MI or cardiac death in patients who underwent vascular surgery (odds ratio >2.7)[54]. In a meta-analysis combining five studies using myocardial perfusion scanning for preoperative risk assessment, HF was the second most important predictor of cardiac events behind reversible perfusion defect (odds ratio 3.6; $P < 0.001$)[55]. In a case-controlled study by Howell et al. in 1999, the only significant risk factor for cardiac death within 30 days of emergency surgery was a history of HF (odds ratio 14.8; 95% CI 2.5–87)[56]. The reason that HF is absent in some models[57] may be that HT and IHD accounted for most cases and these factors were included in the models. Published studies differ in their criteria for diagnosing HF preoperatively. Some rely on history, some on radiological evidence of pulmonary oedema, and others on clinical signs for which there is known interobserver variability[46]. B-type natriuretic peptide may aid in the diagnosis, but is not routinely measured. It is mainly excreted by the ventricles, and is elevated in patients with cardiac disease, and in particular HF. In a prospective study in 204 patients, a preoperative B-type natriuretic peptide level >40 pg ml^{-1} predicted a 7-fold increase in the risk of perioperative cardiac events[58]. The presence of dyspnoea or fatigue in a patient with structural/functional heart disease with or without fluid overload confirms new or worsening HF[59]. If possible, surgery should be postponed until the patient has been adequately evaluated and treatment stabilized[47]. Revascularization and or valve surgery may be indicated. Patients with CAD and impaired LV function are to gain most from revascularization; however, evidence lacks to support preoperative revascularization other than on its own merit. The mainstay of perioperative care is thus to continue anti-failure treatment and consider perioperative beta-blockers[37].

Cerebrovascular disease Stroke and MI share common risk factors and pathological mechanisms, and IHD is an important cause of death in patients with cerebrovascular disease. Approximately 2 to 5% of all stroke patients die from cardiac causes in the first few months after ischaemic stroke[60]. The 5-year risk of MI or fatal cardiac event after stroke is 8.6%[61]. Autonomic and neurohumoral dysfunction may also contribute to cardiac risk in acute stroke populations. Lee and colleagues found a history of stroke and transient ischaemic attack to be independent predictors of perioperative cardiac risk (odds ratio 2.9 and 4.7, respectively)[34].

IHD Detsky added angina at minimal exertion, unstable angina within 6 months, and a history of MI (weighted more heavily if more recent) to their risk index to reflect the importance of severity of IHD[46]. The RCRI found history of IHD to be an independent risk factor with odds ratio 2.4 (95% CI 1.3–4.2)[34]. Ashton and co-workers classified 1487 men >40 years of age, for major surgery, into separate groups, according to their risk for postoperative MI[28]. The high-risk group had a history or ECG evidence of MI, angina, abnormal angiogram, or previous coronary bypass. Just over 4% had an MI, and 2.3%, a cardiac-related death. In contrast, the lesser-risk group had postoperative adverse event rates <1%. Initial findings from the 1986 coronary artery surgery study (CASS) register were that serious cardiac event rates in patients, who remained asymptomatic after coronary bypass surgery, were low and were similar to those among patients without CAD[24]. Ten years on, further data showed non-cardiac surgery involving the thorax, abdomen, vasculature, and head and neck were associated with the highest cardiac risk in patients with known CAD. Prior coronary bypass surgery seemed to reduce risk among patients who had subsequent high-risk surgery, but low-risk surgery yielded good outcomes (risk<1%), regardless of coronary management[62]. The cumulative mortality and morbidity of both the coronary revascularization procedure and the non-cardiac surgery should be weighed carefully when deciding on the best course of action. McFalls and colleagues prospectively investigated the effect of preoperative coronary revascularization (percutaneous coronary intervention or bypass surgery) on long-term outcome in 510 patients undergoing vascular surgery[63]. Patients with severe CAD, poor LV function, or severe aortic stenosis were excluded from randomization. Similar proportions in both groups (11.6% revascularized patients vs. 14.3% of control patients; $P=0.37$) had postoperative MI. At a median follow-up time of 2.7 years, there was no difference in mortality between the groups (22% and 23%, respectively). The results suggested that in patients with stable CAD and normal LV function, prophylactic coronary revascularization before vascular surgery does not improve long-term outcome over good medical therapy[63]. A similar lack of benefit of preoperative revascularization, over best medical management, was found by Poldermans who randomized 101 high-risk patients scheduled for vascular surgery and found to have extensive myocardial ischaemia on stress testing[64]. The outcome of 30-day all-cause death or non-fatal MI after subsequent vascular surgery was similar between the revascularized and medically managed patients at 43% vs. 33% (odds ratio 1.4, 95% CI 0.7–2.8, $P=0.30$), respectively. The indications for preoperative surgical coronary revascularization are essentially identical to those in the non-operative setting[65] and should be recommended on merit rather the fact that an individual is scheduled for non-cardiac surgery. The decision to perform revascularization on a patient before non-cardiac surgery to "get them through" the non-cardiac procedure is appropriate only in a small subset of very-high-risk patients when long-term outcomes are included[47]. Bodenheimer argues that, apart from patients with features consistent with plaque rupture, improved outcomes are more likely to result from limiting oxygen demand after surgery rather than from further investigations[66].

Arrhythmia There is little evidence that preoperative arrhythmia in the absence of IHD and HF adds to cardiac risk. In a prospective study of at-risk patients, preoperative arrhythmias were associated with intraoperative and postoperative arrhythmias but did not predict a higher rate of serious cardiac events[41]. Goldman[45], Detsky[46], and Kumar[29] all found any rhythm other than sinus predictive of risk but Lee[34] and Larsen[35] did not.

Valvular heart disease Aortic stenosis is a progressive disease, and the risk of sudden death increases once symptoms are present. The increased risk of surgery in patients with aortic stenosis has long been recognized[45,46]. Systolic function is often preserved early on but diastolic dysfunction may be a consequence of hypertrophy, and myocardial oxygen supply: demand ratio may be precariously balanced. Patients with aortic stenosis tend to tolerate hypovolaemia, fall in afterload, and atrial fibrillation poorly. In one study, those with significant aortic or mitral valve disease were twice as likely to have a MI (Cl 1.1–3.9) after major vascular surgery[22]. Raymer and Yang found no increase in cardiac risk in 55 patients with aortic stenosis compared to controls[67]. Their sample size was adequate to detect a fourfold increase in risk. However, Kertai, in a larger retrospective case-matched study in 2004, found the chance of MI or death from any cause within 30 days after non-cardiac surgery in patients with severe aortic stenosis rose just over fivefold (CI 1.6–17.0)[68]. In most asymptomatic patients, the risk of aortic valve surgery is greater than the risk of watchful waiting[69]. Symptomatic patients with severe stenosis (calculated valve area <1cm^2 or peak gradient >64 mmHg) ought to be referred for valve surgery prior to elective surgery. It is not uncommon for patients to decrease their activity level below their symptom threshold, and the skill is to ascertain which patients are in fact symptomatic[69]. In the absence of good evidence, prophylactic aortic valve replacement in asymptomatic patients is not recommended.

Age Age demonstrates the relationship between various risk factors clearly. Every risk factor mentioned earlier is more prevalent in the elderly. The incidence of HF, one of the most consistent markers of poor outcome, rises sharply in those >65 years of age and again in those >75 years of age[31]. Advanced age predicted cardiac risk in some studies[24,27,45,54,70] but was only a univariate factor in others[34]. One large prospective cohort study in men found age >75 years of age to be independently associated with postoperative MI (odds ratio 4.8; CI 1.2–19.4)[27]. The risk of death from a perioperative MI is higher with advanced age. In contrast, in a retrospective study, Bai[71] concluded ageing had no influence on perioperative cardiac risk in patients without evidence of MI or ischaemia diagnosed on preoperative stress testing. Other authors have reported that advanced age was not an independent predictor of perioperative outcome[29,72,73]. The most relevant age-related cardiovascular changes are atherosclerosis, systolic and diastolic dysfunction, rigid vasculature, blunted beta-adrenoceptor responsiveness, and impaired autonomic function[2]. These may not matter at rest, but affect the ability to cope with superimposed cardiovascular stress. The elderly are more sensitive to propofol and protein-bound drugs (low albumin) and tend to have more labile perioperative blood pressure. Hypotension on induction of anaesthesia is more common and severe in the elderly because the effects of the anaesthetics are superimposed on impaired cardiovascular compensatory mechanisms[2]. Atrial fibrillation is less well tolerated because of greater reliance on late diastolic LV filling. On balance it appears that age increases the risk of perioperative cardiac risk, independent of the association with CAD and HF. High perioperative risk takes on special significance in someone whose life expectancy may be limited.

Diabetes Diabetes, with or without co-morbid heart disease, is associated with a high prevalence of cardiac risk factors. Cardiovascular risk factors in diabetes include HT, dyslipidaemia, hyperglycaemia, insulin resistance, oxidative/glycoxidative stress, inflammation, endothelial dysfunction, a procoagulant state, and myocardial fibrosis[74]. Vascular, myopathic, and neuropathic alterations may all contribute to the excessive cardiovascular morbidity and mortality. To determine the relationship between pre-operative glucose levels and perioperative mortality in non-cardiac surgery, Noordzij conducted a case-control study in a cohort of over 100 000 patients of whom 989 died within 30 days of surgery[75]. A cardiovascular complication was the primary cause of death in 23%. Elevated preoperative glucose concentrations (>11 mmol L^{-1}) were associated with a 2.1-fold increased risk (95% CI 1.3–3.5; $P<0.001$) of death within 30 days. Lee et al. found a threefold increase (95% CI 1.3–7.1) in perioperative cardiac risk in insulin-treated diabetics [34]. Improved glucose control translates into better cardiovascular outcomes for patients with diabetes in the non-operative setting.

Hypertension Preoperative HT was associated with arrhythmia, myocardial ischaemia, and a labile blood pressure perioperatively[76,77] and Browner[72] and Howell[57] found an association with death, the latter only borderline. However, numerous studies have shown that mild or moderate HT (systolic blood pressure <180 mm Hg and diastolic blood pressure <110 mm Hg) was not an independent risk factor for perioperative car-diovascular complications[47]. There is a marked increase in cardiovascular complica-tions in non-surgical patients with severe HT; however, advice to postpone elective surgery in this subgroup is not based on perioperative evidence[78]. Weksler (2003) randomized patients with a history of HT without other cardiac disease and who had a diastolic blood pressure of 110 to 130 mm Hg preoperatively to postponement of surgery until blood pressure was controlled or to proceeding with surgery after 10 mg intranasal nifedipine; neither group had any postoperative cardiac complications or strokes[79].

Anaemia Perioperative anaemia is a marker of poor outcome but anaemia may only be a surrogate for bleeding and complex surgery. A postoperative haematocrit below 28% was associated with myocardial ischaemia after radical prostatectomy[80] and serious cardiac events after vascular surgery[81]. A low preoperative haemoglobin or a substantial operative blood loss increases the risk of death or serious morbidity more in patients with cardiovascular disease than in those without[82]. However, evidence to demonstrate that perioperative transfusion for anaemia improves outcomes is lacking (see Chapter 14).

Smoking Smoking is a major risk factor for IHD and peripheral vascular disease. Smoking increases myocardial work by increasing heart rate, blood pressure, and myo-cardial contractility. However, it is not clear whether status as an active smoker itself increases the perioperative risk of cardiac events. Most studies have been unable to iden-tify preoperative smoking status as an independent risk factor for major cardiac events.

Pulmonary hypertension Right HF, persistent postoperative hypoxia, and coronary ischaemia are among the potential perioperative complications in patients with pul-monary HT[83]. 12% of patients with systolic pulmonary artery pressures >35 mm Hg who underwent non-cardiac surgery developed significant dysrhythmias or conduc-tion defects and 11% had HF within 30 days. The mortality rate in these patients was 7%. Outcome was worse if pulmonary arterial pressure exceeded two-thirds of sys-temic pressure. Compared with case-matched controls, patients with pulmonary HT were significantly more likely to suffer postoperative HF and in-hospital death[84]. Patients with congenital heart disease are more likely to suffer cardiac complications;

however, they are diverse group, and estimates of risk should be based on the underlying defect, functional reserve, presence of pulmonary HT, and whether palliative or corrective surgery has been performed.

Functional capacity and stress testing Exercise and pharmacological stress testing provide excellent negative predictive values (between 90% and 100%) of cardiac risk but, due to the overall low adverse event rate, poor positive predictive values. Patients with good functional capacity in daily life had very low rates of perioperative cardiac complications[85]. Patients reporting poor exercise tolerance had almost double the incidence of cardiovascular complications (9.6 vs. 5.2%, $P=0.04$) after major surgery[73]. Poor exercise tolerance predicted risk for serious complications, independently of all other patient characteristics, including age (OR 1.9; 95% Cl 1.2–3.2)[73]. The risk of perioperative cardiac events and long-term risks are increased significantly in patients with an abnormal exercise ECG at low workloads[47]. This is the premise on which further testing is based. Patients who were able to raise their heart rate with exercise had a lower risk of complications than patients who could not[86]. For patients who cannot exercise, dobutamine stress echocardiography has become the method of choice. The predictive value of a positive test ranges from 0% to 33% for serious cardiac events. The negative predictive value ranges from 93% to 100%. In the series by Poldermans in 1995[87], a new wall-motion abnormality was a strong predictor for perioperative events. The negative predictive value of a normal stress nuclear myocardial perfusion scan is approximately 99% for MI or cardiac death[47]. However, because of the overall low positive predictive value, it is best used selectively in patients with a high clinical risk of perioperative cardiac events. Using formal cardiopulmonary exercise testing, Older and colleagues[88] demonstrated a clear relationship between preoperative functional reserve, defined by anaerobic threshold, and operative risk. They evaluated patients over 60 years of age before major abdominal surgery. Of 55 patients with anaerobic threshold <11 ml min^{-1} kg^{-1}, 18% died. Only one patient out of 132 with an anaerobic threshold >11 ml min^{-1} kg^{-1}, died ($P < 0.001$). If a low anaerobic threshold was associated with myocardial ischaemia, then the specificity increased, with death in 8 of 19 patients (42%).

Other measures of risk There is a strong association between compromised autonomic nervous function and sudden cardiac death. Heart rate variability measures are widely used to measure alterations in the autonomic nervous system[89]. Studies have shown that decreased heart rate variability can independently predict postoperative long-term mortality, but more studies are needed to establish its role in clinical practice.

Beta-blockers, angiotensin-converting enzyme inhibitors, statins, and aspirin There is very little evidence regarding the use of beta-blockers in low cardiac risk patients. Fleisher and others[90] reviewed the literature on behalf of the AHA and ACC. The majority of evidence suggested a benefit in high-risk patients where beta-blockers may reduce the risk of death and perioperative MI. Therapy should be started days or weeks before elective surgery to aim for a resting heart rate of 50 to 60 beats per min. Beta-blockade should continue into the postoperative period to limit the heart rate to 80 beats per min. Patients taking beta-blockers should continue them up to the day of surgery. The same has not been established for angiotensin-converting enzyme inhibitors, which are integral to treating patients with HT and HF. Angiotensin-converting enzyme inhibitors disable the renin–angiotensin system, and thereby the ability to compensate for reduced sympathetic tone. The induction of anaesthesia may cause severe hypotension, especially in hypovolaemic patients. Several retrospective and prospective studies have shown that statins reduce short- and long-term risk of perioperative cardiac events. The effects are greatest on long-term mortality (>4 years) and in the highest risk (e.g. vascular) patients[91,92]. Patients already receiving statins should continue to take them, and those with established or suspected coronary artery disease undergoing vascular surgery should probably receive statins, but there is insufficient evidence to suggest their routine perioperative use. Extrapolating results from trials on coronary bypass surgery, secondary prevention of CAD and percutaneous coronary intervention, where aspirin nonadherence/withdrawal was associated with three-fold higher risk of major adverse cardiac events[93], Chassot *et al.* recommend antiplatelet medicines should be continued during the perioperative period, except before neurosurgery[94]. For the same reasons, the risk–benefit ratio of preoperative withdrawal of antiplatelet drugs in order to perform neuraxial blockade is not justified.

Surgical factors

Type of surgery The ACC/AHA guidelines[47] stratify risk for cardiac death and nonfatal MI in non-cardiac surgical procedures as high (>5%), intermediate (1–5%), or low (<1%) (Table 13.4). Vascular surgery is consistently associated with high cardiac risk due to high prevalence of IHD and risk factors for IHD and high incidence of non-cardiac complications. Thoracic and major abdominal surgery also carry increased cardiac risks due to prolonged recovery, association with hypoxaemia, and fluid shifts. Minimally invasive techniques may pose a lower cardiovascular risk because of lesser physiological stress and fewer medical complications that may lead to cardiac events, but to what degree is not yet clear[6,95]. Detsky *et al.* reported a postoperative MI rate of 4.8% in patients undergoing major procedures and 0.5% in patients undergoing minor procedures[46]. Warner and colleagues reported a very low rate of myocardial infarction (0.03%) in over 38 000 patients undergoing ambulatory procedures[96]. Several workers have constructed a nomogram to allow estimation of an individual patient's risk for a specific surgical procedure[29,46,54]. The duration of surgery *per se* is not a factor, but longer surgery can be associated with more blood loss or indicate complications.

Urgency of surgery The likelihood of cardiac complications after urgent surgery is more than double[25]. The urgency of surgery sometimes dictates that co-morbidity cannot be adequately addressed or managed. Urgent surgery also increases non-cardiac complications that place added stress on the heart. As many as one-third of surgical procedures are in high-risk populations, such as patients with vascular disease, are performed on an urgent basis[97].

Perioperative factors

Anaesthetic technique

Volatile anaesthetics increase coronary blood flow, reduce myocardial contractility, and reduce afterload. However, as previously mentioned, they may be cardioprotective independently from these actions. Halogenated volatile anaesthetics have a precondi-tioning-like effect, resulting in protection against MI and irreversible myocardial dysfunction. They may also protect against reperfusion injury when administered after the ischaemic insult. Up to now, most clinical studies involved patients undergoing cardiac surgery. Two meta-analyses concluded that there is only some protection with respect to cardiac function and troponin release but no evidence of reduced serious cardiac risk[3,98]. A large retrospective study of over 10 000 consecutive patients under-going single cardiac procedures found patients with preoperative acute coronary syndrome, and thus already preconditioned, did not show any difference in mortality between anaesthetic groups, whereas patients without these predictors showed a lower postoperative mortality after sevoflurane (2.28% v 3.14%, $P = 0.015$)[99]. This could at least partly be explained by a preconditioning-like effect. It is also thought that propofol exerts some protection through its anti-oxidant properties.

Neuraxial anaesthesia

No single randomized trial has shown that postoperative epidural analgesia decreases postoperative MI or death. Because of the low incidence of these complications, indi-vidual studies have been underpowered to show a benefit. Rodgers and colleagues[100] performed a meta-analysis of 141 trials including 9559 patients. Overall mortality was reduced by about one third in patients allocated to neuraxial blockade (2.1% vs 3.1%, odds ratio 0.70, 95% CI 0.54–0.90, $P = 0.006$). Postoperative MI was also reduced by one third. It is thought that the benefits were due to reduction in the surgical stress response. In the subsequent multicentre MASTER trial, adverse outcomes were com-pared in 915 high-risk patients for major surgery under general anaesthesia[101]. There was no difference in 30-day mortality or cardiac risk between patients randomized to the epidural group (intraoperative epidural continued for 72 h) or the control group, who mainly received opioids. A more recent meta-analysis[102] of 11 randomized trials found that there is still insufficient evidence to conclude whether epidural analgesia reduces cardiovascular complications. The greatest potential appears to be with major vascular surgery and in high-risk patients; however, this may become less relevant due to rapid employment of minimally invasive surgical techniques[95].

Perioperative haemodynamic parameters

Intraoperative ischaemia has been reported to predict adverse outcome but less so than ischaemia pre- or postoperatively[19,44]. Postoperative ischaemia is associated with higher risk for later cardiac events[6]. In Mangano's study (1991), all the serious cardiac events noted were preceded by myocardial ischaemia ≥ 24 h before the event[18]. Tachycardia is often a precursor to ischaemia[80,18]. Perioperative hypotension may result in myocardial ischaemia. Charlson and colleagues demonstrated that a decrease of mean arterial pressure >20 mmHg increased postoperative cardiac complications[103].

Level of care

Work by Rao[21] indicated better outcome with close monitoring and high-level post-operative care, although this was not replicated in later studies. Excellent surgical, anaesthetic, and postoperative care may result in a more favourable outcome even in those with high risk. Story and colleagues demonstrated improved postoperative mortality in high-risk surgery after introducing an Anaesthesia Department-led critical care outreach service but this is not the conclusion from other studies[104]. The demand for critical care beds usually outstrips the supply, and resources are usually allocated on the basis of availability, risk factors, and urgency of surgery. The quality of care is probably as relevant, if not more so, than the clinical area in which such care is delivered.

References

1. Buhre, W. and Hoeft, A. (2000). Anaesthesia and the cardiovascular system. In *Cardiovascular Physiology* (H.J. Priebe and K. Skarvan eds.), pp. 331–73, 2nd edition. BMJ Publishing Group, London.

2. Priebe, H.J. (2000). The aged cardiovascular risk patient. *British Journal of Anaesthesia*, **85**, 763–78.

3. Symons, J.A. and Myles, P.S. (2006). Myocardial protection with volatile anaesthetic agents during coronary artery bypass surgery: a meta-analysis. *British Journal of Anaesthesia*, **97**, 127–36.

4. Lee, T.H. and Goldman, L. (1988). The coronary care unit turns 25: Historical trends and future directions. *Annals of Internal Medicine*,**108**, 887–94.

5. Mangano, D.T. and Goldman, L. (1995). Preoperative assessment of patients with known or suspected coronary disease. *New England Journal of Medicine*, **333**, 1750–6.

6. Auerbach, A.D. and Goldman, L. (2006). Assessing and reducing the cardiac risk of noncardiac surgery. *Circulation*, **113**, 1361–76.

7. Lagasse, R.S. (2002). Anesthesia safety: Model or myth? A review of the published literature and analysis of current original data. *Anesthesiology*, **97**, 1609–17.

8. Arbous, M.S., Grobbee, D.E., van Kleef, J.W., *et al.* (2001). Mortality associated with anaesthesia: A qualitative analysis to identify risk factors. *Anaesthesia*, **56**, 1141–53.

9. Sprung, J., Warner, M.E., Contreras, M.G., *et al.* (2003). Predictors of survival following cardiac arrest in patients undergoing noncardiac surgery: a study of 518 294 patients at a tertiary referral center. *Anesthesiology*, **99**, 259–69.

10. Lunn, J.N. and Devlin, H.B. (1987). Lessons from the confidential enquiry into perioperative deaths in three NHS regions. *Lancet*, **2**,1384–6.

11. Devereaux, P.J., Goldman, L., Cook, D.J., *et al.* (2005). Perioperative cardiac events in patients undergoing noncardiac surgery: a review of the magnitude of the problem, the pathophysiology of the events and methods to estimate and communicate risk. *Canadian Medical Association Journal*, **173**, 627–34.

12. Tabib, A., Loire, R., Miras, A., *et al.* (2000). Unsuspected cardiac lesions associated with sudden unexpected perioperative death. *European Journal of Anaesthesiology*, **17**, 230–5.

13. Charlson, M., Peterson, J., Szatrowski, T.P., MacKenzie, R., and Gold, J. (1994). Long-term prognosis after peri-operative cardiac complications. *Journal of Clinical Epidemiology*, **47**, 1389–400.

14. Landesberg, G. (2003). The pathophysiology of perioperative myocardial infarction: facts and perspectives. *Journal of Cardiothoracic and Vascular Anesthesia*, **17**, 90–100.

15. Cohen, M.C. and Aretz, T.H. (1999). Histological analysis of coronary artery lesions in fatal postoperative myocardial infarction. *Cardiovascular Pathology*, **8**, 133–9.

16. Dawood, M., Gupta, D.K., Southern, J., *et al.* (1996). Pathology of fatal perioperative myocardial infarction: Implications regarding pathophysiology and prevention. *International Journal of Cardiology*, **57**, 37–44.

17. Priebe, H.J. (2004). Triggers of perioperative myocardial ischaemia and infarction. *British Journal of Anaesthesia*, **93**, 9–20.

18. Mangano, D.T., Wong, M.G., London, M.J., Tubau, J.F., and Rapp, J.A., and the Study of Perioperative Ischemia Research Group. (1991). Perioperative myocardial ischemia in patients undergoing noncardiac surgery-II: Incidence and severity during the 1st week after surgery. *Journal of the American College of Cardiology*, **17**, 851–7.

19. Mangano, D.T., Browner, W.S., Hollenberg, M., London, M.J., Tubau, J.F., and Tateo, I.M. (1990). Association of perioperative myocardial ischemia with cardiac morbidity and mortality in men undergoing noncardiac surgery. *New England Journal of Medicine*, **323**, 1781–8.

20. Tarhan, S., Moffitt, E.A., Taylor, W.F., and Guiliani, E.R. (1972). Myocardial infarction after general anesthesia. *Journal of the American Medical Association*, **220**, 1451–4.

21. Rao, T.L., Jacobs, K.H., and EI-Etr, A.A. (1983). Reinfarction following anesthesia in patients with myocardial infarction. *Anesthesiology*, **59**, 499–505.

22. Sprung, J., Abdelmalak, B., Gottlieb, A., *et al.* (2000). Analysis of risk factors for myocardial infarction and cardiac mortality after major vascular surgery. *Anesthesiology*, **93**, 129–40.

23. Badner, N.H., Knill, R.L., Brown, J.E., Novick, T.V., and Gelb, A.W. (1998). Myocardial infarction after noncardiac surgery. *Anesthesiology*, **88**, 572–8.

24. Foster, E.D., Davis, K.B., Carpenter, J.A., Abele, S., and Fray, D. (1986). Risk of noncardiac operations in patients with coronary disease. The Coronary Artery Surgery Study (CASS) registry experience. *Annals of Thoracic Surgery*, **41**, 42–9.

25. Mangano, D.T. (1990). Perioperative cardiac morbidity. *Anesthesiology*, **72**, 53–84.

26. Alpert, J.S. and Thygesen, K. (2000). Myocardial infarction redefined—A consensus document of The Joint European Society of Cardiology/American College of Cardiology Committee for the Redefinition of Myocardial Infarction. *European Heart Journal*, **21**, 1502–13.

27. Mangano, D.T. (1998). Adverse outcomes after surgery in the year 2001 – a continuing odyssey. *Anesthesiology*, **88**, 561–4.

28. Ashton, C.M., Petersen, N.J., Wray, N.P., *et al.* (1993). The incidence of perioperative myocardial infarction in men undergoing noncardiac surgery. *Annals of Internal Medicine*, **118**, 504–10.

29. Kumar, R., McKinney, W.P., Raj, G., *et al.* (2001). Adverse cardiac events after surgery-assessing risk in a veteran population. *Journal of General Internal Medicine*, **16**, 507–18.

30. Mangano, D.T., Browner, W.S., Hollenberg, M., *et al.* (1992) for the Study of Perioperative Ischemia Research Group. Long-term cardiac prognosis following noncardiac surgery. *Journal of the American Medical Association*, **268**, 233–9.

31. Cowie, M.R., Wood, D.A., Coats, A.J.S., *et al.* (1999). Incidence and aetiology of heart failure. A population-based study. *European Heart Journal*, **20**, 421–8.

32. Udelsman, R., Norton, J.A., Jelenich, S.E., *et al.* (1987). Responses of the hypothalamic-pituitary-adrenal and renin-angiotensin axes and the sympathetic system during controlled surgical and anesthetic stress. *Journal of Clinical Endocrinology and Metabolism*, **64**, 986–94.

33. Weitz, H.H. (2001). Perioperative cardiac complications. *The Medical Clinics of North America*, **85**, 1151–69.

34. Lee, T.H., Marcantonio, E.R., Mangione, C.M., *et al.* (1999). Derivation and prospective validation of a simple index for prediction of cardiac risk of major noncardiac surgery. *Circulation*, **100**, 1043–9.

35. Larsen, S.F., Olesen, K.H., Jacobsen, E., *et al.* (1987). Prediction of cardiac risk in non-cardiac surgery. *European Heart Journal*, **8**, 179–85.

36. Charlson, M.E., MacKenzie, C.R., Gold, J.P., Ales, K.L., Topkins, M., and Shires, G.T. (1991). Risk for postoperative congestive heart failure. *Surgical Gynecology and Obstetrics*, **172**, 95–104.

37. Hernandez, A.F., Newby, L.K., and O'Connor, C.M. (2004). Preoperative evaluation for major noncardiac surgery focusing on heart failure. *Archives of Internal Medicine*, **164**, 1729–36.

38. Polanczyk, C.A., Goldman, L., Marcantonio, E.R., Orav, E.J., and Lee, T.H. (1998). Supraventricular arrhythmia in patients having noncardiac surgery: clinical correlates and effect on length of stay. *Annals of Internal Medicine*, **129**, 279–85.

39. Mahla, E., Rotman, B., Rehak, P., *et al.* (1998). Perioperative ventricular dysrhythmias in patients with structural heart disease undergoing noncardiac surgery. *Anesthesia and Analgesia*, **86**, 16–21.

40. Amar, D., Zhang, H., and Roistacher, N. (2002). The incidence and outcome of ventricular arrhythmias after noncardiac thoracic surgery. *Anesthesia and Analgesia*, **95**, 537–43.

41. O'Kelly, B., Browner, W.S., Massie, B., *et al.* (1992). Ventricular arrhythmias in patients undergoing noncardiac surgery. The study of perioperative ischaemia research group. *Journal of the American Medical Association*, **268**, 217–21.

42. Waldo, A.L., Henthorn, R.W., Epstein, A.E., and Plumb, V.J. (1984). Diagnosis and treatment of arrhythmias during and following open heart surgery. *Medical Clinics of North America*, **68**, 1153–70.

43. Sloan, S.B. and Weitz, H.H. (2001). Postoperative arrhythmias and conduction disorders. *The Medical clinics of North America*, **85**, 1171–89.

44. Raby, K.E., Goldman, L., Creager, M.A., *et al.* (1989). Correlation between preoperative ischemia and major cardiac events after peripheral vascular surgery. *New England Journal of Medicine*, **321**, 1296–300.

45. Goldman, L., Caldera, D.L., Nussbaum, S.R., *et al.* (1977). Multifactorial index of cardiac risk in noncardiac surgical procedures. *New England Journal of Medicine*, **297**, 845–50.

46. Detsky, A.S., Abrams, H.B., McLaughlin, J.R., *et al.* (1986). Predicting cardiac complications in patients undergoing non-cardiac surgery. *Journal of General Internal Medicine*, **1**, 211–9.

47. Fleisher, L.A., Beckman, J.A., Brown, K.A., *et al.* (2007). ACC/AHA 2007 Guidelines on perioperative cardiovascular evaluation and care for noncardiac surgery: A Report of the American College of Cardiology/American Heart Association Task Force on Practice Guidelines. *Circulation*, **116**, e418–e499.

48. Mantha, S., Roizen, M.F., Barnard, J., Thisted, R.A., Ellis, J.E., and Foss, J. (1994). Relative effectiveness of four preoperative tests for predicting adverse cardiac outcomes after vascular surgery: a meta-analysis. *Anesthesia and Analgesia*, **79**, 422–33.

49. Ali, M.J., Davison, P., Pickett, W., and Ali, N.S. (2000). ACC/AHA guidelines as predictors of postoperative cardiac outcomes. *Canadian Journal of Anaesthesia*, **47**, 10–19.

50. Tyralla, K. and Amann, K. (2003). Morphology of the heart and arteries in renal failure. *Kidney International*, **84**, S80–3.

51. Kertai, M.D., Boersma, E., Bax, J.J., *et al.* (2003). Comparison between serum creatinine and creatinine clearance for the prediction of postoperative mortality in patients undergoing major vascular surgery. *Clinical Nephrology*, **59**, 17–23.

52. Cowie, M.R., Wood, D.A., Coates, A.J.S., *et al.* (2000). Survival of patients with a new diagnosis of heart failure: a population based study. *Heart*, **83**, 505–10.

53. Hernandez, A.F., Whellan, D.J., Stroud, S., Sun, J.L., O'Connor, C.M., and Jollis, J.G. (2004). Outcomes in heart failure patients after major noncardiac surgery. *Journal of the American College of Cardiology*, **44**, 1446–53.

54. L'Italien, G.J., Paul, S.D., Hendel, R.C., *et al.* (1996). Development and validation of a Bayesian model for perioperative cardiac risk assessment in a cohort of 1,081 vascular surgical candidates. *Journal of the American College of Cardiology*, **27**, 779–86.

55. Shaw, L.J., Eagle, K.A., Gersh, B.J., and Miller, D.D. (1996). Meta-analysis of intravenous dipyridamole-thallium-201 imaging (1985 to 1994) and dobutamine echocardiography (1991 to 1994) for risk stratification before vascular surgery. *Journal of the American College of Cardiology*, **27**, 787–98.

56. Howell, S.J., Sear, J.W., Sear, Y.M., Yeates, D., Goldacre, M., and Foëx, P. (1999). Risk factors for cardiovascular death within 30 days after anaesthesia and urgent or emergency anaesthesia: a nested case-control study. *British Journal of Anaesthesia*, **82**, 679–84.

57. Howell, S.J., Sear, Y.M., Yeates, D., Goldacre, M., Sear, J.W., and Foëx, P. (1998). Risk factors for cardiovascular death after elective surgery under general anaesthesia. *British Journal of Anaesthesia*, **80**, 14–9.

58. Cuthbertson, B.H., Amiri, A.R., Croal, B.L., *et al.* (2007). Utility of B-type natriuretic peptide in predicting perioperative cardiac events in patients undergoing major non-cardiac surgery. *British Journal of Anaesthesia*, **99**, 170–6.

59. ACC/AHA 2005 Guideline Update for the Diagnosis and Management of Chronic Heart Failure in the Adult. (2005). *Journal of the American College of Cardiology*, **46**, 1116–43.

60. Adams, R.J., Chimowitz, M.I., Alpert, J.S., *et al.* (2003). Coronary risk evaluation in patients with transient ischemic attack and ischemic stroke: a scientific statement for healthcare professionals from the Stroke Council and the Council on Clinical Cardiology of the American Heart Association/American Stroke Association. *Stroke*, **34**, 2310–22.

61. Dhamoon, M.S., Sciacca, R.R., Rundek, T., Sacco, R.L., and Elkind, M.S.V. (2006). Recurrent stroke and cardiac risks after first ischemic stroke: the Northern Manhattan Study. *Neurology*, **66**, 641–6.

62. Eagle, K.A., Rihal, C.S., Mickel, M.C., *et al.* (1997). Cardiac risk of noncardiac surgery. Influence of Coronary Disease and Type of Surgery in 3368 Operations. *Circulation*, **96**, 1882–7.

63. McFalls, E.O., Ward, H.B., Moritz, T.E., *et al.* (2004). Coronary-artery revascularization before elective major vascular surgery. *New England Journal of Medicine*, **351**, 2795–804.

64. Poldermans, D., Schouten, O., Vidakovic, R., *et al.* (2007). A clinical randomized trial to evaluate the safety of a noninvasive approach in high-risk patients undergoing major vascular surgery: the DECREASE-V Pilot Study. *Journal of the American College of Cardiology*, **49**, 1763–9.

65. Eagle, K.A., Guyton, R.A., Davidoff, R., *et al.* (2004). ACC/AHA 2004 guideline update for coronary artery bypass graft surgery: a report of the American College of Cardiology/American Heart Association Task Force on Practice Guidelines (Committee to Update the 1999 Guidelines for Coronary Artery Bypass Graft Surgery). *Circulation*, **110**, e340–e437.

66. Bodenheimer, M.M. (1996). Noncardiac surgery in the cardiac patient: what is the question? *Annals of Internal Medicine*, **124**, 763–6.

67. Raymer, K. and Yang, H. (1998). Patients with aortic stenosis: cardiac complications in non-cardiac surgery. *Canadian Journal of Anaesthesia*, **45**, 855–9.

68. Kertai, M.D., Bountioukos, M., Boersma, E., *et al.* (2004). Aortic stenosis: an underestimated risk factor for perioperative complications in patients undergoing noncardiac surgery. *American Journal of Medicine*, **116**, 8–13.

69. Otto, C.M. (2006). Valvular aortic stenosis: disease severity and timing of intervention. *Journal of the American College of Cardiology*, **47**, 2141–51.

70. Shah, K.B., Kleinman, B.S., Rao, T.L.K., *et al.* (1990). Angina and other risk factors in patients with cardiac diseases undergoing noncardiac operation. *Anesthesia and Analgesia*, **70**, 240–7.

71. Bai, J., Hashimoto, J., Nakahara, T., Suzuki, T., and Kubo, A. (2007). Influence of ageing on perioperative cardiac risk in non-cardiac surgery. *Age and Ageing*, **36**, 68–72.

72. Browner, W.S., Li, J., Mangano, D.T., *et al.* (1992) for the Study of Perioperative Ischemia Research Group. In-hospital and long-term mortality in male veterans following non-cardiac surgery. *Journal of the American Medical Association*, **268**, 228–32.

73. Reilly, D.F., McNeely, M.J., Doerner, D., *et al.* (1999). Self-reported exercise tolerance and the risk of serious perioperative complications. *Archives of Internal Medicine*, **159**, 2185–92.

74. Candido, R., Srivastava, P., Cooper, M.E., and Burrell, L.M. (2003). Diabetes mellitus: a cardiovascular disease. *Current Opinion in Investigational Drugs*, **4**, 1088–94.

75. Noordzij, P.G., Boersma, E., Schreiner, F., *et al.* (2007). Increased preoperative glucose levels are associated with perioperative mortality in patients undergoing noncardiac, nonvascular surgery. *European Journal of Endocrinology*, **156**, 137–42.

76. Forrest, J.B., Rehder, K., Goldsmith, C.H., *et al.* (1990). Multicenter study of general anesthesia. I. Design and patients demography. *Anesthesiology*, **72**, 252–61.

77. Prys-Roberts, C., Meloche, R., and Foex, P. (1971). Studies of anaesthesia in relation to hypertension. I. Cardiovascular responses of treated and untreated patients. *British Journal of Anaesthesia*, **43**, 122–37.

78. Howell, S.J., Sear, J.W. and Foëx, P. (2004). Hypertension, hypertensive heart disease and perioperative cardiac risk. *British Journal of Anaesthesia*, **92**, 570–83.

79. Weksler, N., Klein, M., Szendro, G., *et al.* (2003). The dilemma of immediate preoperative hypertension: to treat and operate, or to postpone surgery. *Journal of Clinical Anesthesia*, **15**, 179–83.

80. Hogue, C.W. Jr., Goodnough, L.T., and Monk, T.G. (1998). Perioperative myocardial ischemic episodes are related to hematocrit level in patients undergoing radical prostatectomy. *Transfusion*, **38**, 924–31.

81. Nelson, A.H., Fleisher, L.A., and Rosenbaum, S.H. (1993). Relationship between postoperative anemia and cardiac morbidity in high-risk vascular patients in the intensive care unit. *Critical Care Medicine*, **21**, 860–6.

82. Carson, J.L., Duff, A., Poses, R.M., *et al.* (1996). Effect of anaemia and cardiovascular disease on surgical mortality and morbidity. *Lancet*, **348**, 1055–60.

83. Ramakrishna, G., Sprung, J., Ravi, B.S., Chandrasekaran, K., and McGoon, M.D. (2005). Impact of pulmonary hypertension on the outcomes of noncardiac surgery: predictors of perioperative morbidity and mortality. *Journal of the American College of Cardiology*, **45**, 1691–9.

84. Lai, H.C., Lai, H.C., Wang, K.Y., Lee, W.L., Ting, C.T., and Liu, T.J. (2007). Severe pulmonary hypertension complicates postoperative outcome of non-cardiac surgery. *British Journal of Anaesthesia*, **99**, 184–90.

85. Morris, C.K., Ueshima, K., Kawaguchi, T., Hideg, A., and Froelicher, V.F. (1991). The prognostic value of exercise capacity: a review of the literature. *American Heart Journal*, **122**, 1423–31.

86. McPhail, N., Calvin, J.E., Shariatmadar, A., Barber, G.G., and Scobie, T.K. (1988). The use of preoperative exercise testing to predict cardiac complications after arterial reconstruction. *Journal of Vascular Surgery*, **7**, 60–8.

87. Poldermans, D., Arnese, M., Fioretti, P.M., *et al.* (1995). Improved cardiac risk stratification in major vascular surgery with dobutamine-atropine stress echocardiography. *Journal of the American College of Cardiology*, **26**, 648–53.

88. Older, P., Smith, R., Courtney, P., and Hone, R. (1993). Preoperative evaluation of cardiac failure and ischaemia in elderly patients by cardiopulmonary exercise testing. *Chest*, **104**, 701–4.

89. Laitio, T., Jalonen, J., Kuusela, T., and Scheinin, H. (2007). The role of heart rate variability in risk stratification for adverse postoperative cardiac event. *Anesthesia and Analgesia*, **105**, 1548–60.

90. Fleisher, L.A., *et al.* (2006). AHA/ACC 2006 guideline update on perioperative cardiovascular evaluation for non-cardaca surgery: focused update on peri-operative beta-blocker update. *Journal of the American College of Cardiology*, **47**, 2343–55.

91. Feringa, H.H., Schouten, O., Karagiannis, S.E., *et al.* (2007). Intensity of statin therapy in relation to myocardial ischemia, troponin T release, and clinical cardiac outcome in patients undergoing major vascular surgery. *Journal of the American College of Cardiology*, **50**, 1649–56.

92. Poldermans, D., Bax, J.J., Kertai, M.D., *et al.* (2003). Statins are associated with a reduced incidence of perioperative mortality in patients undergoing major noncardiac vascular surgery. *Circulation*, **107**, 1848–51.

93. Biodi-Zoccai, G.G.L., Lotrionte, M., Agostini, P., *et al.* (2006). A systematic review and meta-analysis on the hazards of discontinuing or not adhering to aspirin among 50 279 patients at risk for coronary artery disease. *European Heart Journal*, **27**, 2667–74.

94. Chassot, P.G., Delabays, A., and Spahn. DR. (2007). Perioperative antiplatelet therapy: the case for continuing therapy in patients at risk of myocardial infarction. *British Journal of Anaesthesia*, **99**, 316–28.

95. Sheehan, M.K., Marone, L., and Makaroun, M.S. (2005). Use of endoluminal aortic stent-grafts for the repair of abdominal aortic aneurysms. *Perspectives in Vascular Surgery and Endovascular Therapy*, **17**, 289–96.

96. Warner, M.A., Shields, S.E., and Chute, C.G. (1993). Major morbidity and mortality within 1 month of ambulatory surgery and anesthesia. *Journal of the American Medical Association*, **270**, 1437–41.

97. Munoz, E., Cohen, J., Chang, J., *et al.* (1989). Socioeconomic concerns in vascular surgery: A survey of the role of age, resource consumption, and outcome in treatment cost. *Journal of Vascular Surgery*, **9**, 479–86.

98. Yu, C.H. and Beattie, W.S. (2006). The effects of volatile anesthetics on cardiac ischemic complications and mortality in CABG: a meta-analysis. *Canadian Journal of Anaesthesia*, **53**, 906–18.

99. Jakobsen, C.J., Berg, H., Hindsholm, K.B., Faddy, N., and Sloth, E. (2007). The influence of propofol versus sevoflurane anesthesia on outcome in 10,535 cardiac surgical procedures. *Journal of Cardiothoracic and Vascular Anesthesia*, **21**, 664–71.

100. Rodgers, A., Walker, N., Schug, S., *et al.* (2000). Reduction of postoperative mortality and morbidity with epidural or spinal anaesthesia: results from overview of randomised trials. *British Medical Journal*, **321**, 1493.

101. Rigg, J.R.A., Jamrozik, K., Myles, P.S., *et al.* (2002). Epidural anaesthesia and analgesia and outcome of major surgery: a randomised trial. *Lancet*, **359**, 1276–82.

102. Liu, S.S. and Wu, C.L. (2007). Effect of postoperative analgesia on major postoperative complications: a systematic update of the evidence. *Anesthesia and Analgesia*, **104**, 689–702.

103. Charlson, M.E., MacKenzie, C.R., Gold, J.P., et al. (1990). Intraoperative blood pressure: What patterns identify patients at risk for postoperative complications? *Annals of Surgery*, **50**, 567–80.

104. Story, D.A., Shelton, A.C., Poustie, S.J., Colin-Thome, N.J., McIntyre, R.E., and McNicol, P.L. (2006). Effect of an anaesthesia department led critical care outreach and acute pain service on postoperative serious adverse events. *Anaesthesia*, **61**, 24–8.

105. Kim, L.J., Martinez, E.A., Faraday, N., *et al.* (2002). Cardiac troponin I predicts short-term mortality in vascular surgery patients. *Circulation*, **106**, 2366–71.

106. Landesberg, G., Mosseri, M., Zahger, D., *et al.* (2001). Myocardial infarction after vascular surgery: the role of prolonged stress-induced, ST depression-type ischemia. *Journal of the American College of Cardiology*, **37**, 1839–45.

107. Pasternak, P.F., Grossi, E.A., Baumann, G., *et al.* (1992). Silent myocardial ischemia monitoring predicts late as well as perioperative cardiac events in patients undergoing vascular surgery. *Journal of Vascular Surgery*, **16**, 171–80.

108. Boersma, E., Poldermans, D., Bax, J.J., *et al.* (2001). Predictors of cardiac events after major vascular surgery: role of clinical characteristics, dobutamine echocardiography, and beta blocker therapy. *Journal of the American Medical Association*, **285**, 1865-73.

109. Baron, J.F., Mundler, O., Bertrand, M., *et al.* (1994). Dipyridamole-thallium scintigraphy and gated radionuclide angiography to assess cardiac risk before abdominal aortic surgery. *New England Journal of Medicine*, **330**, 663–9.

110. Rinfret, S., Goldman, L., Polanczyk, C.A., Cook, E.F., and Lee, T.H. (2004). Value of immediate postoperative electrocardiogram to update risk stratification after major noncardiac surgery. *American Journal of Cardiology*, **94**, 1017–22.

Chapter 14

Haematological risk

Henry J Skinner & Iain K Moppett

Patients undergoing surgery and anaesthesia are at risk of three main haematological problems: excessive bleeding, venous thromboembolism, and risk associated with blood transfusion.

Bleeding

Anaesthesia *per se* does not cause bleeding. However, interventions or omissions by the anaesthetist may promote or inhibit bleeding during and after surgery. Invasive procedures performed by anaesthetists may also carry risks from bleeding. Patient and surgical factors contribute most to the risk of bleeding in the perioperative period.

Excessive bleeding is a serious surgical complication which increases perioperative morbidity, mortality and intensive care stay[1]. Cardiac surgical bleeding requiring more than 5 units blood was associated with an eightfold increase in the risk of death[2]. A meta-analysis of trials of thromboprophylaxis in general, orthopaedic, and urological surgery found that in around 3% of operations, bleeding was considered to be excessive[3]. Bleeding during and after surgery is usually of a technical nature but can be aggravated by pre-existing or acquired coagulation disorders.

Patient factors

Pre-existing bleeding disorders can usually be identified on the basis of history. A history of bruising, epistaxis, gingival bleeding, menorrhagia, bleeding in joints, and excess bleeding with visible bruises, purpura or petechiae, is the cornerstone of identifying patients at risk. A coagulopathy should be considered on clinical grounds if there is bleeding from several sites, oozing from an unseen source, or if bleeding is delayed after initially adequate clotting. Bleeding from a single site or sudden onset of massive bleeding is probably due to a local structural defect[4,5]. Routine coagulation tests were not designed as a screening test for coagulopathy and lack the sensitivity for this purpose[4,6]. Thromboelastography performed better with a negative predictive value, for postoperative bleeding after cardiac surgery, of >80%[7]. The British Committee for Standards in Haematology do not recommend routine screening in the absence of a suspicious history[8]. The risk of postpartum haemorrhage is high in women with inherited bleeding disorders. In one centre, the incidence of primary and secondary postpartum haemorrhage was between 11% and 24% in carriers of haemophilia, von Willenbrand disease, or Factor XI deficiency[9]. History of a bleeding disorder predicted an increased risk of 30-day mortality after surgical treatment for appendicitis (OR 3.5)[10]. In less severe bleeding disorders, pharmacological treatment may be sufficient, but in patients with severe bleeding disorders, there is always a need for clotting factor concentrates. Mishra demonstrated that patients with severe bleeding disorders, including patients with inhibitors, can be treated safely, provided that the patients receive adequate treatment with clotting factor concentrates[11].

Causes of excessive bleeding

Inherited coagulopathy
Haemophilia A and B

Patients with severe haemophilia usually have a dramatic bleeding history and the diagnosis is confirmed by reduced factor VIII or IX levels. Appropriate replacement therapy is usually effective in preventing surgical bleeding[11,12]. Target levels for surgery depend on the likelihood of bleeding, how easy it is to achieve haemostasis, and whether bleeding would compromise the surgical result. A large proportion of haemophiliacs develop antibody inhibitors against coagulant activity and recombinant factor VIIa provides a valuable treatment alternative[13,14]; reported rates of bleeding complications do not appear particularly high when managed appropriately (2/27[15] and 2/53[16] patients).

Von Willebrand's disease

Von Willebrand's disease (vWD) is the most common inherited bleeding disorder and is due to quantitative or qualitative defects of von Willebrand factor. Milder forms of the disease may affect >1% of the population[5]. Two series[17,18] of over 200 procedures found bleeding complications in around 9% of procedures when vWD was appropriately managed, and in over 60% of cases where vWD was previously unknown.

Rare clotting disorders

Prevalences in the general population vary between 1 in 500 000 and 1 in 2 000 000 for the homozygous forms. There are no suitable clinical trials to supply good evidence for how these patients are best treated[19].

Liver disease

The bleeding tendency in liver disease is complex and includes reduced synthesis of clotting factors and inhibitors of fibrinolysis, abnormal fibrinogen, abnormal platelet function, and thrombocytopaenia[20]. Although patients with severe liver disease may have marked coagulopathy, milder disease (platelet count $50–99 \times 10^9 \, L^{-1}$ and/or prothrombin and partial thromboplastin times 1–1.5 times normal) may not be associated with a particularly increased risk, at least for moderately invasive procedures such as liver biopsy[21].

Thrombocytopaenia and platelet dysfunction

Thrombocytopaenia may be due to insufficient production or increased consumption, either congenital or acquired. Platelet dysfunction may also be congenital or acquired with uraemia, myeloproliferaive disorders, and dysproteinaemias[20]. The British Committee for Standards in Haematology recommends prophylactic platelet infusion to cover spinal or epidural anaesthesia if the level is less than 50×10^9 L^{-1}. A level above 100×10^9 L^{-1} is advised for neurosurgery and eye surgery. In the actively bleeding patient, a platelet transfusion trigger of 75×10^9 L^{-1} should provide a margin of safety to ensure the count does not fall below the generally accepted critical level of 50×10^9 L^{-1}. In multiple or central nervous system trauma, levels $> 100 \times 10^9$ L^{-1} are desirable[22]. The evidence for these platelet counts is poor, particularly for spinal and epidural anaesthesia, where the rate of bleeding complications is too low for the reported case series to rule out increased risks with lower platelet counts.

Critical illness

Patients who are critically ill have a relatively high risk of bleeding both due to surgical or traumatic injury and spontaneously due to sepsis. One study found bleeding unexplained by local or surgical factors in 13.6% of patients admitted to an adult intensive care unit[23]. Two-thirds of patients had a prothrombin time ratio ≥1.5 and 38% had a platelet count $<100 \times 10^9$ L^{-1}. Both factors were predictive of excessive bleeding and poor outcome. The incidence of acute bleeding with percutaneous dilatational tracheotomy was independent of the coagulation variables tested[24], but chronic bleeding was more common with an activated partial thromboplastin time > 50 s (OR 3.7; 95% CI 1.1–12.7) or a platelet count $< 50 \times 10^9$ L^{-1} (OR 5.0; 95% CI 1.4–17.2). Low-dose heparin treatment did not significantly increase the risk of chronic bleeding.

A study of over 1,000 critically ill patients whose lungs were ventilated for at least 48 h randomized patients to stress ulcer prophylaxis with intravenous ranitidine or nasogastric sucralfate. Independent predictors of upper gastrointestinal bleeding included higher serum creatinine (OR 1.2; 95% CI 1.0–1.3); enteral nutrition (OR 0.3; 95% CI 0.1–0.7]), and ranitidine administration (OR 0.4; 95% CI 0.2–0.8) were protective[25].

Thromboembolic prophylaxis

Patients taking warfarin have an increased risk of spontaneous and traumatic bleeding. Elective surgery can be carried out safely if warfarin is stopped 4–5 days prior to surgery and INR is less than 1.5[20]. Overzealous anticoagulation around the time of surgery more often led to unnecessary bleeding rather than prevented further thrombosis[26]. In patients who have atrial fibrillation (AF), use anticoagulants, and undergo a surgical procedure, there is a 3.6-fold increased risk for all bleeding complications within 1 month after surgery, compared with the control period (95% CI 1.1–12.0)[27]. In another study of patients with atrial fibrillation, the rate of postoperative bleeding was 4.8% in patients who had prophylactic low–molecular-weight heparin, and 17.6% in those who had therapeutic unfractionated heparin ($P < 0.001$). Postoperative anticoagulation with therapeutic unfractionated heparin in patients with AF was associated with an increased rate of bleeding without reducing the risk of thromboembolism[28]. Conversely, the stroke risk for patients in non-valvular AF without anticoagulation is between 1 and 6% per year (average 5%), which translates to around 1 in 1,000 per week[29]. Serious bleeding complications were rare in a review of 33 randomized trials of deep venous thrombosis prophylaxis trials[30].

Antiplatelet drugs

A large review and meta-analysis of 474 studies on the impact of low-dose aspirin on surgical blood loss showed that patients on aspirin alone have an average intra-operative haemorrhagic risk increased by a factor of 1.5, without an increase in surgical mortality or morbidity[31]. The risk of a perioperative cardiac event after stopping antiplatelet therapy probably offsets any benefits in reduction in bleeding, and these drugs are often continued right up to surgery especially in at-risk patients[32]. The continuation of aspirin in patients undergoing surgery where small haematomata could be catastrophic, such as neurosurgery, is controversial.

Clopidogrel is being taken by an increasing number of patients presenting for surgery. For those patients who have drug-eluting coronary stents, the risk of stent occlusion (around 20% in one study[33]) following stopping of clopidogrel is very high, so surgery should be deferred if possible, or clopidogrel continued after due consideration of the risks and benefits.

Surgical factors

Surgery associated with substantial bleeding includes cardiothoracic, major vascular, hepatobiliary, spinal and major joint surgery, radical prostatectomy, and craniotomy. Cardiothoracic surgery accounts for 13% of all blood used in the United Kingdom[34]. Excessive bleeding after cardiac surgery is related to many factors. Haemodilution, hypothermia, excessive activation of coagulation by the extracorporeal circuit, consumption of platelets and clotting factors, and a high proportion of patients on antiplatelet and antithrombotic agents are the most significant. Bleeding during liver transplantation is mainly due to existing end-stage liver disease.

Perioperative factors

Trauma and bleeding Early coagulopathy is common after trauma and independently predicts mortality[35]. Abnormal prothrombin time (PT) was found to have an OR for mortality of 1.35 and partial thromboplastin time (PTT) an OR of 4.26 in one cohort of over 14 000 U.S. trauma patients. Platelet count was not found to be an independent risk factor. Substantial tissue factor exposure results in early clot formation. Widespread activation and subsequent fibrinolysis consume and deplete clotting factors[36]. Uncontrolled bleeding lowers the haemoglobin concentration, dilutes platelets and clotting factors, and may cause shock and diffuse intravascular coagulation. If not addressed early, a bloody downward spiral may ensue.

Hypothermia and acidosis Hypothermia is known to reduce platelet function and impair enzymes of the coagulation cascade. Hypothermia has been shown to increase activated clotting time *in vitro*[37]. A recent meta-analysis and systematic review concluded that even mild hypothermia (a decrease of 1°C) significantly increases blood loss by approximately 16% (4–26%), and increases the relative risk for transfusion by approximately 22% (3–37%)[38]. Deep hypothermic circulatory arrest results in significant derangement of the coagulation system and a high incidence of postoperative bleeding[39].

Acidosis and hypothermia have been found to increase the risk for coagulopathy and are complicating factors in trauma[40]. It has been proposed that acidosis impairs ionic interaction between the coagulation factors and negatively charged phospholipids at high concentrations of hydrogen ions, accounting for lower activity[41].

Hypertension Hypertension increases the transmural pressure gradient and blood vessel wall tension and increases bleeding along vascular suture lines. Perioperative hypertension is a known risk factor for bleeding in cardiac surgery[42]. End-stage renal disease and hypertension combined with preoperatively decreased haemoglobin concentration were the risk factors associated with transfusion after tonsillectomy[43].

Anaesthetic technique and blood loss Anaesthetic technique may influence surgical blood loss. Regional techniques have been associated with less operative blood loss than general anaesthesia alone for some procedures[44]. This is seen both for absolute volume of blood loss[44] and for volume of blood transfusion[45]. The reduction in blood loss may be greater with spinal anaesthesia than with epidural anaesthesia. This effect has been demonstrated in Caesarean section[46], and in abdominal, pelvic, and lower-extremity surgery[44]. A meta-analysis of hip fracture surgery found no benefit of regional technique over general anaesthesia with regard to blood loss[47]. Some of this effect is due to the greater degree of arterial and venous hypotension with regional techniques, compared to general anaesthesia. There is no good evidence that the reduction in blood loss associated with regional techniques impacts upon major morbidity or mortality. This may reflect the fact that the mean difference in blood loss is relatively small (200–300 ml).

Use of antifibrinolytics and local agents In a recent meta-analysis, tranexamic acid, aminocaproic acid, and aprotinin were effective in reducing blood loss and transfusion after cardiac surgery. However, high-dose aprotinin was associated with a statistically significant increased risk of renal dysfunction[48,49]. There are currently serious questions regarding the safety of aprotinin[50]. Various locally applicable agents including bone wax, gelatin, collagen, oxidized regenerated cellulose, fibrin sealant glues, and synthetic glues are used with varying success. Some evidence from randomized controlled trials exists regarding the use of fibrin sealants on their own or combined with collagen fleece[51].

Transfusions

The risks from blood transfusion are diminishing in the United Kingdom. During 2005, almost a decade after the first report of Serious Hazards of Transfusion, only five deaths were caused by transfusions[52]. Considering that the national blood service issues more than 3 000 000 units of blood products annually, blood transfusion in the United Kingdom is very safe. Incorrect blood component transfuion is the most frequent serious complication (1 in 600 000 units transfused). It follows a sequence of failures to correctly identify the blood product or patient. The most serious consequence of this is ABO-incompatibility. Even a small amount of incompatible blood may elicit acute and often fatal intravascular haemolysis. Other serious complications include transmission of infective agents. The risk of catching hepatitis B from a blood transfusion is 1 in 900 000 and less than 1 in 30 000 000 for hepatitis C. The chance of HIV infection is less than 1 in several million. As yet, we do not know the level of risk of variant Creutzfeldt–Jakob disease being transmitted by blood. Transfusion-related acute lung injury is caused by antibodies in the transfused component that react with neutrophil antigens in the recipient. Pulmonary oedema ensues in the absence of circulatory overload. Lung injury occurs 5–6 times more frequently following transfusion with platelets or fresh frozen plasma than red cells. These and other known complications of transfusion, and a national shortage of blood have led to calls for more restrictive transfusion practice than Allen's 10/30 rule[53] (haemoglobin of 10 g dL^{-1} and haematocrit of 30% as transfusion triggers) to be adopted. Anaemia has been shown to be a marker of poor outcome. Carson and colleagues (1996) performed a retrospective cohort study in 1958 patients who underwent surgery and declined blood tranfusion for religious reasons[54]. The mortality was 1.3% (95% CI 0.8–2.0) in patients with preoperative haemoglobin $\geq$12 g dL^{-1}, but 33% for patients with preoperative haemoglobin <6 g dL^{-1}. The risk was greatest in patients with a history of angina, myocardial infarction, heart failure, or peripheral vascular disease (P<0.03). Not surprisingly, blood loss was also better tolerated in those who had higher preoperative haemoglobin levels (P< 0.001). Decisions about transfusion should take account of cardiovascular status and operative blood loss as well as the haemoglobin concentration[54]. Postoperative haematocrit <28% was associated with myocardial ischaemia after radical prostatectomy[55] and serious cardiac events after vascular surgery[56]. What is less clear, however, is whether transfusing blood improves outcome. In a large retrospective study, Waggoner and co-workers found that, compared with historical controls, there was no change in the incidences of perioperative stroke and myocardial infarction following carotid endarterectomy after they had agreed to a lower acceptable transfusion trigger[57].

At what plasma haemoglobin concentration do the risks of anaemia outweigh the potential risks of blood transfusion? It is not known if increased oxygen delivery after transfusion promotes increased oxygen consumption to relieve tissue hypoxia. The Canadian Critical Care Trials Group conducted a large multicentre, randomized, controlled trial in critical care[58]. The investigators enlisted 838 patients with haemoglobin concentration <9 g dL^{-1} unless they were actively bleeding, had chronic anaemia, or had cardiac surgery. Patients were randomized to a restrictive transfusion strategy (transfusion trigger of 7 g dL^{-1} and a maintenance range of 7–9 g dL^{-1}) or a liberal strategy (transfusion trigger of 10 g dL^{-1} and a maintenance range of 10–12 g dL^{-1}). They found a restrictive transfusion strategy decreased transfusion by 54%, transfusion exposure by 33%, and was associated with decreases in hospital mortality, multiple organ dysfunction, and cardiovascular complications. They recommended the restrictive strategy as best practice in patients with cardiovascular disease unless there was evidence of ongoing myocardial ischaemia. Reservations about a restrictive strategy in all patients were supported by later subgroup analysis, which suggested that patients with severe cardiac disease randomized to the restrictive strategy group had a nonsignificant increase in 30-day all-cause mortality[59]. A later meta-analysis by Carson *et al.*[60] confirmed that mortality, rates of cardiac events, morbidity, and length of hospital stay were unaffected by restrictive transfusion triggers. However, the effects of conservative transfusion triggers on functional status, morbidity, and mortality, particularly in patients with cardiac disease, need to be tested in further large clinical trials.

Venous thromboembolism

Venous thromboembolism (VTE) encompasses deep venous thrombosis (DVT) and pulmonary embolism (PE) and is an important and preventable cause of perioperative morbidity and mortality. The 1991–1992 National Enquiry into Perioperative Deaths found that pulmonary embolism was responsible for 7% of perioperative deaths[61]. DVT of the lower limb is the most important cause for PE but upper-limb DVT and right atrial thrombus are also known sources. In patients in AF, thromboembolism was associated with increased perioperative mortality (OR 9.5; 95% CI 2.5–35.8)[62]. Anaesthesia and surgery directly or indirectly perpetuate Virchow's triad of venous stasis, abnormal coagulation, and intimal damage. Venous pooling associated with ischaemia gives rise to local hypercoagulability[63]. Several risk factors for VTE have been included in the recent NICE guideline (Table 14.1)[64]. The incidence of VTE depends on the presence of risk factors, history of VTE, and type of surgery. Roughly one in five of patients have venographic evidence of thrombosis after neurosurgery, one in four after abdominal surgery, and as many as one is two after orthopaedic surgery[65]. The incidence of DVT after hip and knee surgery is particular is high. The true benefit of treating asymptomatic, venographic thromboses is not yet clear and data about cost-effectiveness are still lacking. Patients undergoing total hip or knee replacement or colorectal resections have the highest rates (0.7%) of PE[66]. Of almost a quarter of a million patients who underwent knee replacement, 0.4% developed pulmonary embolism within 3 months. Perioperative PE carries a high mortality (30%)[63]. Outcome depends on early diagnosis and treatment, the size of the embolus, and cardiopulmonary co-morbidity.

Modifiable factors

Mechanical methods and low-molecular-weight heparin NICE recommends that graduated stocking be offered to all inpatients, that low-molecular-weight heparin be given prophylactically for orthopaedic surgery and neurosurgery (delay pharmacological prophylaxis in ruptured cranial or spinal vascular malformations until after surgery), and other surgery where patients have one or more risk factors [Table 14.1]. Graduated stockings are not without risk, and if not fitted properly, may increase the risk of VTE[67]. Due to the high incidence and late presentation of DVT after hip replacement and surgery for hip fracture, low-molecular-weight heparin therapy should be continued for 4 weeks after surgery.

Intermittent pneumatic compression (IPC) devices are also effective at reducing DVT. However, there is no good evidence to suggest that they are more effective than graduated stockings alone or prophylactic heparin. To be effective, they need to be worn continuously whilst in bed. This may not be achievable in clinical practice.

Anaesthetic technique

Rogers, in a meta-analysis in 2000, found neuraxial block (without thromboprophylaxis) reduces the odds of PE by 55% and DVT by 44%[45]. However, thromboprophylaxis is now more commonly used after hip and knee surgery, and low-molecular-weight heparins have considerably decreased the incidence of DVT. A meta-analysis of 15 randomized studies of hip fracture repair reported that regional anaesthesia decreased

Table 14.1 Risk factors for venous thromboembolism

- Active cancer or cancer treatment
- Active heart or respiratory failure
- Acute medical illness
- Age over 60 years
- Antiphospholipid syndrome
- Behçet's disease
- Central venous catheter in situ
- Continuous travel of more than 3 hours approximately 4 weeks before or after surgery
- Immobility (for example, paralysis or limb in plaster)
- Inflammatory bowel disease (for example, Crohn's disease or ulcerative colitis)
- Myeloproliferative diseases
- Nephrotic syndrome
- Obesity (body mass index >30 kg/m^2)
- Paraproteinaemia
- Paroxysmal nocturnal haemoglobinuria
- Personal or family history of VTE
- Pregnancy or puerperium
- Recent myocardial infarction or stroke
- Severe infection
- Use of oral contraceptives or hormonal replacement therapy
- Varicose veins with associated phlebitis
- Inherited thrombophilias, for example:
  - High levels of coagulation factors (for example, Factor VIII)
  - Hyperhomocysteinaemia
  - Low activated protein C resistance (for example, Factor V Leiden)
  - Protein C, S, and antithrombin deficiencies

Prothrombin 2021A gene mutation

the relative risk of DVT (0.41; 95% CI 0.23–0.72), but had no significant impact on other postoperative complications or on the 1-year mortality rate[68].

References

1. Prytherch, D.R., Whiteley, M.S., Higgins, B., *et al.* (1998). POSSUM and Portsmouth POSSUM for predicting mortality. Physiological and Operative Severity Score for the enumeration of Mortality and morbidity. *British Journal of Surgeiry*, **85**, 1217–20.

2. Karkouti, K., Wijeysundera, D.N., Yau, T.M., *et al.* (2004). The independent association of massive blood loss with mortality in cardiac surgery. *Transfusion*, **44**, 1453–62.

3. Collins, R., Scrimgeour, A., Yusuf, S., and Peto, R. (1988). Reduction in fatal pulmonary embolism and venous thrombosis by perioperative administration of subcutaneous heparin. Overview of results of randomized trials in general, orthopedic, and urologic surgery. *New England Journal of Medicine*, **318**, 1162–73.

4. Bombeli, T. and Spahn, D.R. (2004). Updates in perioperative coagulation: physiology and management of thromboembolism and haemorrhage. *British Journal of Anaesthesia*, **93**, 275–87.

5. Baker, R. (2002). Pre-operative hemostatic assessment and management. *Transfusion and Apheresis Science*, **27**, 45–53.

6. Eckman, M.H., Erban, J.K., Singh, S.K., and Kao, G.S. (2003). Screening for the risk for bleeding or thrombosis. *Annals of Internal Medicine*, **138**, 15–24.

7. Cammerer, U., Dietrich, W., Rampf, T., *et al.* (2003). The predictive value of modified computerized thromboelastography and platelet function analysis for postoperative blood loss in routine cardiac surgery. *Anesthesia and Analgesia*, **96**, 51–7.

8. Chee, Y.L., Crawford, J.C., Watson, H.G., and Greaves, M. Guideline on the assessment of bleeding risk prior to surgery or invasive procedures http://www.bcshguidelines.com/pdf/Coagscreen200107.pdf (last accessed 16th January 2009).

9. Kadir, R.A. and Aledort, L.M. (2000). Obstetrical and gynaecological bleeding: a common presenting symptom. *Clinical and Laboratory Haematology*, **22**, S12-16.

10 Margenthaler, J.A., Longo, W.E., Virgo, K.S., *et al.* (2003). Risk factors for adverse outcomes after the surgical treatment of appendicitis in adults. *Annals of Surgery*, **238**, 59–66.

11 Mishra, V., Paus, A.C., and Tjønnfjord, G.E. (2005). Surgery in patients with bleeding disorders-expensive treatment for a small group of patients. *Tidsskr Nor Laegeforen*, **125**, 883–5.

12. Habermann, B., Eberhardt, C., Hovy, L., Zichner, L., Scharrer, I., and Kurth, A.A. (2007). Total hip replacement in patients with severe bleeding disorders. A 30 years single center experience. *International Orthopaedics (SICOT)*, **31**, 17–21.

13. Kubisz, P. and Stasko, J. (2004). Recombinant activated factor VII in patients at high risk of bleeding. *Hematology*, **9**, 317–32.

14. Siddiqui, M.A. and Scot, L.J. (2005). Recombinant factor VIIa (Eptacog Alfa): a review of its use in congenital or acquired haemophilia and other congenital bleeding disorders. *Drugs*, **65**, 1161–77.

15. Rodriguez-Merchan, E.C., Quintana, M., Jimenez-Yuste, V., and Hernandez-Navarro, F. (2007). Orthopaedic surgery for inhibitor patients: a series of 27 procedures (25 patients). *Haemophilia*, **13**, 613–9.

16. Hvid, I. and Rodriguez-Merchan, E.C. (2002). Orthopaedic surgery in haemophilic patients with inhibitors: an overview. *Haemophilia*, **8**, 288–91.

17. Blombäck, M., Johansson, G., Johnsson, H., Swedenborg, J., and Wabo, E. (1989). Surgery in patients with von Willebrand's disease. *British Journal of Surgery*, **76**, 398–400.

18. von Auer, C., Lotter, K., and Scharrer, I. (2007). Bleeding complications in surgical patients with von willebrand's disease. *Journal of Thromb Haemost* **5** Supplement 2, P–W–175. http://www.blackwellpublishing.com/isth2007/abstract. asp?id=67427.

19. Peyvandi, F., Kaufman, R.J., Seligsohn, U., *et al.* (2006). Rare bleeding disorders. *Haemophilia*, **12**, S137–S142.

20. Francis, C.W. and Kaplan, K.L. (2000). Hematological problems in the surgical patients: bleeding and thrombosis. In *Hematology – Basic Principles and Practice* (R. Hoffman, E.J. Benz, S.J. Shattl, et al., eds.), pp. 2381–91. Churchill Livingstone. New York.

21. Davenport, R.D. (1992). Predicting post-procedure bleeding in liver disease. *Hepatology*, **15**, 735–7.

22. British Committee for Standards in Haematology, Blood Transfusion Task Force. Guidelines for the use of platelet transfusions. (2003). *British Journal of Haematology*, **122**, 10–23.

23. Chakraverty, R., Davidson, S., Peggs, K., Stross, P., Garrard, C., and Littlewood, T.J. (1996). The incidence and cause of coagulopathies in an intensive care population. *British Journal of Haematology*, **93**, 460–3.

24. Beiderlinden, M., Eikermann, M., Lehmann, N., Adamzik, M., and Peters, J. (2007). Risk factors associated with bleeding during and after percutaneous dilational tracheostomy. *Anaesthesia*, **62**, 342–6.

25. Cook, D., Heyland, D., Griffith, L., *et al.* (1999) for the Canadian Critical Care Trials Group. Risk factors for clinically important upper gastrointestinal bleeding in patients requiring mechanical ventilation. *Critical Care Medicine*, **27**, 2812–7.

26. Kearon, C. and Hirsh, J. (1997). Management of anticoagulation before and after elective surgery. *New England Journal of Medicine*, **336**, 1506–11.

27. Vink, R., Rienstra, M., Van Dongen, C.J., *et al.* (2005). Risk of thromboembolism and bleeding after general surgery in patients with atrial fibrillation. *American Journal of Cardiology*, **96**, 822–4.

28. Beldi, G., Beng, L., Siegel, G., Bisch, K.S., and Candinas, D. (2007). Prevention of perioperative thromboembolism in patients with atrial fibrillation. *British Journal of Surgery*, **94**, 1351–5.

29. Quality Standards Subcommittee of the American Academy of Neurology. Practice Parameter: Stroke prevention in patients with nonvalvular atrial fibrillation. (1998). *Neurology*, **51**, 671–3.

30. Leonardi, M.J., McGory, M.L., and Ko, C.Y. (2006). The rate of bleeding complications after pharmacologic deep venous thrombosis prophylaxis: a systematic review of 33 randomized controlled trials. *Archives of Surgery*, **141**, 790–7.

31. Burger, W., Chemnitius, J.M., Kneissl, G.D., and Rücker, G. (2005). Low-dose aspirin for secondary cardiovascular prevention—cardiovascular risks after its preoperative withdrawal versus bleeding risks with its continuation—review and meta-analysis. *Journal of Internal Medicine*, **257**, 399–414.

32. Chassot, P-G., Delabays, A., and Spahn, D.R. (2007). Perioperative antiplatelet therapy: the case for continuing therapy in patients at risk of myocardial infarction. *British Journal of Anaesthesia*, **99**, 316–28.

33. Conroy, M. Bolsin, S. N. C., Black, S. A., and Orford, N. (2007). Perioperative complications in patients with drug-eluting stents: a three-year audit at Geelong Hospital. *Anaesthesia and Intensive Care*, **35**, 939–44.

34. http://blood.co.uk/pages/e18used.html

35. MacLeod, J.B., Lynn, M., McKenny, M.G., Cohn, S.M., and Murtha, M. (2003). Early coagulopathy predicts mortality in trauma. *Journal of Trauma*, **55**, 39–44.

36. Rossaint, R., Cerny, V., Coats, T.J., *et al.* (2006). Key issues in advanced bleeding care in trauma. *Shock*, **26**, 322–31.

37. Kmiecik, S.A., Liu, J.L., Vaadia, T.S. *et al.* (2001).Quantitative evaluation of hypothermia, hyperthermia, and hemodilution on coagulation. *Journal of Extra-corporeal Technology*, **33**, 100–5.

38. Rajagopalan, S., Mascha, E., Na, J.M., and Sessler, D.I. (2008). The effects of mild perioperative hypothermia on blood loss and transfusion requirement. *Anesthesiology*, **108**, 71–7.

39. Mossad, E.B., Machado, S., and Apostolakis, J. (2007). Bleeding following deep hypothermia and circulatory arrest in children. *Seminars in Cardiothoracic and Vascular Anesthesia*, **11**, 34–46.

40. Cosgriff, N., Moore, E.E., Sauaia, A., *et al.* (1997). Predicting life-threatening coagulopathy in the massively transfused trauma patient: Hypothermia and acidoses revisited. *Journal of Trauma*, **42**, 857–861.

41. Meng, Z.H, Wolberg, A.S., Monroe, D.M. III, *et al.* (2003). The effect of temperature and pH on the activity of factor VIIa: Implications for the efficacy of high-dose factor VIIa in hypothermic and acidotic patients. *Journal of Trauma*, **55**, 886–91.

42. Leslie, J.B. (1993). Incidence and aetiology of perioperative hypertension. *Acta Anaesthesiologica Scandinavica*. **Suppl 99**, 5–9.

43. Meyer, J.E., Jeckström, W., Ross, D.A., Rudack, C., and Maune, S. (2004). Incidence and clinical background of posttonsillectomy bleeding related blood transfusion over 12 years. *Otolaryngology Polska*, **58**, 1065–9.

44. Richman, J.M., Rowlingson, A.J., Maine, D.N., *et al.* (2006). Does neuraxial anesthesia reduce intraoperative blood loss? A meta-analysis. *Journal of Clinical Anesthesia*, **18**, 427–35.

45. Rodgers, A., Walker, N., Schug, S., *et al.* (2000). Reduction of postoperative mortality and morbidity with epidural or spinal anesthesia: results from overview of randomised trials. *British Medical Journal*, **321**, 1493–7.

46. Afolabi, B.B., Lesi, F.E.A., and Merah, N.A. (2006). Regional versus general anaesthesia for caesarean section. *Cochrane Database of Systematic Reviews*, Issue **4**. Art. No.: CD004350. DOI: 10.1002/14651858.CD004350.pub2.

47. Sorenson, R.M. and Pace, N.L. (1992). Anesthetic techniques during surgical repair of femoral neck fractures. A meta-analysis. *Anesthesiology*, **77**, 1095–104.

48. Brown, J. R., Birkmeyer, N.J.O., and O'Connor, G.T. (2007). Meta-analysis comparing the effectiveness and adverse outcomes of antifibrinolytic agents in cardiac surgery. *Circulation*, **115**, 2801–13.

49. Henry, D.A., Carless, P.A., Moxey, A.J., *et al.* (2001). Anti-fibrinolytic use for minimising perioperative allogeneic blood transfusion. *Cochrane Database of Systematic Reviews*, Issue **1**. Art. No.: CD001886. DOI: 10.1002/14651858.CD001886.pub2.

50. Shaw, A.D., Stafford-Smith, M., White, W.D. *et al.* (2008). The effect of aprotinin on outcome after coronary-artery bypass grafting. *New England Journal of Medicine*, **358**, 784–93.

51. Bechstein, W.O. and Strey, C. (2007). Local and systemic hemostasis in surgery. *Chirurg*, **78**, 95–6.

52. Stainsby, D., Cohen, H., Jones, H., *et al.* (2005). Serious Hazards of Transfusion Annual Report.

53. Allen, J.B. and Allen, F.B. (1982). The minimum acceptable level of hemoglobin. *International Anesthiology Clinics*, **20**, 1–22.

54. Carson, J.L., Duff, A., Poses, R.M., *et al.* (1996). Effect of anaemia and cardiovascular disease on surgical mortality and morbidity. *Lancet*, **348**, 1055–60.

55. Hogue, C.W. Jr., Goodnough, L.T., and Monk, T.G. (1998). Perioperative myocardial ischemic episodes are related to hematocrit level in patients undergoing radical prostatectomy. *Transfusion*, **38**, 924–31.

56. Nelson, A.H., Fleisher, L.A., and Rosenbaum, S.H. (1993). Relationship between postoperative anemia and cardiac morbidity in high-risk vascular patients in the intensive care unit. *Critical Care Medicine*, **21**, 860–6.

57. Waggoner, J.R., Waas, C.T., Polis, T.Z., *et al.* (2001). The effect of changing transfusion practice on rates of perioperative stroke and myocardial infarction in patients undergoing carotid endarterectomy: A retrospective analysis of 1114 Mayo Clinic patients. *Mayo Clinic Proceedings*, **76**, 376–83.

58. Hebert, P.C., Wells, G., Blajchman, M.A., *et al.* (1999). A multicenter, randomised, controlled clinical trial of transfusion requirements in critical care. *New England Journal of Medicine*, **340**, 409–17.

59. Hebert, P.C., Yetisir, E., Martin, C., *et al.* (2001). Is a low transfusion threshold safe in critically ill patients with cardiovascular diseases? *Critical Care Medicine*, **29**, 227–33.

60. Carson, J.L., Hill, S., Carless, P., Hebert, P., and Henry, D. (2002). Transfusion triggers: a systematic review of the literature. *Transfusion Medicine Reviews*, **16**, 187–99.

61. 1991–92 National Enquiry into Perioperative Deaths.

62. Beldi, G., Beng, L., Siegel, G., Bisch-Knaden, S., and Candinas, D. (2007). Prevention of perioperative thromboembolism in patients with atrial fibrillation. *British Journal of Surgery*, **94**, 1351–5.

63. Kroegel, C. and Reissig, A. (2003). Principle mechanisms underlying venous thromboembolism: epidemiology, risk factors, pathophysiology and pathogenesis. *Respiration*, **70**, 7–30.

64. National Institute for Health and Clinical Excellence. Venous thromboembolism. Reducing the risk of venous thromboembolism (deep vein thrombosis and pulmonary embolism) in patients undergoing surgery. NICE London, 2007.

65. Arcelus, J.I., Caprini, J.A., Motykie, G.D., *et al.* (1999). Matching risk with treatment strategies in deep vein thrombosis. *Blood Coagulation Fibrinolysis*, **10**, S37–43.

66. Mahid, S.S., Polk, H.C. Jr., Lewi, J.N., and Turina, M. (2008). Opportunities for improved performance in surgical specialty practice. *Annals of Surgery*, **247**, 380–8.

67. Best, A.J., Williams, S., Crozier, A., *et al.* (2000). Graded compression stockings in elective orthopaedic surgery. An assessment of the in vivo performance of commercially available stockings in patients having hip and knee arthroplasty. *Journal of Bone and Joint Surgery. British Volume.* **82**, 116–118.

68. Urwin, S.C., Parke, M.J., and Griffiths, R. (2000). General versus regional anaesthesia for hip fracture surgery: a meta-analysis of randomized trials. *British Journal of Anaesthesia*, **84**, 450–5.

Chapter 15

Nervous system and regional anaesthesia

Jonathan G Hardman

Introduction

The first part of this chapter will deal with complications relating to anaesthesia that impact the central nervous system, particularly cerebrovascular accident, seizures, intracranial haemorrhage, and spinal cord infarction. This chapter will not cover the psychological complications of general anaesthesia, including delirium and post-operative cognitive dysfunction; these are dealt with in detail in Chapter 16.

The second part of the chapter will deal with complications arising during regional anaesthesia. These include systemic effects of local anaesthetic agents, inadequate and excessive block, and injury to nerves, the spinal cord, arteries, and pleura.

Brain injury

Cerebral infarction is caused by inadequate oxygenation of an area of brain tissue, secondary to embolus, haemorrhage, arterial constriction, or hypoxaemia. Focal cerebrovascular accident (CVA) or 'stroke' is reported to occur around the time of 1% of surgical procedures[1]. Only 17% occur during anaesthesia, while 83% occur during the 10 days following surgery[1,2]. The risk for each patient is dependent upon his or her existing pathology (e.g. atherosclerosis) and upon his or her operative procedure (Table 15.1). Pre-existing atrial fibrillation (giving a predisposition to the formation of emboli) greatly increases the risk of CVA. A history of prior transient ischaemic attacks (TIAs) or strokes indicates possible cerebral or carotid arterial disease and increases the risk of perioperative CVA tenfold[2], while pre-existing hypertension increases the risk of perioperative CVA fourfold. Symptomatic carotid artery disease carries a substantially increased risk of perioperative CVA and prophylactic carotid endarterectomy should be considered[3]. Carotid surgery and bypass cardiac surgery are associated with a greatly increased risk of perioperative CVA[4]. In view of the factors that appear to modify the incidence of perioperative CVA, the quoted rate of 1% should be viewed as not applicable to otherwise uncomplicated cases; indeed, in a large prospective study of patients undergoing ambulatory surgery, no increase (compared to a non-operative population) was observed in the rate of perioperative CVA following 45 000 procedures[5].

Diffuse, hypoxic brain injury may occur following severe or prolonged hypoxaemia, hypotension, or restriction of cerebral blood flow (e.g. carotid compression).

Table 15.1 The risk of perioperative cerebrovascular accident

Injury	Risk(%)
Perioperative CVA	
Total	1
Intra operative	0.17
Postoperative	0.83
In hypertensive patients	4
In patients with a history of CVA/TIA	10
During head/neck surgery	5

Note: CVA; cerebrovascular accident. TIA; transient ischaemic attack.

Mild insults may cause subtle postoperative personality changes or memory impairment. Severe insults are very rare, but are usually catastrophic, resulting in lifelong care-dependency. Severe injury is unlikely if cardiac output is maintained; in this scenario, hypoxaemia and/or hypotension must be very severe and prolonged or the patient must have a predisposition to cerebral injury (e.g. carotid artery disease). However, cardiac arrest produces diffuse brain injury very rapidly, and cardiac standstill lasting 3 min or more will inevitably result in significant, diffuse brain injury.

Severe hypocapnia is considered to present a risk of cerebral hypoperfusion through widespread cerebral vasoconstriction. In situations of deranged cerebrovascular autoregulation (e.g. following head injury), such vasoconstriction may aggravate brain injury, but it is unlikely that injury will result to the healthy brain from mild to moderate hyperventilation, even if prolonged.

Seizures

Seizures may occur during regional anaesthesia due to the exposure of the brain to local anaesthetic through intravascular injection, rapid local uptake or overdose. These are discussed later in this chapter. Seizures are uncommon during general anaesthesia because most general anaesthetic agents are anti-convulsant, with the exception of ketamine. Seizures occur occasionally postoperatively. Patients known to be epileptic are most at risk, while patients who have undergone intracranial surgery or who have suffered a recent head injury are also at risk[6]. Seizures may also occur in the context of alcohol withdrawal, and the extra stress of surgery combined with withdrawal is a fairly common cause of postoperative convulsions.

A number of drugs in anaesthetic practice are pro-convulsant, and they should be used with caution (or avoided) in patients at risk of seizures. These drugs include doxapram, ketamine, enflurane propofol, and methohexitone.

Intracranial haemorrhage

In patients at risk of intracranial bleeding (those with a history of CVA or with an intracranial aneurysm), severe surges in arterial pressure may cause intracranial haemorrhage and brain injury. Such complications are rare.

Spinal cord infarction

The anterior portion of the thoracolumbar spinal cord has a relatively tenuous blood supply via the anterior spinal artery. Patients with atherosclerosis or patients suffering prolonged or severe hypotension or hypoxaemia may suffer infarction of the spinal cord. Such injury is also associated with abdominal aortic aneurysm surgery, but this may not be properly considered a risk of anaesthesia. There may be an association between epidural analgesia and spinal cord infarction[7], although the number of cases reported makes it difficult to be certain.

Nerve injury during general anaesthesia

Nerve injury is a relatively common complication of anaesthesia, occurring during 0.1–0.3% of anaesthetics (1 in 300–1000)[8–10]. The ulnar nerve is the most commonly injured nerve; indeed, it is reported to be injured 3–5 times as commonly as any other nerve during general anaesthesia[8]. It is at greater risk than other nerves because it runs close to the skin surface and is easily trapped by external compression against the medial epicondyle of the humerus. Other commonly injured nerves include the common peroneal nerve at the knee, the lateral femoral cutaneous nerve and the brachial plexus. The majority of nerve injuries arising during general anaesthesia are temporary; recovery is expected over weeks to months.

Nerves may be injured through direct trauma, but this is often obvious (e.g. transection at surgery). Position-related nerve injury usually occurs through compression or stretching of the nerve and its surrounding tissues; this causes reduction in blood supply to the nerve, and over a period of time, the nerve suffers ischaemic damage. It is not clear how long a nerve must be deprived of its blood supply to cause damage, but very prolonged ischaemia is likely to lead to permanent injury, while brief ischaemia is more likely to produce temporary injury.

Arterial tourniquets, which are in common use in surgical practice, are often inflated for up to 2 h, producing near-complete nerve ischaemia. Nerve injury is uncommon after the use of such tourniquets, but several reports have indicated no other risk factors for nerve injuries arising during general anaesthesia, and tourniquets are accepted as being an occasional cause of intra-operative neurological injury. As for muscular injury, inflation duration and inflation pressure determine the severity and likelihood of injury.

Risk factors for nerve injury arising during general anaesthesia include diabetes, male sex, old age, illness, and thin build[9]. Some patients have an anatomical predisposition to ischaemia of the ulnar nerve, placing them at higher risk of intra operative ulnar injury. Such a predisposition may be indicated by previous or current ulnar nerve symptoms in the arm (e.g. experiencing pins and needles or occasionally a numb hand, especially the little finger). These symptoms may represent a pre-existing ulnar compression neuropathy. Some researchers have indicated that mobility of the ulnar nerve places patients at risk of its injury during anaesthesia. This mobility, which occurs in 16% of the population, allows the nerve to escape the groove behind the medial epicondyle and become compressed against the medial aspect of the medial epicondyle.

Table 15.2 Positional factors affecting the risk and severity of nerve injury arising during general anaesthesia

Nerve	Positional factor increasing risk of injury
Ulnar	The prone (face-down) position with the arms abducted This is associated with an increase in the pressure in the ulnar groove, even without external compression
	Supine, with the elbows extended, the shoulder abducted and hands pronated (facing towards the floor) with the arms resting on arm-boards
	Supine, with the elbows flexed and resting against a solid surface
Brachial plexus	Excessive stretch (arm in abduction with lateral rotation of the head to the opposite side)
	Compression (upward movement of the clavicle and sternal retraction)
	Forced downward movement of shoulders (e.g. in head-down tilt while using shoulder braces)
Radial	Compression of the nerve against the humerus (e.g. elbow slipping off table side or in lateral position with arm in gutter)
Sciatic	Elevation of opposite buttock (e.g. hip surgery)
	In lithotomy position, external rotation of the leg may damage the nerve by stretch-induced ischaemia
Common peroneal	Compression against the head of the fibula in the lithotomy position or between the fibula and the operating table in the lateral position

Certain positions have been associated with injury to the peripheral nerves and nerve plexuses; these are detailed in Table 15.2[11].

Arterial tourniquets, hypoxaemia, dehydration, and hypotension make nerve injury more likely. In medicolegal situations, a position of *res ipsa loquitor* existed for some time regarding intra-operative nerve injury; the fact of injury was considered to indicate that care must have been sub-standard. However, it is clear that some patients do have a predisposition to nerve injury (especially the ulnar nerve). In Sawyer's review article[12], he states: '*Intra-operative ulnar nerve compression can result in lesions of quite remarkable severity and recovery can be slow and often incomplete. Nevertheless, it seems quite likely that postoperative ulnar nerve palsy can occur without apparent cause and despite accepted methods of positioning and padding.*'

Postoperative visual loss

Blindness is a rare but devastating complication of general anaesthesia. Loss of vision in a single eye occurs following 0.0008% of general anaesthetics (1 in 125 000)[13]. Binocular loss of vision occurs in around 50% of cases of postoperative visual loss, and has even greater implications for the patient's future life.

The most frequent cause of loss of vision following general anaesthesia is ischaemic optic neuropathy[14]. Optic nerve ischaemia may be generated by external compression of the eye, arterial hypotension, elevated venous or intra-ocular pressure, increased resistance to flow (e.g. dehydration), or decreased oxygen delivery (e.g. anaemia, hypoxaemia). If intraocular pressure exceeds 60 mmHg, blood flow to the optic nerve at the optic disc ceases, but flow is maintained in the choroidal and retinal circulations. Infarction at this watershed leads to anterior ischaemic neuropathy, with a visual field defect, a pale oedematous optic disc, and oedema of the optic nerve in the posterior scleral foramen. The posterior part of the optic nerve is more vulnerable to ischaemia in the event of a fall in perfusion pressure or anaemia, because of the limited autoregulatory capacity of its arterial supply; ischaemia here may lead to posterior ischaemic optic neuropathy, causing mild optic disc oedema and a visual field defect of later onset. Postoperative visual loss may also be caused by occlusion of the retinal artery, through embolization or external compression. Postoperative fundoscopy reveals a pale retina with a 'cherry red spot'[15].

Several factors have been associated with postoperative visual loss. These include external compression of the globe; in the prone position, the choice of headrest can influence the risk of visual injury, and horseshoe-type headrests have been implicated in the majority of reported cases. Concurrent pathophysiological factors are known to increase the risk of postoperative visual loss; these include diabetes, hypertension, smoking, and polycythaemia. The prone position is associated with postoperative visual loss, and it has been shown that this posture doubles intraocular pressure[16]. Surgery associated with major bleeding or systemic emboli (e.g. spinal, cardiac, and carotid procedures) are associated with an increase in the risk of postoperative visual loss. In particular, spinal surgery, which is most often performed with the patient in the prone position, has been associated with the majority of the reported cases of post-operative visual loss and cardiac surgery accounts for 10% of cases[17].

Vision that is lost during anaesthesia is rarely recovered. Early treatment may allow small improvements if the cause is central retinal artery occlusion, but infarction in the optic nerve almost always results in permanent loss of visual acuity.

Postoperative hearing loss

Following cardiac bypass surgery, hearing loss may occur in 0.1% of patients[18]. In non-cardiac surgery, hearing loss is very rare and is usually temporary. Nitrous oxide, which diffuses into the middle ear during general anaesthesia, inevitably causes some minor and temporary distortion of hearing postoperatively. Sudden hearing loss has been reported on several occasions following neuraxial block, and subarachnoid (spinal) anaesthesia in particular[19]. Such auditory disturbance is probably caused by acute changes in cerebrospinal fluid (CSF) pressure.

Regional anaesthesia

This section deals in detail with injuries to peripheral nerves and to the spinal cord and its surroundings during regional anaesthesia. The reader is recommended to refer to an excellent and recent review article by Brull, McCartney, Chan, and El-Beheiry[20]. Within this section, systemic toxicity related to local anaesthetics and the issues of failed and excessive block are discussed.

Table 15.3 Complications of regional anaesthesia

Complication	Risk	
Failed block	1–20%	1 in 5–100
Peripheral nerve injury		
Temporary	0.34–2.84%	1 in 35–294
Permanent	0.003–0.006%	1 in 17 000–33 000
Spinal cord and nerve root injury		
Permanent paraplegia	0.001–0.0001%	1 in 100 000–1 000 000
Neurological injury (all)	0.03%	1 in 3300
Neurological injury (obstetric)	0.005%	1 in 20 000
Cauda equina injury	0.0002–0.01%	1 in 10 000–50 000
Epidural collections		
Abscess (non-obstetric)	0.05%	1 in 2000
Abscess (obstetric)	0.0007%	1 in 143 000
Haematoma (after spinal)	0.0005%	1 in 200 000
Haematoma (after epidural)	0.0007%	1 in 143 000
Seizure	0.01–0.7%	1 in 143–10 000
Cardiac arrest		
Spinal anaesthesia	0.06%	1 in 1700
Epidural or nerve block anaesthesia	0.01%	1 in 10,000
Ophthalmic block		
Globe puncture	0.01–0.1%	1 in 1000–10 000
Central spread of local anaesthetic	0.002–0.1%	1 in 1000–50 000

The complications of regional anaesthesia are summarized in Table 15.3.

Peripheral nerve injury during regional anaesthesia

The risk of permanent nerve damage following peripheral nerve blockade is uncertain; its incidence varies widely among practitioners and among patients, and depends upon the techniques used. In a prospective survey in France, Auroy estimated that nerve injury (temporary and permanent) occurred in 1 in 5000 nerve blocks[21], while Brull's review of contemporary literature[20] indicated that temporary neuropathy occurred in 0.34–2.84% of peripheral nerve and plexus blocks. According to the American Society of Anesthesiologists' *Closed Claims study*, temporary nerve injury is *at least* 2½ times more common than permanent nerve injury following peripheral nerve blockade[22]; this ratio may well be even larger, and the litigation bias (where temporary injury is less likely to be litigated upon) may cause permanent injury to be over-represented. Indeed, Auroy's series indicated that after all regional techniques, temporary injury was six times as common as permanent injury. Therefore, we may estimate that permanent nerve injury occurs after 1 in 15 000 to 35 000 nerve blocks (0.003–0.006%). In Brull's contemporary review, only a single case of permanent neurological injury followed peripheral nerve or plexus block in 65 000 procedures.

Neurological complications following peripheral nerve block can be caused by extrinsic trauma to the nerve (e.g. by a needle), injection into the nerve (intraneural), nerve ischaemia (e.g. caused by an arterial tourniquet or by scarring and contracture around a nerve), neurotoxicity of local anaesthetics, or drug error (injection of wrong drug).

Injuries to peripheral nerves after intraneural injection are well documented and are generally considered to represent the great majority of permanent nerve injuries. Extrinsic nerve injury is an uncommon cause of persisting neuronal dysfunction; it is more common when a long-bevelled needle is used[23], and use of a short-bevelled needle has become a widely-accepted standard of care. However, nerve injuries caused by sharp (long-bevelled) needles tend to heal more quickly and more completely than those caused by blunt (short-bevelled) needles[24]. In general, local anaesthetics administered correctly do not carry a risk of nerve injury through local neurotoxicity[25]; of course, a great variety of substances may be injected inadvertently instead of local anaesthetics, and reports exist of horrific injuries following intra-plexal administration of thiopentone. Arterial tourniquets are recognized as having the capacity to injure nerves through compression ischaemia. Laboratory data demonstrate that ischaemia damages the sciatic nerve irreversibly in less than 4 h. However, the rarity of nerve damage, despite the widespread use of arterial tourniquets, demonstrates that nerves are relatively resistant to *in vivo* ischaemia. However, the combination of increased intraneural pressure caused by intraneural injection, reduced blood flow (due to injected adrenaline), and the use of an arterial tourniquet could result in severe nerve injury; consequently, it may be wise to avoid placing a tourniquet directly over the site of injection.

There is no evidence that the use of a nerve stimulator is safer than using paraesthesia (in the awake patient) to locate nerves. However, most practitioners agree that paraesthesia indicates close proximity to a nerve and may confer greater risk. Nerve stimulation (muscle twitching) obtained at a current of 0.5 mA or less allows confidence of adequate proximity to a nerve for reliable nerve blockade. However, when twitching occurs with currents less than 0.2 mA, there is the possibility that the needle is touching or is inside the nerve; in this situation, the needle should be withdrawn until the twitch disappears. High injection pressure may indicate intraneural injection, and a large-capacity syringe (e.g. 20 mL) is recommended for all injections during regional techniques; this reduces the risk of excessive pressure being exerted and allows the operator to gain a feel for the impeded and unimpeded injections during regional techniques. Pain may indicate intraneural injection, and should cause immediate cessation of injection and repositioning of the needle tip. Consequently, some experts advise against performing peripheral nerve blockade in patients under deep sedation or anaesthesia, although this does not represent a consensus[26,27]. Consensus is growing that properly performed ultrasound guidance reduces the risks of intravascular and intraneural injections; there is little published literature to support this[28], but this should not be taken as evidence against the assertion, because the use of ultrasound for this purpose is still in its infancy.

Spinal cord and spinal nerve root injury during regional anaesthesia

Subarachnoid (spinal) anaesthesia, epidural anaesthesia, and peri-spinal blocks (e.g. paravertebral, intercostal, lumbar plexus) have been reported to cause spinal cord and nerve root injury[29,30]. Paraplegia is very rare after subarachnoid anaesthesia (1 in 100 000–1 000 000)[31,32], but other neurological injuries are more common (3 in 10 000)[20,21]. Severe neurological injury is 5–7 times less likely in the obstetric population than in the general population[31,33]. Injury may be caused by direct needle trauma, intra-cord injection, or disturbance of the blood supply to the spinal cord. Recovery following spinal cord injury is slow and usually incomplete. Residual defects often include bowel and bladder disturbance and lower limb weakness or sensory disturbance. Lifestyle is frequently affected.

Spinal cord injury during subarachnoid (spinal) anaesthesia is often the result of insertion of the needle at too cephalad a level. The spinal cord terminates in adults at around the level of the second lumbar vertebra; insertion at or above this level is seldom justified, even if difficulty is encountered at lower levels, and is almost never justified as a site of first attempt[34–36]. Difficulty of palpation of landmarks at the more appropriate, lower levels is not adequate justification for high placement of a subarachnoid injection. This is particularly true if the patient is unconscious, and cannot warn the anaesthetist of the pain of the proximity of needle to nerves. Spinal cord injury by needles and by the injection of local anaesthetic into the cord can produce widespread neurological lesions, but with very subtle clinical signs because nerve fibres transmitting only one or two sensory modalities may be affected.

Anaesthetists' estimation of the spinal level for insertion of needles has been shown to be inaccurate. The actual lumbar interspace identified by anaesthetists was one space higher than the interspace which the anaesthetist believed to have been identified in 51% of cases, and two spaces higher in 15.5%[37]. It is likely that, in the past, many injuries associated with spinal anaesthesia which were thought to be nerve root injuries or whose cause could not readily be explainedresulted from damage to the spinal cord; the introduction of magnetic resonance (MR) imaging has revolutionized the diagnosis of neurological injury. One of the editors has seen 25 cases of spinal cord injury associated with spinal anaesthesia in the last 10 years, all caused by insertion of the needle inadvertently at too high a level and all confirmed by MR scans. It is recommended that subarachnoid injections should be performed only below the third lumbar vertebra to avoid injury to the spinal cord[34].

Pencil-point needles are often referred to as 'atraumatic,' but this only has relevance to their effect on the dura and headaches following subarachnoid injection (see following paragraphs). Pencil-point needles may be more traumatic than their counterparts (cutting needles) with respect to spinal cord injury[36]. However, this additional risk with respect to spinal cord injury (which is uncommon) is outweighed by the advantages they bring with respect to dural injury (see following paragraphs).

Pain during needle insertion and subarachnoid injection may indicate proximity of the needle to a nerve root; subsequent injection or deeper insertion risks damage to the nerve. Clearly, patients who are anaesthetized cannot inform the anaesthetist that they are experiencing pain during subarachnoid injection. There is a clear argument for ceasing needle insertion or injection if the patient complains of pain. There is also an argument that the loss of such a warning caused by performing the subarachnoid injection after induction of general anaesthesia or deep sedation may make neurological injury more likely. The current broad consensus is that such techniques are better performed in conscious patients, but there is little evidential support.

Cranial nerve palsies may follow neuraxial anaesthesia as a result of reduced cerebrospinal fluid-pressure. In obstetric patients, the incidence has been reported as 1–3.7 in 100 000, with the 6th cranial nerve most commonly affected[38].

Cauda equina injury

Cauda equina syndrome is a rare neurological complication of subarachnoid (spinal) anaesthesia; back pain, leg weakness, and bowel and bladder dysfunction may occur. Its reported incidence following subarachnoid (spinal) anaesthesia has ranged between 1 in 10 000 and 1 in 500 000[21,31,32]. Historically, it was associated with the use of 5% lidocaine solutions[39,40] and has been linked to the use of microcatheters for subarachnoid local anaesthetic infusion. It is very rare after single injections of local anaesthetic, but has been reported[41]. Concurrent spinal pathology, such as herniated intervertebral disc or spinal canal stenosis may place patients at increased risk of cauda equina pathology. Although the pathogenesis of cauda equina syndrome is poorly understood, there is agreement on the neurotoxicity of local anaesthetics, particularly of 5% hyperbaric lidocaine.

Epidural abscess

Deep infection and abscess in the epidural space risks permanent paraplegia. Onset is typically with painless limb weakness and occurs within a few days of performance of an epidural or, more, rarely, subarachnoid (spinal) anaesthetic[42]. The incidence of epidural abscess in epidural anaesthesia has been reported as 1 in 1930 in the non-obstetric population[43] and 1 in 145 000 in the obstetric population[44]. It is not a rare complication in non-obstetric patients, and careful monitoring of sensory and motor block, and a high index of suspicion, are essential if the condition is to be diagnosed and treated in time to prevent permanent neurological damage.

Epidural haematoma

The incidence of spinal or epidural haematoma associated with regional anaesthesia was found in the early 1990s to be 1 in 150 000 for epidural anaesthesia and 1 in 220 000 for subarachnoid anaesthesia[45]. The risk factors identified include insertion difficulty, use of an epidural, catheter, coagulopathy, and timing in relation to anticoagulant administration[46]. Insertion or removal during anticoagulation increases the risk of epidural bleeding and haematoma, and larger doses of prophylactic anticoagulation (e.g. low-molecular-weight heparin) are associated with increased risk.

Dural injury

Subarachnoid (spinal) anaesthesia requires puncture of the dura. Headache, caused by loss of CSF and CSF hypotension, follows in around 1% of cases[47] when a 25-gauge, pencil-point needle is used; larger needles and those with a cutting tip produce headache more frequently. Accidental dural injury occurs during around 1% of epidurals[48]. Headache follows dural puncture with an epidural needle in 70–90% of cases. Most headaches occur within 48 h of dural injury and last for 3–6 days. Treatment may be by bed rest, intravenous fluids, epidural saline infusion, or epidural blood patch. Most headaches resolve with no long-term sequelae, but subdural haemorrhage within the skull can occur as a result of the reduced CSF pressure.

Back pain

Despite patients' frequent reports of back pain following epidural anaesthesia, no association has been identified in large prospective surveys[49]. It appears that post-partum or post-surgical back pain (which is common) may be blamed upon an epidural, leading to an apparent but fictitious association.

Failed block

Attempts at regional anaesthesia fail (i.e. produce insufficient anaesthesia for the intended procedure) in 0.1–20% of cases. The rate is very variable and depends upon operator expertise, the surgical procedure, the type of block and the drug used. This complication of regional anaesthesia is common enough to warrant its inclusion in every patient's consent process when regional anaesthesia is planned.

Extensive block during subarachnoid (spinal) and epidural anaesthesia

Excessively extensive block may occur following injection of local anaesthetic. Intended epidural injection, in particular, may travel in the subdural space, generating a very high block. The incidence is uncertain.

Systemic toxicity of local anaesthetics

All local anaesthetic techniques have the potential for systemic adverse effects resulting from intravascular injection or rapid absorption into the systemic circulation. Dysphoria, circum oral tingling, light-headedness, and twitching are relatively common, early signs. Their incidence is dependent upon the site of injection, the dose injected, the rate of administration, and the patient's susceptibility; the large majority of patients experiencing these symptoms have no further problems. Seizures occur during or after 0.1–7 in 1000 regional blocks[50]. Epidural administration of local anaesthetic seemed the least likely to cause seizures in this large study, whereas local anaesthetic administration around the neck (e.g. interscalene, supraclavicular)or caudal injections seemed the most likely to cause convulsions. In Brown's study (which used data collected between 1985 and 1992), 26 seizures were observed in 25 697 blocks, but no patient proceeded to suffer severe cardiovascular depression or cardiac arrest. It is well known that the plasma concentration of local anaesthetic required to produce cardiovascular depression is several times higher than that required to produce central nervous system symptoms, and it is likely that with careful, modern care, cardiac arrest due to local anaesthetic toxicity will be extremely rare.

Cardiac arrest during regional anaesthesia

Cardiac arrest occurs most commonly during subarachnoid (spinal) anaesthesia (0.06%), followed by epidural (0.01%) and peripheral nerve blocks (0.01%)[21]. Factors leading to cardiac arrest include hypotension due to vasodilatation and systemic spread of local anaesthetic. Sedation during regional anaesthesia, especially in the context of inadequate monitoring of the cardiovascular system and adequacy of ventilation, has been implicated in fatalities.

Injury to nearby structures

Regional anaesthetic techniques make use of a needle, and structures near the intended target of the needle risk injury. Such structures include the pulmonary pleura, arteries, veins, lymph ducts, bowel, the fetal head, and the ureters. The most common complication, vascular puncture, usually causes no long-term sequelae, but haematoma formation or distal embolization may occur. Pneumothorax has been reported to occur as frequently as in 6% of supraclavicular brachial plexus blocks[51]. The use of ultrasound in regional anaesthesia promises to reduce the incidence of local injury during needling[28], but evidential support is, as yet, slight.

Ophthalmic block

During local anaesthetic techniques intended to provide an insensate and/or immobile eye, ocular injury may occur. The major, recognized hazards of peribulbar and retrobulbar block include globe perforation, optic nerve injury, orbital haemorrhage, and central (brain) spread of local anaesthetic. Globe perforation may be very painful and may cause subsequent intra-ocular scarring, retinal detachment, and possible blindness. It is rare (0.01–0.1%) and is associated with a long eye (more than 25 mm, and usually occurring in short-sighted patients), a deeply-sunken eye in a narrow orbit, a mobile eye during performance of the block, an inexperienced operator, and pain during needle insertion[52]. Severe pain during needle advancement and the finding of a very soft eye after injection may indicate globe perforation. Loss of vision may occur immediately, but often does not occur until later[52]. Optic nerve injury is relatively rare and is often caused by injury to or obstruction of the central retinal artery, but may be caused also by direct injury through passing the needle into the optic nerve. Optic nerve injury is most likely in patients with a mobile eye during performance of the block (especially looking away from the needle insertion), an inexperienced operator, deep insertion of the needle (>30 mm), and attempted retrobulbar block (vs. peribulbar). Orbital haemorrhage is common and usually recovers without serious sequelae; on occasion, it may cause restriction of the blood supply and drainage of the globe (through compression of the vessels), risking retinal injury. It is more likely in patients taking aspirin or anti-coagulants (e.g. warfarin).

Central (brain) spread of local anaesthetic is rare but has been reported to cause severe hypotension, loss of consciousness, convulsions, bilateral temporary blindness, and cardiac arrest; it is caused by injection of local anaesthetic into the sheath surrounding the optic nerve.

Central spread of local anaesthetic agent occurs more commonly following retrobulbar block, where an incidence of 0.002–0.1% is reported[52]. Such spread may cause convulsions, loss of consciousness and cardiac arrest. More minor effects (e.g. dysphoria, dizziness) are more common.

Risk minimization in ophthalmic block is achieved currently through maintaining a fixed gaze, ceasing needle advancement or injection in the presence of pain and the use of a relatively short needle (<30 mm). Sub-tenon anaesthesia is a relatively new approach that offers the potential for reduced risk of penetrative ocular injury. There is little evidence as yet of any superiority to traditional approaches to ophthalmic regional anaesthesia.

References

1. Hart, R. and Hindman, B. (1982). Mechanisms of perioperative cerebral infarction. *Stroke*, **13**, 766–73.
2. Jenkins, K. and Baker, A.B.(2003). Consent and anaesthetic risk. *Anaesthesia*, **58**, 962–84.
3. Gerraty, R.P., Gates, P.C., and Doyle, J.C. (1993). Carotid stenosis and perioperative stroke risk in symptomatic and asymptomatic patients undergoing vascular or coronary surgery. *Stroke*, **24**, 1115–8.
4. Roach, G.W., Kanchuger, M., Mangano, C.M., *et al.* (1996). Adverse cerebral outcomes after coronary bypass surgery. Multicenter Study of Perioperative Ischemia Research Group and the Ischemia Research and Education Foundation Investigators. *New England Journal Medicine*, **335**(25), 1857–63.
5. Warner, M.A., Shields, S.E., and Chute, C.G. (1993). Major morbidity and mortality within 1 month of ambulatory surgery and anesthesia. *Journal of the American Medical Association*, **270**(12), 1437–41.
6. Kofke, W.A., Tempelhoff, R., and Dasheiff, R.M. (1997). Anesthetic implications of epilepsy, status epilepticus, and epilepsy surgery. *Journal of Neurosurgical Anesthesiology*, **9**(4), 349–72.
7. Weinberg, L., Harvey, W.R., and Marshall, R.J. (2002). Postoperative paraplegia following spinal cord infarction. *Acta Anaesthesiologica Scandinvica*, **46**(4), 469–72.
8. Dhuner, K.G. (1950). Nerve injuries following operations: survey of cases during a 6 year period. *Anesthesiology*, **11**, 289–93.
9. Kroll, D.A., Caplan,R.A., Posner, K., Ward, R.J., and Cheney, F.W. (1990). Nerve injury associated with anaesthesia. *Anesthesiology*, **73**, 202–7.
10. Warner, M.A., Warner, D.O., Matsumoto, J.Y., Harper, C.M., Schroeder, D.R., and Maxson, P.M. (1999). Ulnar neuropathy in surgical patients. *Anesthesiology*, **90**, 54–9.
11. Knight, D.J.W. and Mahajan, R.P. (2004). Patient positioning in anaesthesia. *Continuing Education in Anaesthesia, Critical Care & Pain*, **4**, 160–3.
12. Sawyer, R.J., Richmond, M.N., Hickey, J.D., and Jarratt, J.A. (2000). Peripheral nerve injuries associated with anaesthesia. *Anaesthesia*, **55**, 980–91.
13. Warner, M.E., Warner, M.E., Garrity, J.A., Mackenzie, R.A., and Warner, D.O. (2001). The frequency of perioperative vision loss. *Anesthesia and Analgesia*, **93**, 1417–21.

14. White, E. Care of the eye during anaesthesia. (2004). *Anaesthesia and Intensive Care,* **5**, 302–3.

15. Werrett, G. (2003). Nerve injury. In *Oxford Handbook of Anaesthesia*(K.G. Allman and I.H. Wilson eds.), pp. 948–52.Oxford University Press, Oxford.

16. Cheng, M.A., Todorov, A., Tempelhoff, R., McHugh, T., Crowder, C.M., and Lauryssen, C., (2001). The effect of prone positioning on intraocular pressure in anesthetized patients. *Anesthesiology,* **95**(6), 1351–5.

17. Sweeney, P.J., Breuer, A.C., Selhorst, J.B. *et al.* (1982). Ischemic optic neuropathy: a complication of cardiopulmonary bypass surgery. *Neurology,* **32**, 560–2.

18. Evan, K.E., Tavill, M.A., Goldberg, A.N., and Silverstein, H. (1997). Sudden sensorineural hearing loss after general anesthesia for non-otologic surgery. *Laryngoscope,* **107**, 747–52.

19. Lamberg, T., Pitkanen, M.T., Marttila, T., Rosenberg, P.H. (1997). Hearing loss after continuous or single shot spinal anesthesia. *Regional Anesthesia,* **22**, 539–42.

20. Brull, R., McCartney, C.J., Chan, V.W. and El-Beheiry, H. (2007). Neurological complications after regional anesthesia: contemporary estimates of risk. *Anesthesia and Analgesia,* **104**(4), 965–74.

21. Auroy, Y., Narchi, P., Messiah, A., *et al.* (1997). Serious complications related to regional anesthesia: results of a prospective survey in France. *Anesthesiology,* **87**, 479–86.

22. Lee, L.A., Posner, K.L., Domino, K.B., Caplan, R.A., Cheney, F.W. (2004). Injuries associated with regional anesthesia in the 1980s and 1990s: a closed claims analysis. *Anesthesiology,* **101**(1), 143–152.

23. Selander, D., Dhuner, K.G., and Lundborg, G. (1977). Peripheral nerve injury due to injection needles used for regional anesthesia. An experimental study of the acute effects of needle point trauma. *Acta Anaesthesiologica Scandinavica,* **21**(3), 182–8.

24. Rice, A.S. and McMahon, S.B. (1992). Peripheral nerve injury caused by injection needles used in regional anaesthesia: influence of bevel configuration, studied in a rat model. *British Journal of Anaesthesia,* **69**(5), 433–8.

25. Kalichman, M.W, Powel, H.C,, and Myers, R.R. (1988). Pathology of local anesthetic-induced nerve injury. *Acta Neuropathologica,* **75**, 583–9.

26. Fischer, H.B.J. (1998). Regional anaesthesia – before or after general anaesthesia? *Anaesthesia,* **53**, 727–9.

27. Bogdanov, A. and Loveland, R. (2005). Is there a place for interscalene block performed after induction of general anaesthesia? *European Journal of Anaesthesiology,* **22**, 107–10.

28. Hopkins, P.M. (2007). Ultrasound guidance as a gold standard in regional anaesthesia. *British Journal of Anaesthesia,* **98**(3), 299–301.

29. Hamandi, K., Mottershead, J., Lewis. T., Ormerod, I.C., and Ferguson, I.T. (2002). Irreversible damage to the spinal cord following spinal anesthesia. *Neurology,* **59**(4), 624–6.

30. Rajakulendran, Y., Rahman, S. and Venkat, N. (1999). Long-term neurological complication following traumatic damage to the spinal cord with a 25 gauge Whitacre spinal needle. *International Journal of Obstetric Anesthesia,* **8**, 626.

31. Moen, V., Dahlgren, N., Irestedt, L. (2004). Severe neurological complications after central neuraxial blockades in Sweden 1990–1999. *Anesthesiology,* **101**, 950–9.

32. Aromaa, U., Lahdensuu, M., and Cozanitis, D.A. (1997). Severe complications associated with epidural and spinal anaesthesias in Finland 1987–1993. A study based on patient insurance claims. *Acta Anaesthesiologica Scandinavica,* **41**, 445–52.

33. Auroy, Y., Benhamou, D., Bargues, L., *et al.* (2002). Major complications of regional anesthesia in France: the SOS regional anesthesia hotline service. *Anesthesiology,* **97**, 1274–80.

34. Reynolds, F. (2001). Damage to the conus medullaris following spinal anaesthesia. *Anaesthesia*, **56**(3), 238–47.

35. Reynolds, F. (2000). Logic in the safe practice of spinal anaesthesia. *Anaesthesia*, **55**(11), 1045–6.

36. Fettes, P.D. and Wildsmith, J.A. (2002). Somebody else's nervous system. *British Journal of Anaesthesia*, **88**(6), 760–3.

37. Broadbent, C.R., Maxwell, W.B., Ferrie, R., Wilson, D.J., Gawne-Cain, M., and Russell, R. (2000). Ability of anaesthetists to identify a marked lumbar interspace. *Anaesthesia*, **55**, 1106–26.

38. Scott, D.B. and Hibbard, B.M. (1990). Serious non-fatal complications associated with extradural block in obstetric practice. *British Journal of Anaesthesia*, **64**, 537–41.

39. Johnson, M.E. (2004). Neurotoxicity of lidocaine: implications for spinal anesthesia and neuroprotection. *Journal of Neurosurgical Anesthesiology*, **16**, 80–3.

40. Zaric, D., Christiansen, C., Pace, N.L., and Punjasawadwong, Y. (2005). Transient neurologic symptoms after spinal anesthesia with lidocaine versus other local anesthetics: a systematic review of randomized, controlled trials. *Anesthesia and Analgesia*, **100**, 1811–16.

41. Moussa, T., Abdoulaye, D., Youssouf, C., Oumar, G.C., Karim, T.S., and Traore, T.J. (2006). Cauda equina syndrome and profound hearing loss after spinal anesthesia with isobaric bupivacaine. *Anesthesia and Analgesia*, **102**, 1863–4.

42. Kindler, C.H., Seeberger, M.D., and Staender, S.E. (1998). Epidural abscess complicating epidural anesthesia and analgesia. An analysis of the literature. *Acta Anaesthesiologica, Scandinavica*, **42**, 614 –20.

43. Wang, L.P., Hauerberg, J., and Schmidt, J.F. (1999). Incidence of spinal epidural abscess after epidural analgesia. *Anesthesiology*, **91**, 1928–36.

44. Ruppen, W., Derry, S., McQuay, H., and Moore, R.A. (2006). Incidence of epidural hematoma, infection, and neurologic injury in obstetric patients with epidural analgesia/anesthesia. *Anesthesiology*, **105**(2), 394–9.

45. Tryba, M. (1993). Epidural regional anesthesia and low molecular heparin: Pro. *Anasthesiologie, Intensivmedizin, Notfallmedizin, Schmerztherapie*, **28**, 179–81.

46. Vandermeulen, E.P., Van Aken, H., and Vermylen, J. (1994). Anticoagulants and spinal-epidural anesthesia. *Anesthesia and Analgesia*, **79**, 1165–77.

47. Turnbull, D.K. and Shepherd, D.B. (2003). Post-dural puncture headache: pathogenesis, prevention and treatment. *British Journal of Anaesthesia*, **91**(5), 718–29.

48. Reynolds, F. (1993). Dural puncture and headache. *British Medical Journal*, **306**, 874–6.

49. Russell, R., Dundas, R., and Reynolds, F. (1996). Long term backache after childbirth: prospective search for causative factors. *British Medical Journal*, **312**, 1384–8.

50. Brown, D.L., Ransom, D.M., Hall, J.A., Leicht, C.H., Schroeder, D.R., and Offord, K.P. (1995). Regional anesthesia and local anesthetic-induced systemic toxicity: seizure frequency and accompanying cardiovascular changes. *Anesthesia and Analgesia*, **81**, 321–8.

51. Brand, L. and Papper, E.M. (1961). A comparison of supraclavicular and axillary techniques for brachial plexus blocks. *Anesthesiology*, **22**, 226–9.

52. Rubin, A.P. (1995). Complications of local anaesthesia for ophthalmic surgery. *British Journal of Anaesthesia*, **75**(1), 93–6.

Chapter 16

Psychiatric risk

Michael H Nathanson

Psychiatric complications following anaesthesia and surgery are feared by both patients and anaesthetists. Patients are fearful of 'losing control' and embarrassing or injuring themselves, whereas for anaesthetists, these complications may appear difficult to diagnose, prevent, or manage. Many patients are frightened of developing postoperative cognitive dysfunction and can recall family stories of an uncle or aunt who was 'never the same' after his/her operation. Furthermore, all psychiatric conditions still have a stigma attached to them.

Many doctors will have faced a combative postoperative patient, unsure what to do and hesitant of giving any medication that may make the situation worse. Many of these complications are due to an underlying cause (Table 16.1) that in some cases can be easily remedied. However, some are idiosyncratic reactions or associated with much more complicated underlying conditions. This chapter describes in detail two problems: postoperative delirium and postoperative cognitive dysfunction, the risk of developing these complications, and the factors that can be modified. Neurocognitive problems after cardiac surgery are also described.

Introduction

In 1955, Bedford reviewed 18 patients whom he had known both prior to and after surgery and anaesthesia and who developed what he termed 'extreme dementia'[1]. He commented that while it was difficult from his figures to determine the exact incidence of this condition, he believed that operations on elderly people should be undertaken only in 'unequivocally necessary cases'. He cautioned against the use of preoperative and postoperative medication—especially 'narcotic and potent analgesic drugs'. He believed that, during and after surgery, the blood pressure, haemoglobin concentration, and oxygenation should be kept at 'optimal levels'. Hypotensive surgery was absolutely contraindicated in elderly patients in his opinion. Finally, he stated that complications of surgery should be anticipated, prevented, and treated. Was he right?

Delirium

Delirium is an acute onset of disturbed mental function (an acute confusional state, ACS). The clinical picture includes impaired cognition and disorganized thinking, fluctuating levels of consciousness, altered psychomotor activity, and a disturbed sleep/wake cycle. Many patients have hallucinations, anxiety, and distress. The symptoms are

Table 16.1 Specific causes of altered mental status after anaesthesia and surgery

Alcohol or drug withdrawal
Bladder distension
High-dose steroids
Hypoglycaemia
Ketamine
Pain
Perioperative cerebrovascular accident
Porphyria
Recovery from anaesthesia in children after use of short-acting anaesthetic agents, e.g. sevoflurane
Seizures
Shock
Tight dressings
TURP syndrome

often worse at night. Delirium may be an 'agitated' variant or a 'quiet' variant which can be easily missed or misdiagnosed as depression[2]. It often manifests after a lucid interval, usually of one day[3]. Delirium is often poorly documented by doctors and nurses[4].

Most of the literature on delirium is related to elderly patients and there is a significant risk of developing delirium in all elderly patients admitted to hospital—not just those undergoing anaesthesia and surgery. Delirium may lead to increased morbidity including urinary problems, decubitus ulcers, and feeding problems[5], delayed functional recovery and prolonged hospital stay, and increased mortality[6]. The total cost to the healthcare system of delirium is huge—in hospitalized patients, it inevitably leads to increased length of stay and increases costs after discharge from the acute unit with the need for long-term care in some sufferers. Although risk factors in the perioperative period have been identified (see following paragraphs) the influence of the type of anaesthesia seems negligible. However, other modifiable factors have been identified.

Differential diagnosis

In elderly patients, it may be difficult to differentiate between delirium and pre-existing dementia. Dementia is a chronic, irreversible condition. There is a global deterioration in cognitive ability in the absence of clouding of consciousness. It may be associated with failure of cholinergic transmission, and these patients may be sensitive to anticholinergic drugs[7]. Further diagnostic confusion may arise because patients with dementia are at increased risk of delirium. The features described in Table 16.2 may help to differentiate dementia from delirium.

Table 16.2 Differential diagnosis of patient with altered cognition after surgery

	Delirium	Dementia
Onset	Sudden	Insidious
24-h course	Fluctuating	Stable
Consciousness	Reduced	Clear
Attention	Globally disordered	Normal except in advanced cases
Cognition	Globally disordered	Globally impaired
Hallucinations	Usually visual	Often absent
Delusions	Fleeting, poorly systematized	Often absent
Orientation	Usually impaired	Often impaired
Psychomotor	Increased, reduced	Often normal
Speech	Often incoherent, slow or rapid	Perseveration, difficulty finding words
Physical illness or drug toxicity	Often present	Often absent, especially in Alzheimer's type

Source: Modified from Gosney, M.A. (2005). Acute confusional states and dementia's: perioperative considerations. Current Anaesthesia and Critical Care, **16**, 34–9. With permission.

Incidence

The exact incidence of delirium in any population depends on which diagnostic criteria and methods of surveillance are used. As a result, it is difficult to compare studies in which the methodology, in this respect, is often different.

The incidence of delirium in elderly patients admitted to a general medical ward is 15–50%[8,9]. The incidence in general surgical patients of all ages is 5–10%[9], and the incidence in some populations of elderly postoperative patients is up to 61% (see following paragraphs).

A study of 51 patients undergoing bilateral total knee replacement found that the incidence of postoperative delirium was 41% (21 patients), although only 11 of these had 'overt' delirium that would have been diagnosed by the patients' normal attending medical and nursing staff[10]. The incidence of delirium in 70 elderly patients without pre-existing cognitive dysfunction undergoing major abdominal surgery was 25%[11]. A much larger study of 1341 elective surgery patients, aged 50 years or more, undergoing mostly orthopaedic (43%), vascular, abdominal, or non-cardiac thoracic procedures[12] found that the overall incidence of delirium was 9%. In 701 elderly (≥65 years of age; mean age 73 years) patients undergoing elective orthopaedic or urological surgery, the incidence of delirium was 5.1%[13].

The incidence of delirium appears to be greater after non-elective surgery and is particularly high in patients with a hip fracture. Ní Chonchubhair and colleagues[14] found the incidence of postoperative delirium to be 23% in elderly (>65 years of age) orthopaedic patients (mostly hip fractures) and 9% after non-orthopaedic surgery.

In 111 hip fracture patients, aged ≥65 years(mean age 79 years), 68 (61%) had an acute confusional state either on admission or during their ward stay[5], and in a study of 105 hip surgery patients aged ≥60 years (mean age 75 years), the overall incidence of delirium was 23.8%, with 40.5% in the hip fracture patients and 14.7% in the elective hip replacement surgery patients[3].

Risk factors

Many predisposing factors for the development of delirium have been identified including urinary and chest infections, alcohol withdrawal, anticholinergic drugs or drops (including those with a weak anticholinergic action such as digoxin, thiazide diuretics, and corticosteroids), metabolic disturbances (for example disturbances of sodium and glucose), increasing age, re-operation, pathological brain states, drug interactions, alcohol and sedative withdrawal, depression, dementia, sleep deficiency, anxiety, gender, fat embolism, and impaired vision.

Tsutsui et al[15]. showed that delirium in a general surgical unit was more likely with increasing age and after emergency surgery. Dai et al[13]. studied elective surgical patients and found age (age ≥ 80 years, relative risk 2.75) and pre-existing cognitive impairment (relative risk 4.4) to be 'vulnerability factors' (that is, factors present on admission), and use of psycho-active drugs (including opioids, sedatives, H_2-receptor antagonists, anti-Parkinson agents, and anticholinergice drugs) during hospitalization (relative risk 6.56), a 'precipitating factor' (that is, a noxious insult or hospitalization-related factors). Williams-Russo et al[10]. studied patients undergoing bilateral total knee replacement and found, using logistic regression analysis, that increasing age, chronic alcohol use, and male gender were associated factors. A study of elective surgery patients aged 50 years or more undergoing major non-cardiac surgery examined the relationship between intra-operative events including type of anaesthesia, hypotension, and blood loss, and the onset of delirium on day 2 or later after surgery[12]. The occurrence of intra-operative hypotension did not predict delirium. However, blood loss and the requirement for postoperative blood transfusion did predict delirium. Of course, it is not clear if early transfusion would have prevented any of the cases of delirium. Hearing loss, opioid usage, and greater postoperative pain have also been found to be associated factors[16,17].

Hip fracture

Galankis and colleagues[3]. studied delirium in elderly hip surgery patients (elective and hip fracture) and found the risk factors (determined by multivariate analysis) to be age, pre-existing cognitive impairment, depression, low educational state, and abnormal preoperative sodium status (<135 or >145 mmol/l). Berggren[18] found risk factors for delirium after hip fracture surgery to be pre-existing depression and use of anticholinergic drugs. Gustafson and colleagues.[5] investigated elderly (aged ≥65 years) hip fracture patients and reported the following risk factors for delirium: increasing age, dementia, depression, and cerebrovascular or cardiovascular diseases. 85% of patients receiving regular anticholinergic medication developed delirium, and 12 of 13 patients whose systolic blood pressure fell to 80 mmHg or lower, developed delirium after surgery. A later study from the same group[19] found that age and male gender predicted development of ACS.

Marcantonio[6] developed a clinical prediction rule for preoperative factors (Table 16.3) by studying elective, major non-cardiac surgical patients (orthopaedic 45%) aged over 50 years (mean age 68 years). This rule can be used preoperatively to stratify patients into risk groups. However, the usefulness of a prediction system that utilizes a scoring scheme for cognitive status that will not be known to most practitioners is probably limited. The Telephone Interview for Cognitive Status (TICS) is an 11-point screening test for cognitive impairment that takes approximately 10 min to perform, either by phone or face-to-face, and correlates with the more commonly used mini-mental examination.

Effect of type of anaesthesia and analgesia

There is no convincing evidence that the type of anaesthesia or postoperative pain relief influences the likelihood of postoperative delirium. After hip fracture surgery, there was no difference in the incidence of delirium in those receiving halothane general anaesthesia, compared with those who received epidural anaesthesia[18]. Urwin, Parker and Griffiths' meta-analysis of general versus regional anaesthesia for hip fracture surgery[20] found a tendency towards a lower incidence of delirium in patients receiving regional anaesthesia. However, a study[12] of over 1000 elective

Table 16.3 Clinical prediction rule for postoperative delirium

Risk factor	points
Age ≥70 years	1
Alcohol abuse	1
TICS score <30[a]	1
SAS class IV[b]	1
Abnormal preoperative sodium, potassium or glucose[c]	1
Aortic aneurysm surgery	2
Non-cardiac thoracic surgery	1
Total points	*Risk of delirium (%)*
0	2
1 or 2	11
≥3	50

a TICS—Telephone Interview for Cognitive Status (<30 indicates cognitive impairment).

b SAS—Specific Activity Scale (class IV indicates severe physical impairment).

c Sodium <130 or >150 mmol/l; potassium <3.3 or >6 mmol/l; glucose <3.3 or >16.7 mmol/l.

Source: Adapted from Marcantonio, E.R., Goldman, L., Mangione, C.M., *et al.* (1994). A clinical prediction rule for delirium after elective noncardiac surgery. *Journal of the American Medical Association*, **271**, 134–9. With permission.

surgery patients, aged 50 years or more, undergoing orthopaedic, vascular, abdominal or non-cardiac thoracic procedures found no difference in the incidence of delirium between patients who received general anaesthesia, general anaesthesia combined with an epidural, epidural alone, or subarachnoid (spinal) block. Mann *et al.*[11] studied 70 elderly patients undergoing major abdominal surgery and found no difference in the incidence of delirium in those receiving general anaesthesia followed by morphine patient-controlled analgesia (PCA), compared with those who had combined general and epidural anaesthesia and postoperative patient-controlled epidural analgesia with bupivacaine and sufentanil. In patients undergoing bilateral total knee replacement surgery, there was no difference in the incidence of delirium between those who received intravenous fentanyl and those who received epidural fentanyl and bupivacaine for postoperative pain relief[10].

Constituent parts of an anaesthetic technique such as the use of anticholinergic medication may, however, have a large effect on the incidence of delirium.

Efficacy of techniques to modify risk factors

It is likely that the cause of delirium in most patients is multifactorial and it is no surprise, therefore, that techniques that adopt a variety of measures to reduce delirium have some benefit. Inouye and colleagues[8] developed a programme for the management of cognitive impairment, sleep deprivation, immobility, visual impairment, hearing impairment, and dehydration in elderly medical (that is, non-surgical) patients which reduced the likelihood of delirium from 15% to 10%. Another study of active geriatric care with daily visits and targeted recommendations based on a structured protocol, reduced the incidence of delirium after hip fracture surgery from 50 to 32%[21];however, length of stay in hospital was not changed. Gustafson and colleagues[19] used a programme of pre- and postoperative assessments, oxygen therapy, early surgery, prevention and treatment of perioperative hypotension, and treatment of postoperative complications to reduce delirium after hip fracture (compared with historical control); the incidence was reduced from 61% to 48%. Finally, Milisen and colleagues[22] reported on a nurse-led programme; the incidence of delirium in hip fracture patients was not changed, although the severity of the delirium was less and the duration was shorter.

It appears that for many patients the risk of delirium is dependent on factors that cannot be modified such as their age, pre-existing dementia, and the need for emergency surgery. Clearly, avoiding anticholinergic medication is advisable, as is careful observation for and prevention of the problems listed in Table 16.1. For patients in whom delirium seems an almost inevitable risk, some form of multidisciplinary approach may offer some benefit, but there is no convincing evidence that one particular anaesthetic technique is better than any other.

Postoperative cognitive dysfunction

An exact working clinical definition of postoperative cognitive dysfunction (POCD) does not exist although it has been described as 'a long-term, possibly permanent, disabling deterioration in cognitive function following surgery'[7]. However, determining what degree of loss of cognitive function equates to a diagnosis of POCD, requires the use of a statistical test—for example, it can be defined as a deterioration in performance of a battery of neuropsychological tests expected in <3.5% of controls. Research is further complicated by the different tests used by different workers and the fact that, in the (usually elderly) population used as controls, there will be a decline in cognitive ability over time, in any event. Changes in mental function do not occur only in elderly patients after anaesthesia and surgery[23]. One other difficulty in determining the exact incidence of POCD is that patients' own reports of problems such as poor memory after anaesthesia and surgery tend to be more common than can be identified by objective testing[24]. A number of large, well-conducted studies into POCD have been published in the last decade and are described in the following paragraphs.

The incidence of POCD depends on the type of surgery, patient age, method of detection, preoperative level of education, co-existing disease, and preoperative cognitive performance[25]. Possible aetiologies include hypotension, cerebral hypoxia, effects of long-acting sedatives or anaesthetics, metabolic disturbances, and cerebral embolism. However, an effect of regional anaesthesia (as compared with general anaesthesia) in reducing the incidence of persistent POCD has not been proven.

The ISPOCD studies

The first International Study of Postoperative Cognitive Dysfunction (ISPOCD) reported in 1998[26]. This international, multicentre study followed more than 1000 patients aged 60 years or more after major non-cardiac (abdominal, thoracic, or orthopaedic) surgery under general anaesthesia. There was no restriction on the anaesthetic technique used, but normocapnia was maintained throughout the operative period. A number of neuropsychological tests were performed before surgery, and at one week and three months afterwards. The incidence of POCD was 25.8% (95% CI 23.1–28.5) at one week and 9.9% (8.1–12.0) at three months. In the control group, 3.4% of participants had scores suggestive of cognitive dysfunction at 1 week, and 2.8% at three months. The risk factors for POCD at one week were increasing age, duration of anaesthesia, little education, a second operation (odds ratio 2.7), postoperative infection (OR 1.7), and respiratory complications (OR 1.6). The only risk factor for POCD at three months was increasing age. Perioperative hypoaxaemia (during the first 24 h and the second and third postoperative nights) and hypotension (during the first 24h) were not risk factors.

A long-term follow up of a subset (determined geographically) of the patients investigated in ISPOCD was reported by Abildstrom and colleagues in 2000[27]. These patients were re-studied after 1–2 years and the rate of POCD was 10.4% (vs. 10.3% in this subset at 3 months). The risk factors for POCD at 1–2 years were increasing age, infective complications (OR 2.61), and POCD detected at one week (OR 2.84). The rate of similar deterioration in cognitive function in a small ($n=47$) control group was 10.6% (CI 1.7–19.4%). Only 0.9% of patients had POCD at all three tests (one week, three months, and 1–2 years). It is notable that many of the patients with impaired cognitive function at 1–2 years did not demonstrate impaired cognitive function at either one or both of the earlier assessments.

The second ISPOCD study reported in 2002[28] on the incidence of POCD in middle-aged (40–59 years) patients undergoing major abdominal or orthopaedic surgery.

General anaesthesia was again used (with preservation of normocapnia), and the use of epidural analgesia was optional. The incidence of POCD was 19.2% (CI 15.7–23.1) at one week and 6.2% (4.1–8.9) at three months (vs. 4% and 4.1% in the control groups, respectively). This is a lower incidence than that reported in the earlier ISPOCD study of patients aged more than 60 years. POCD at one week was associated with use of supplementary epidural analgesia (OR 2.47) and avoidance of alcohol (as reported by the patient) (OR 1.81). The latter effect may be because patients who avoid alcohol are more vulnerable to the effects of sedative drugs perioperatively. The reason for the association with the use of epidural local anaesthetic-based analgesia was not clear. It may have been because patients who received epidural analgesia were more likely to have had more major operations, or, perhaps, because infusions of local anaesthetics can impair the ability to complete neuropsychological tests.

Effect of general versus regional anaesthesia

In 1980, Hole and colleagues[29] reported their study of 60 patients who underwent total hip replacement surgery and compared general anaesthesia maintained with nitrous oxide and fentanyl with epidural anaesthesia. The patients who received general anaesthesia had lower arterial blood oxygen tensions on days 1 and 3. Patients who received epidural anaesthesia had greater falls of blood pressure perioperatively. One patient in each group had signs of central cholinergic syndrome, which improved after administration of physostigmine. Seven of the remaining 30 general anaesthesia patients had evidence of mental changes on interview, compared with none of the remaining 28 epidural patients. The mean preoperative arterial oxygen tension (PaO_2) in the seven patients with mental changes was 11.6 kPa, and the mean PaO_2 on day 1 was 9.2 kPa. There was no significant change in PaO_2 in the epidural patients. One the seven patients died and, of the remaining six, only two thought that they had recovered completely when assessed several months later. Eight patients in each group who did not have mental changes detected during their in-hospital stay, later complained of slight mental changes after discharge from hospital. This study has been subsequently criticized for the somewhat subjective determination of POCD.

Williams-Russo and colleagues.[30] studied 262 patients who underwent total knee replacement surgery. Patients were allocated randomly to receive either general anaesthesia (maintenance with fentanyl and isoflurane) or epidural anaesthesia (plain lidocaine or bupivacaine without any adjuvants, or with opioids added). The epidural group received a postoperative epidural infusion, and the general anaesthesia patients received intravenous opioid analgesia. In all patients, there was a generalized decline in cognitive function at one week, which returned to (or near to) baseline by 6 months in most patients. The overall incidence of POCD at 6 months was 5%, with no significant difference between general anaesthesia (4%) and epidural anaesthesia (6%).

The ISPOCD group examined the effect of general versus regional (spinal or epidural) anaesthesia in elderly patients (aged >60 years) who underwent non-cardiac surgery (predominantly major joint replacement)[31]. Approximately one-third of the patients who received regional anaesthesia also received 'light' sedation with propofol. There was no difference in the incidence of cognitive dysfunction at three months. At one week, there was no difference when the data were analysed on an 'intention to treat' basis, but on a per protocol analysis, there was a greater incidence of POCD at one week in the general anaesthesia patients (21.2% vs. 12.7% for general and regional anaesthesia, respectively).

Other factors

Rosenberg and Kehlet[32] examined the relationship between postoperative confusion and hypoxaemia after major abdominal surgery. They found a correlation between mental function on the third day after surgery and mean peripheral blood oxygen saturation on the second postoperative night. In a small (60 patients) observational study, the incidence of cerebral desaturation detected by near-infrared spectroscopy (NIRS) was found to be 26% in elderly (aged >65 years) patients after major abdominal, non-vascular surgery[33]. Patients with cerebral desaturation were four times more likely to show a decline in cognitive function postoperatively. In none of the patients was desaturation identified on standard peripheral blood oxygen saturation monitoring (pulse oximetry).

It seems that the incidence of early POCD may be increased in patients having general (as opposed to regional) anaesthesia, but there is no long term-difference in rates of POCD. Furthermore, given the changes in cognitive function which occur in the elderly over a period of time, it is not clear how much of the POCD seen several years later is due to anaesthesia and surgery, and how much would have happened in any event. Fines and Severn have listed the predisposing factors for POCD (Table 16.4).

Cardiac surgery

After cardiac surgery requiring cardiopulmonary bypass, early POCD may be present in up to 80% of patients[25], and may persist in up to 42% five years later[34]. The exact incidence is difficult to determine because of problems in identifying suitable control groups. Open heart (i.e., mitral or aortic valve surgery) is associated with a greater

Table 16.4 Predisposing factors for POCD

Early POCD
Increasing age
General anaesthesia (vs. regional anaesthesia)
Increasing duration of anaesthesia
Respiratory complications
Lower level of education
Re-operation
Postoperative infection
Prolonged POCD
Increasing age

Source: Modified from Fines, D.P., Severn, A.M. (2006). Anaesthesia and cognitive disturbance in the elderly. *British Journal of Anaesthesia – Continuing Education in Anaesthesia, Critical Care and Pain,* **6,** 37–40. With permission.

incidence of postoperative decline in neurocognitive tests than coronary artery surgery, and combined valve and coronary artery surgery is associated with the greatest risk.

Possible causative factors include emboli, generalized cerebral hypoperfusion, systemic inflammation, genetic predisposition, rapid rewarming or hyperthermia after bypass. Selnes[35] reviewed this topic and concluded that short-term decline (1 week to 1 month) was associated with increasing age, low education, and increased numbers of emboli as measured by carotid ultrasound. Long-term decline was associated with the presence of diabetes and the severity of arteriosclerotic disease of the aorta.

One recent intriguing finding is that there may be a genetic predisposition to POCD after cardiac surgery. Patients with the apolipoprotein E ε4 (APOE ε4) allele had a significantly greater incidence of POCD at discharge and six weeks after surgery[36]. However, later studies have failed to confirm this association.

References

1. Bedford, P.D. (1955). Adverse effects of anaesthesia on old people. *Lancet ii*, 259–63.

2. Gosney, M.A. (2005). Acute confusional states and dementia's: peri-operative considerations. *Current Anaesthesia and Critical Care*, **16**, 34–9.

3. Galanakis, P., Bickel, H., Gradinger, R., Von Gumppenberg, S., and Förstl, H. (2001). Acute confusional state in the elderly following hip surgery: incidence, risk factors and complications. *International Journal of Geriatric Psychiatry*, **16**, 349–55.

4. Gustafson, Y., Brännström, B., Norberg, A., Bucht, G., and Winblad, B. (1991). Underdiagnosis and poor documentation of acute confusional states in elderly hip fracture patients. *Journal of the American Geriatrics Society*, **39**, 760–5.

5. Gustafson, Y., Berggren, D., Brännström, B., *et al.* (1988). Acute confusional states in elderly patients treated for femoral neck fracture. *Journal of the American Geriatrics Society*, **36**, 525–30.

6. Marcantonio, E.R., Goldman, L., Mangione, C.M., *et al.* (1994). A clinical prediction rule for delirium after elective noncardiac surgery. *Journal of the American Medical Association*, **271**, 134–9.

7. Fines, D.P., Severn, A.M. (2006). Anaesthesia and cognitive disturbance in the elderly. *British Journal of Anaesthesia – Continuing Education in Anaesthesia, Critical Care and Pain*, **6**, 37–40.

8. Inouye, S.K., Bogardus, S.T. Jr., Charpentier, P.A., *et al.* (1999). A multicomponent intervention to prevent delirium in hospitalized older patients. *New England Journal of Medicine*, **340**, 669–76.

9. Parikh, S.S. and Chung, F. (1995). Postoperative delirium in the elderly. *Anesthesia and Analgesia*, **80**, 1223–32.

10. Williams-Russo, P., Urquhart, B.L., Sharrock, N.E., and Charlson, M.E. (1992). Post-operative delirium: predictors and prognosis in elderly orthopaedic patients. *Journal of the American Geriatric Society*, **40**, 759–67.

11. Mann, C., Pouzeratte, Y., Boccara, G., *et al.* (2000). Comparison of intravenous or epidural patient-controlled analgesia in the elderly after major abdominal surgery. *Anesthesiology*, **92**, 433–41.

12. Marcantonio, E.R., Goldman, L., Orav, E.J., Cook, E.F., and Lee, T.H. (1998). The association of intraoperative factors with the development of postoperative delirium. *American Journal of Medicine*, **105**, 380–4.

13. Dai, Y.T., Lou, M.F., Yip, P.K., and Huang, G.S. (2000). Risk factors and incidence of postoperative delirium in elderly Chinese patients. *Gerontology*, **46**, 28–35.

14. Ní Chonchubhair, Á., Valacio, R., Kelly, J., and O'Keeffe, S. (1995). Use of the abbreviated mental test to detect postoperative delirium in elderly people. *British Journal of Anaesthesia*, **75**, 481–2.

15. Tsutsui, S., Kitamura, M., Higashi, H., Matsuura, H., and Hirashima, S. (1996). Development of postoperative delirium in relation to a room change in the general surgical unit. *Surgery Today*, **26**, 292–4.

16. Knill, R.L., Rose, E.A., and Berko, S.L. (1989). Idiopathic postoperative delirium in the elderly. *Canadian Journal of Anesthesia*, **36**, S90–1.

17. Lynch, E.P., Lazor, M.A., Gellis. J,E., Orav, J., Goldman, L., and Marcantonio, E.R. (1998). The impact of postoperative pain on the development of postoperative delirium. *Anesthesia and Analgesia*, **86**, 781–5.

18. Berggren, D., Gustafson, Y., Eriksson, B., *et al.* (1987). Postoperative confusion after anesthesia in elderly patients with femoral neck fractures. *Anesthesia and Analgesia*, **66**, 497–504.

19. Gustafson, Y., Brännström, B., Berggren, D., *et al.* (1991). A geriatric-anesthesiologic program to reduce acute confusional states in elderly patients treated for femoral neck fractures. *Journal of the American Geriatric Society*, **39**, 655–62.

20. Urwin, S.C., Parker, M.J., and Griffiths, R. (2000). General versus regional anaesthesia for hip fracture surgery: a meta-analysis of randomized trials. *British Journal of Anaesthesia*, **84**, 450–5.

21. Marcantonio, E.R., Flacker, J.M., Wright, R.J., and Resnick, N.M. (2001). Reducing delirium after hip fracture: a randomized trial. *Journal of the American Geriatrics Society*, **49**, 516–22.

22. Milisen, K., Foreman, M.D., Abraham, I.L., *et al.* (2001). A nurse-led interdisciplinary intervention program for delirium in elderly hip-fracture patients. *Journal of the American Geriatrics Society*, **49**, 523–32.

23. Smith, R.J., Roberts, N.M., Rodgers, R.J., and Bennett, S. (1986). Adverse cognitive effects of general anaesthesia in young and elderly patients. *International Clinical Psychopharmacology*, **1**, 253–9.

24. Dijkstra, J.B. and Jolles, J. (2002). Popstoperative cognitive dysfunction versus complaints: a discrepancy in long-term findings. *Neuropsychology Review*, **12**, 1–14.

25. Mackensen, G.B. and Gelb, A.W. (2004). Postoperative cognitive deficits: more questions than answers. *European Journal of Anaesthesiology*, **21**, 85–8.

26. Moller, J.T., Cluitmans, P., Rasmussen, L.S., *et al.* (1998). Long-term postoperative cognitive dysfunction in the elderly: ISPOCD 1 study. *Lancet*, **351**, 857–61.

27. Abildstrom, H., Rasmussen, L.S., Rentowl, P., *et al.* (2000). Cognitive dysfunction 1-2 years after non-cardiac surgery in the elderly. *Acta Anaesthesiologica Scandinavica*, **44**, 1246–51.

28. Johnson, T., Monk, T., Rasmussen, L.S., *et al.* (2002). Postoperative cognitive dysfunction in middle-aged patients. *Anesthesiology*, **96**, 1351–7.

29. Hole, A., Terjesen, T., Breivik, H. (1980). Epidural versus general anaesthesia for total hip arthroplasty in elderly patients. *Acta Anaesthesiologica Scandinavica*, **24**, 279–87.

30. Williams-Russo, P., Sharrock, N.E., Mattis, S., Szatrowski, P., and Charlton, M.E. (1995). Cognitive effects after epidural vs general anesthesia in older adults. A randomized trial. *Journal of the American Medical Association*, **274**, 44–50.

31. Rasmussen, L.S., Johnson, T., Kuipers, H.M., *et al.* (2003). Does anaesthesia cause postoperative dysfunction? A randomized study of regional versus general anaesthesia in 438 elderly patients. *Acta Anaesthesiologica Scandinavica*, **47**, 260–6.

32. Rosenberg, J. and Kehlet, H. (1993). Postoperative mental confusion – association with postoperative hypoxemia. *Surgery*, **114**, 76–81.

33. Casati, A., Fanelli, G., Pietropaoli, P., Protietti, R., Tufano, R., and Montanini, S. (2007). Monitoring cerebral oxygen saturation in elderly patients undergoing general abdominal surgery: a prospective cohort study. *European Journal of Anaesthesiology*, **24**, 59–65.

34. Newman, M.F., Kirchner, J.L., Phillips-Bute, B., *et al.* (2001). Longitudinal assessment of neurocognitive function after coronary-artery bypass surgery. *New England Journal of Medicine*, **344**, 395–402.

35. Selnes, O.A., Goldsborough, M.A., Borowicz, L.M., and McKhann, G.M. (1999). Neurobehavioural sequelae of cardiopulmonary bypass. *Lancet*, **353**, 1601–6.

36. Tardiff, B.E., Newman, M.F., Saunders, A.M., *et al.* (1997). Preliminary report of a genetic basis for cognitive decline after cardiac surgery operation. The Neurologic Outcome Research Group of the Duke Heart Center. *Annals of Thoracic Surgery*, **64**, 715–20.

Chapter 17

Endocrine and renal surgery

Felicity S Plaat & Scott Wallace

Anaesthesia for thyroid surgery

Introduction

The specific risks of anaesthesia for thyroid surgery arise from the potentially compromised, difficult, and shared airway in patients who may have significant co-morbidities.

The position of the thyroid accounts for many risks associated with surgery. The thyroid gland lies anteriorly and inferiorly in the neck. The two lobes are connected by an isthmus that commonly overlies the second and third tracheal rings. The recurrent laryngeal nerve lies between the thyroid and the oesophagus posteriorly. Posterolaterally, the lobes abut onto the carotid sheath.

The pathological features and the type of surgery undertaken obviously influence the type and magnitude of associated risks; total thyroidectomy, for whatever reason, is associated with an increased risk of recurrent laryngeal nerve damage (2.5% compared to <1% for partial surgery[1] and permanent, postoperative hypoparathyroidism in 8% compared to 1.5% for partial thyroidectomy[2]).

Risk of difficult intubation

The estimated incidence of difficult tracheal intubation associated with this type of surgery is 6%. Minor difficulties were encountered in 57% patients in one study. Thyroid size was not correlated with difficulty, and tracheal compression did not predict difficulty in passing the tracheal tube. The variables that were independently associated with difficult intubation were thyroid malignancy and a Cormack and Lehane score of 3 or 4[3].

Induction of anaesthesia as well as intubation are more difficult in the patient who already has stridor or is unable to lie flat. The larynx may be distorted by an enlarging gland, making the view at laryngoscopy difficult. The trachea may be significantly narrowed due to external compression or local infiltration. Infiltrating carcinomas may limit neck extension, increasing difficulties with intubation. Asymmetrical enlargement can distort the bronchial tree such that the left main bronchus is intubated. Endobronchial intubation is more likely because reinforced, uncut tubes are used commonly. Retrosternal goitres are not usually associated with problems during intubation but may be associated with obstruction of the superior vena cava and more demanding surgery with an increased risk of haemorrhage.

Failure to intubate may necessitate the use of the laryngeal mask airway but this may increase surgical difficulty. If airway obstruction (e.g. laryngospasm), occurs, venous congestion can present significant difficulties to the surgeon. The stridulous patient may desaturate extremely rapidly.

Imaging (chest X-ray, lateral thoracic inlet views, CT scan) may reveal deviation of the larynx or trachea. Although the degree of compression may look alarming on imaging, intubation with a modest-sized tube (e.g. 7.5mm reinforced) is rarely a problem in the absence of symptoms. However, CT scanning is recommended if there is >50% narrowing on plain X-ray[4].

Awake fibreoptic intubation may be unsuccessful if there is significant tracheal compression or narrowing. If there is severe preoperative airway obstruction, inhalational induction using sevoflurane in oxygen/helium has been used successfully. In a selected group of patients, regional anaesthesia comprising deep and superficial cervical plexus blocks and local infiltration has been used to avoid the need for general anaesthesia[5], This technique has not been found suitable for large goitres, in the obese patient, or when communication is difficult.

Haemorrhage/haematoma

Risk of major haemorrhage in this type of surgery is estimated to be 1 in 500 cases. The risk is reduced in skilled hands, or during the excision of simple nodules. The risk is increased when there has been previous surgery, if vascularity is increased (in the thyrotoxic patient) and when the gland is retrosternal. Excision of retrosternal thyroid may involve splitting the sternum, which significantly increases the risk of haemorrhage. Patients who take anti-platelet medication, and possibly non-steroidal anti-inflammatory drugs, are at increased risk of bleeding. Bleeding is decreased by infiltration with solutions containing epinephrine, head-up position and mildly hypotensive anaesthesia.

Haematoma is estimated to occur in 1% of cases, is more common after repeat surgery and may cause life-threatening respiratory embarrassment due to laryngeal oedema and compression. Surgical decompression is required in 0.03% of cases. When surgical haemostasis is tested by temporarily putting the patient in a head-down position and simulating a Valsalva manoeuvre, the incidence of life-threatening postoperative haematoma is reduced[6].

Postoperative airway obstruction

This may be caused by bilateral recurrent laryngeal nerve damage, oedema, haematoma, or tracheomalacia, and commonly occurs within 12 h of surgery.

If there is bilateral recurrent laryngeal nerve damage, the vocal cords are adducted and complete airway obstruction may occur. The need for permanent tracheostomy has been described. If surgery is prolonged, a single dose of dexamethasone and smooth extubation in the sitting position are recommended to reduce postoperative swelling. Humidified oxygen may be required. The risk of haematoma has been discussed above.

Tracheomalacia (floppy, collapsible trachea) is more likely to occur when a goitre is very long-standing and/or malignant. In the United Kingdom, it is extremely rare, but in one series from Sudan, five cases were identified among 103 patients. The absence of a leak around the deflated cuff of the tracheal tube at the end of the procedure should alert the anaesthetist to the possibility of tracheomalacia.

Pneumothorax may complicate dissection of a retrosternal goitre. The use of a double lumen tube in order to collapse one lung has been recommended to avoid this complication.

Postoperative voice change

Temporary hoarseness is extremely common following thyroid surgery. Permanent change to the voice occurs in 3–4% of patients due to unilateral nerve damage. Bilateral nerve damage occurs in less than 1% of cases[6]. The risk of damage is greater when there has been previous surgery. Some surgeons use preoperative nasendoscopy to identify abnormal vocal cord mobility[7]. Some ask for laryngoscopic examination before extubation of the trachea; the tracheal tube may be replaced by a laryngeal mask airway to allow continued ventilatory support in the deeply anaesthetized, non-paralysed patient. The effect of intra-operative electrophysiological monitoring of the recurrent laryngeal nerves on the incidence of damage to the vocal cords is currently being evaluated[8].

Hypocalcaemia

This occurs in up to 20% of patients who undergo thyroidectomy. The most common time is 36 h postoperatively. Calcium supplementation is required, but usually only temporarily, although 3% of patients require ongoing replacement. Untreated hypocalcaemia can lead to tetany, seizures, and arrhythmias. Unintentional parathyroidectomy occurred in >10% of patients in one series.

Hypothyroidism can complicate partial thyroidectomy, and all patients need to be aware of the possible need for postoperative replacement. Thyroid crisis or storm can be precipitated by surgery in the thyrotoxic patient.

Thyroid storm

This rare complication of thyrotoxicosis is associated with a mortality of 10–25%. It may be precipitated by surgery (or trauma) in a patient with partially or untreated thyrotoxicosis. Other precipitating factors include infection, diabetic ketoacidosis, myocardial infarction, and pulmonary embolism. Thyroid storm has been associated with radioiodine treatment and amiodarone[9]. The incidence of this complication has fallen as the proportion of patients presenting for surgery with severe biochemical and clinical features of hyperthyroidism has reduced.

Other complications

Approximately 0.1% of patients undergoing anaesthesia suffer eye injury, most commonly corneal abrasion. Due to the features of thyroid-related eye disease, (exophthalmos, lid lag, and lid retraction) and the need to drape the face, the incidence is likely to be higher during thyroid surgery. The risk is reduced by ensuring that the eye is shut, the conjunctiva is not exposed and the orbit is padded (against compression trauma).

Mortality associated with thyroid surgery is quoted as <1%. This is 100 times higher than the overall perioperative mortality in ASA 1 & II patients, although in one specialist centre there have been no deaths in >3000 cases[10].

Parathyroid surgery

In contrast to thyroid surgery, most of the risks associated with this type of surgery arise from the underlying medical condition. Hyperparathyroidism occurs most commonly in women >45 years of age (1 in 500). Approximately one-quarter of cases require surgery and one quarter would die within 10 years if left untreated.

Hypercalcaemia has multi-system effects. Decreased bone density is associated with increased incidence of fracture. Cardiac dysfunction and hypertension have been linked to increased cardiovascular mortality[11]. In patients with chronic renal failure and secondary hyperparathyroidism, 5% will require parathyroidectomy (although serum calcium concentration may be within the normal range). Hyperparathyroidism may be associated with impaired glucose tolerance and 24% of patients with the condition have evidence of peptic ulcer disease. Depression and, rarely, psychosis add to the risks of surgery and anaesthesia[12]. Surgical complications arise from the wide distribution of parathyroid glands in the neck. The upper glands may be as high as the bifurcation of the carotid artery or as low as the anterior mediastinum. Parathyroid tissue may occur within the carotid sheath.

Although removal of all four parathyroids and re-exploration generally require general anaesthesia with tracheal intubation, the risks of general anaesthesia in these often unwell, elderly patients may be avoided through the use of local anaesthesia if scanning has localized disease to one or two glands. A minimally invasive approach can reduce operating time to as little as 20 min, although in 4% of cases, conversion to open surgery is required[13]. Superficial cervical nerve blocks and local infiltration, with or without sedation, have been employed successfully, as have hypnosis and acupuncture[12].

Exploration using a conventional surgical technique is successful in 97% of cases—a higher success rate than with the minimally invasive technique. Complications such as recurrent laryngeal nerve damage, haematomas, and seromas are rarer than the incidences associated with thyroid surgery.

Serum calcium concentration occasionally dips temporarily postoperatively, but this rarely requires treatment. If possible, supplementation should be avoided as it can stimulate the regeneration of any residual parathyroid tissue. Occasionally, however, patients develop 'hungry bone disease' and require massive, long-term calcium and vitamin D therapy.

Postoperative morbidity and mortality may be due to the effects of long-standing hypercalcaemia, e.g. renal disease, even though surgery has restored a normal serum calcium concentration. Postoperative pancreatitis has been reported.

Adrenal surgery

Introduction

The risks associated with surgery to this gland arise from surgical and medical factors.

Surgically, even if the tumour is non-secreting, (often picked up unexpectedly and known as an *incidentaloma*), access may be difficult. A transabdominal approach is recommended for larger phaeochromocytomas or if the likelihood of multiple tumours is high. Surgery to the right gland is associated with greater risk of haemorrhage from the inferior vena cava. This approach is associated with a higher incidence of poor wound healing and dehiscence and with postoperative ileus; insertion of a nasogastric tube is advisable[14]. The posterior approach requires the patient to be prone, and resection of part of the twelfth rib, with the risk of pneumothorax. If breach of the pleura occurs, a postoperative chest drain is required. Nevertheless, this approach is associated with less risk of postoperative complications, particularly infection, and is the one recommended in cases of Cushing's disease and for unilateral small tumours. A thoraco-abdominal approach is reserved for very large tumours or evidence of invasion of the inferior vena cava. Postoperative morbidity is related to high analgesic requirements, the need to breach the dura, and in the case of malignant tumours, occasionally significant blood loss.

Cushing's disease

Untreated Cushing's disease is associated with 50% 5-year mortality. Anaesthetic problems are associated with practical challenges of obesity, osteoporosis, skin fragility, and occasionally florid psychiatric symptoms. Obesity-associated sleep apnoea, kyphoscoliosis, and muscle weakness impair respiratory function, which must be evaluated preoperatively. Perioperative steroid cover is required. Hypertension, cardiac failure, hypernatraemia, hypokalaemia, and diabetes can complicate the perioperative period. Postoperatively, hypercoagulability[15], poor healing, and increased susceptibility to infection may occur. Postoperative respiratory function may be impaired by the residual effects of anaesthetic drugs and non-depolarizing neuromuscular blockers, to which patients exhibit enhanced sensitivity. Postoperative care should initially be in a high dependency unit. Surgery for resistant Cushing's disease requires bilateral removal of the adrenal glands. Postoperatively, there is a need for both glucocortcoids and mineralocorticoids.

Phaechromocytoma

'Few medical conditions pose such a severe yet unpredictable threat to the patient's life'[16]. The risks associated with surgery, the only definitive form of management, have to be viewed in the context of the hazards of the condition itself.

Although phaeochromocytoma is extremely rare, with the peak incidence in the third and fourth decades, and affects both sexes equally, it is responsible for approximately 1% of cases of hypertension. Approximately one-third of patients have a cardiomyopathy. Patients without treatment are at risk of ventricular failure, pulmonary oedema, stroke, and death. In one series, 50% of diagnoses were made post-mortem[17]. Phaeochromocytoma may be associated with multiple endocrine neoplasia (MEN) syndromes. MEN 1 syndromes are exceptionally rare outside Tasmania. In MEN 2A (Sipple's) syndrome, medullary thyroid carcinoma is associated with phaeochromocytoma in about 50% of cases, and with hyperparathyroidism. In MEN 2B syndrome, medullary carcinoma of the thyroid occurs together with ganglioneuromatosis with hypertrophic corneal nerves, neurofibromatosis, von Hippal–Lindau disease and, at a late stage, phaechromocytoma.

Mortality and morbidity associated with the phaeochromocytoma has decreased as a result of more accurate and earlier diagnosis (including the knowledge of associated conditions), preoperative pharmacological preparation, and careful perioperative anaesthetic management. In Prys–Roberts' series of 50 patients, the only death within 31 days of surgery occurred in a patient in whom the tumour appeared inoperable. No major postoperative complications were reported[18]. The type of surgery required depends on the size, nature, and distribution of the tumour. Approximately 10% of phaeochromocytomas are malignant, and the same proportion is extra-adrenal or bilateral. In recent years, small (5 cm on imaging) tumours have generally been removed laparoscopically, a technique used recently for bilateral as well as single tumours. Larger and extra-adrenal tumours may necessitate an open retroperitoneal or occasionally transabdominal approach.

Preoperative adrenoreceptor blockade and restoration of intravascular volume decrease the risk of potentially fatal changes in blood pressure, heart rate, and arrhythmias perioperatively. Full α-receptor blockade should be achieved prior to β-blockade to avoid paradoxical hypertension. Drugs that stimulate catecholamine release and precipitate hypertension should be avoided (e.g. metoclopramide, antidepressants, phenothiazines). The side-effects of non-selective α-blockade (somnolence, headaches, and stuffy nose) may be avoided using a selective α_1-inhibitor, e.g. prazosin, or the competitive antagonist doxazosin. The three major hazards are haemodynamic instability, arrhythmias, and bleeding. Hypertension during tumour manipulation is more likely if full α-blockade has not been achieved. Pre- and perioperative use of magnesium has recently become used more widely than adrenoreceptor blocker or vasodilators such as sodium nitroprusside in the management of perioperative instability[19]. Neuraxial blockade is advocated, even when laparoscopic surgery is undertaken. Irreversible blockade and down-regulation of the adrenoreceptors can cause refractory hypotension after removal of the tumour, necessitating large volumes of intravenous fluid replacement, an increased incidence of peripheral oedema, a risk of pulmonary oedema, and prolonged need for intensive care postoperatively. These risks may be minimized by the use of competitive α-blockade, short-acting vasodilators (e.g. magnesium) and adequate preoperative intravascular volume normalization. Although laparoscopic surgery may be associated with longer periods of tumour manipulation and associated hypertension than open techniques, patients can leave hospital 48–72 h after uncomplicated surgery.

After surgery, 75% of patients can expect normalization of blood pressure, although as many as 5% may become temporarily hypotensive. In one series of 142 patients, there were no ventricular arrhythmias or intra operative deaths[20]. In this series, the median length of hospital stay was 6 days (the surgery was open, not laparoscopic). Postoperative complications included pulmonary embolism (0.7% of patients), renal or biliary dysfunction (1.4% and 0.7% respectively), and sepsis (0.7%). The most common problem was prolonged tracheal intubation (4.2%: of the 41% patients admitted to the intensive therapy unit (ITU), the median length of stay was 24 h). However the mortality associated with malignant disease is significant, with only a 44% 5-year survival.

Adrenal insufficiency has been noted to be an adverse prognostic feature in high-risk surgical patients who require intensive care. Rivers identified a cohort of such patients, suffering postoperative hypotension. Those treated with hydrocortisone had a lower mortality and were weaned more quickly from vasopressor treatment[21].

Pituitary surgery

Although the trans-sphenoidal approach means that surgery should be straightforward, over- or undersecretion of pituitary hormones result in specific anaesthetic problems for this type of surgery.

Acromegaly may result from excess growth hormone or growth hormone releasing hormone, associated usually with a pituitary adenoma. Hypertension is present in 40% of patients and 45% have impaired glucose tolerance. Cardiomyopathy may be complicated by cardiac failure[22]. Anatomical changes (macroglossia; osteoarthritis involving neck, larynx, and spine; goitre; prognathia; overgrowth of nasal tissue including turbinates; and narrowing of the glottic inlet) result in a threefold increase in death from respiratory causes[23]. These include difficulties with tracheal intubation; 26% of patients had a grade 3 intubation in a series of 100 patients[24]. Obstructive sleep apnoea, postoperative upper airway obstruction, and respiratory failure are all more common. Careful preoperative assessment of the airway and pulmonary function is essential. The need for fibre-optic intubation, or even transtracheal ventilation, should be anticipated[25]. A history of obstructive sleep apnoea is associated with particular risk of cardiac impairment and airway problems. This can be improved by treatment with octreotide and may justify a 3-month delay to surgery in high-risk cases. Pre- and postoperative nasal continuous positive airway pressure (CPAP) may improve right ventricular function.

Table 17.1 Complications of pituitary surgery

Complication	Incidence (%)
Hormonal	
Diabetes insipidus; transient or permanent	3.8–17
SIADH—usually transient, occurs within 7–10 days	
Cerebral salt-wasting syndrome	
Pituitary insufficiency	19
Other	
Haematoma	2
Haemorrhage	1–2
Ophthalmoplegia	1
Loss of vision	1
Meningitis	0.5
Sinusitis	0.5
CSF fistulae	3–4
Carotid artery injury	1–2
Supra-alveolar nerve injury (sublabial approach)	6

Complications of surgery are listed in Table 17.1. Both mortality (<1%) and morbidity have been shown to improve if only specialists working in nominated centres carry out the procedure.

Diabetes mellitus

3% of the UK population (1.8 million people) are diagnosed with diabetes and possibly half that number again have undiagnosed Type 2 diabetes. The incidence is rising rapidly. Type 1 diabetes may be associated with other autoimmune disorders and Type 2 with obesity (the risk increases 10-fold with a BMI >30 kg.m^{-2})[26]. Life expectancy is shortened by 20 years in Type 1 and by 10 years in Type 2 diabetics and cardiovascular disease accounts for 80% of deaths. Approximately one-quarter of patients admitted to ITU suffer from diabetes.

Diabetics commonly present for surgery due to the complications of diabetes, e.g. peripheral vascular surgery, coronary artery bypass surgery (28% of all patients undergoing such surgery are diabetic), and cataract extraction. About half of all diabetics will require surgery during their life[27].

Although the evidence is missing in the case of elective non-cardiac surgery, diabetics have a 50% greater perioperative mortality rate following coronary artery bypass grafting and a much higher rate of morbidity than their non-diabetic counterparts. Type 1 diabetics are particularly at risk of postoperative complications[28],

The increased risks are due to the following:

1. Non-metabolic effects of hypoglycaemia (acute: cerebral damage) and hyperglycaemia (impaired wound healing and increased breakdown of surgical anastomoses, increased infection, exacerbation of cerebral and myocardial ischaemia).

2. Dehydration, electrolyte loss, (K^+, Mg^{++}, PO_4^-), acidaemia (results of hyperglycaemia).

3. Lipolysis and increased catabolism (common in Type 1, occurs in the presence of physiological stresses, e.g. infection, dehydration, in type 2).

4. Cardiovascular disease including hypertension, ischaemic heart disease, peripheral vascular disease, congestive cardiac failure, valvular abnormalities (some degree of cardiovascular disease should be assumed in all long-standing diabetics).

5. Autonomic neuropathy (gastric stasis, cardiovascular instability).

6. Renal disease.

7. Obesity.

8. Respiratory problems (decreased FVC and FEV_1 in poorly controlled Type 1 diabetics, stiff-neck syndrome).

Preoperative optimization may attenuate some of the factors mentioned in the list, if time is available. One study showed that asymptomatic Type 1 diabetics with renal failure benefited from preoperative screening for coronary artery disease with revascularization when indicated, prior to renal transplantation[29]. General measures include, where relevant, smoking cessation, weight reduction, and optimizing glycaemic control. Patients randomized to receive a glucose-insulin-potassium infusion to maintain blood glucose at <10 mmol.L^{-1} showed an 11%

improvement in long-term survival after 3–4 years compared to a group with glucose <12 mmol.L^{-1}[30].

Recent studies suggest that tight blood pressure control (<140/80mmHg) using angiotensin-converting enzyme (ACE) inhibitors or β-blockers significantly reduced mortality from cardiovascular disease and the incidences of stroke, myocardial infarction, and congestive cardiac failure in Type 2 diabetics[31]. ACE inhibitors also appear to have a renal protective effect in Type 1 diabetics[32]. The use of lipid-lowering agents for at least one year has been shown to decrease the incidences of stroke, major vascular events and death from vascular disease by around 25%. The maximum protective effect occurs after 5–6 years of treatment and benefits both sexes and all ages.

During preoperative assessment it should be borne in mind that the incidences of microvascular complications (retinopathy, nephropathy) and neuropathies (autonomic, peripheral) are the same in Type 1 and Type 2 diabetics, when quality of glycaemic control and duration of disease are taken into account. The cumulative life-time incidence of such complications in diabetics is approximately 50%. Cardiovascular mortality is also similar between the two types. Preoperative assessment of glycosylated haemoglobin should be undertaken as an indication of the quality of recent glycaemic control. If the HbA1c is <6.2%, it is likely that fluid and electrolyte balance is normal. Levels persistently above 8% make it likely that complications are present. Levels of between 12 and 15% indicate that ketoacidosis is imminent.

Diabetic autonomic neuropathy should be suspected in the presence of hypertension, and if there are symptoms of sweating, diarrhoea, postural hypotension, impotence, or urinary problems (although symptoms are rare). Autonomic neuropathy increases the risks of regurgitation and cardiovascular instability. There is impairment of heart rate variability that may be responsible for an increased incidence of ventricular arrhythmia and sudden death. Presence of the stiff-neck syndrome increases the risk of difficult intubation. If regional analgesia is planned, the presence, extent and severity of pre-existing neuropathy should be documented carefully.

Perioperative metabolic control has been shown to influence mortality and morbidity. A study by Furnary and colleagues showed a lowering of mortality associated with coronary artery bypass surgery from 5.3% to 2.5% when blood glucose concentration was controlled with intravenous rather than subcutaneous insulin[33]. Preoperative starvation, the stress response to surgery, and immobilization all increase the risk of poor control of blood glucose concentration. Current recommendations are that blood glucose concentration should be kept between 6 and 12 mmol.L^{-1} perioperatively. With bedside measurement of concentrations, this is not associated with an increased risk of hypoglycaemia as was previously feared. Control is made easier by minimizing the period of preoperative fasting (although the possibility of gastric stasis must also be taken into account). For major surgery, all diabetics should receive intravenous insulin. The sliding scale has the advantage of flexibility in comparison to the Alberti regimen. Problems can be minimized by ensuring that one method is uniformly adopted in any unit.

Anaesthetic technique

There is no evidence that a specific anaesthetic technique affects perioperative morbidity and mortality in diabetic patients overall. The following discussion is therefore concerned with potential risks and benefits for individual patients.

Regional techniques attenuate the stress response to surgery, and may therefore allow better glycaemic control. Because consciousness is maintained, the symptoms of impending hypoglycaemia are not lost. Blood loss and the risk of thromboembolism are reduced. Regional anaesthesia is associated with a shorter recovery period, with better analgesia and less nausea or vomiting, allowing earlier resumption of a normal diet and usual diabetic medication.

One of the risks of regional anaesthesia that is potentially greater in diabetics is infection[34]. In addition, in the presence of autonomic neuropathy, cardiovascular instability may be more likely. The consequences of periods of profound hypotension with co-existing micro and macrovascular disease are likely to be worse than in non-diabetic patients. Careful preoperative examination of the peripheral nervous system should avoid pre-existing lesions being blamed on the regional technique[35].

Drugs used as part of a general anaesthetic technique may affect glucose metabolism in either beneficial or deleterious ways. Benzodiazepines reduce the glycaemic response to surgery through inhibition of adrenocorticotrophic hormone (ACTH) secretion and reduction of sympathetic stimulation, although it is unlikely that these effects occur at the doses used during sedation or induction of anaesthesia. High-dose opiate techniques that block the stress response to surgery (and allow a high degree of haemodynamic stability) may be beneficial in diabetic patients[36]. Etomidate reduces the glycaemic response to surgery in non-diabetic patients through its effect on steroid production, but its use in diabetic patients is not established. Because diabetic patients have reduced ability to clear lipids from the plasma, prolonged infusions of propofol should be avoided. The clinical significance of the *in vitro* ability of halothane, enflurane, and isoflurane to inhibit insulin secretion is unknown.

Perioperative volume replacement requires close monitoring of fluid balance and should involve invasive monitoring in major surgery or when renal dysfunction is present. Fluid replacement should be with 0.9% sodium chloride to offset the hyponatraemia that results from infusion of glucose–insulin–potassium regimens. The lactate content of 1–2 litres of Hartmann's solution, (29 mmol.L^{-1}), probably has a minimal effect on blood glucose concentration. However, transfusion with packed red cells results in rapid increases in glucose and potassium concentrations.

Postoperatively, diabetic patients should be monitored more intensively than their non-diabetic counterparts. The aim is tight glycaemic control, excellent analgesia to attenuate catabolism, with as rapid as possible a return to normal diet and medication.

Anaesthesia for renal surgery and patients with renal disease

The associations between surgery, anaesthesia, and renal dysfunction are complex. Surgery, and major procedures in particular, present a challenge to renal function and patients with renal disease present for major surgery quite frequently. In those who are critically ill and/or with pre-existing renal insufficiency, there is a significant risk of postoperative deterioration in renal function or acute renal failure (ARF).

The multi-system effects of chronic renal failure increase the risks associated with surgery and anaesthesia, whether or not the surgery is coincidental or related directly to the renal condition, e.g. transplantation. Estimating the magnitude of anaesthetic or surgical risk associated with renal failure is hampered by the lack of universal definitions of acute or chronic renal failure[37].

Recently, it has been argued that there are two distinct populations with renal problems. 'Medical' renal failure patients tend to have single organ disease resulting from a specific insult (e.g. autoimmune disease), are stable, and have a low mortality associated with renal dysfunction. In contrast, in the postoperative/critically ill patient, ARF is commonly part of multi-organ dysfunction of multi factorial origin; sepsis often plays a significant role. In this patient population, mortality is high[38]. Approximately 200–223 patients per million develop ARF per year and one-third will require intensive care[39]. Ten to twenty-five percent of ITU patients suffer ARF, mainly of the 'non-medical' variety. Their mortality has been reported to be 40–70%. Higher values are associated with the need for intermittent positive pressure ventilation and when ARF develops late. In a study of 1,000 patients, those admitted to ITU in ARF did better than those who developed it following admission as part of multi-system failure[40]. Mortality is especially high in patients who require dialysis.

Risk factors for the development of postoperative renal failure in the general surgical population include pre-existing renal dysfunction, age >65 years, and poor left ventricular function. The overwhelming perioperative factor is hypotension associated with hypovolaemia and/or preoperative dehydration. Hypotension was the sole factor in one-third of patients developing ARF on one ITU, and implicated in 85%[41]. ARF is common following cardiac arrest, especially if resuscitation is prolonged and the total dose of epinephrine is high[42].

Many conditions that predispose to ARF also require intervention for diagnosis and management that itself increases the risk of renal failure (e.g. contrast media or major surgery). If mortality is related mainly to the predisposing condition, and renal failure can be as successfully managed as it is in the stable 'medical' patients described earlier, then such interventions are generally justified. However when Levy *et al.* compared mortality in patients who developed contrast media-associated renal failure with a matched cohort, who also received contrast media but did not develop renal failure, they found that mortality in the study group was 34% compared to 7% amongst controls. For any given co-morbidity, e.g. diabetes, hypertension, or acute myocardial infarction, mortality was higher in the patients with renal failure. Acute renal failure was associated with an odds ratio of dying of 5.5, after adjustment for differences in co-morbidities. If renal failure *per se* increases mortality, the value of anaesthetic and surgical interventions which increase the risk of renal failure should be carefully considered[43].

The risk of developing postoperative ARF depends on the type of surgery. Less than 0.6% of general surgical patients develop ARF requiring dialysis. In contrast, 15% of patients develop a degree of renal dysfunction following coronary artery bypass graft surgery, with 1.1% developing ARF. In a study of 42 500 patients, mortality in those with ARF was 63.7% compared with 4.3% in those not affected[44]. Controversy exists over the effect of cardiopulmonary bypass. Some authorities maintain that a bypass time of >3 h increases the risk of ARF whilst others point out that rates are not significantly different between bypass and beating heart surgery.

Vascular surgery, particularly if it involves the thoracic aorta or suprarenal aortic cross-clamping, is associated with an enhanced risk of ARF (5.5% of patients required dialysis in one series)[45].

In the presence of obstructive jaundice, renal failure develops in 10–60% of surgical patients. The incidence may be even higher in those with severely impaired hepatic function, for example those undergoing liver transplantation.

Apart from significantly increased mortality, ARF is associated with gastrointestinal haemorrhage, respiratory infection, sepsis and, not surprisingly, increased hospital stay.

Preoperatively, the anaesthetist, as well as participating in the risk analysis described earlier, needs to identify the high-risk patient, and reduce the risk when possible. Omitting angiotensin-converting enzyme inhibitors for 12 h preoperatively appears to ameliorate the increased risk associated with long-term treatment with these drugs[46]. Potentially nephrotoxic drugs, such as the aminoglycosides should be avoided or given in divided doses. Non-steroidal anti-inflammatory analgesics were used in 18% of patients who developed ARF compared with 11% of controls[47]. If contrast media are used, the dose should be minimized and adequate hydration ensured. There is some work to suggest that pre treatment with N-acetylcysteine reduces the risk of ARF[48].

The fluid and electrolyte status of patients on diuretic therapy should be assessed carefully. Hypokalaemia predisposes to arrhythmias and fluid depletion increases the likelihood of ARF.

The selection of anaesthetic technique has not been shown to influence the risk of developing ARF. The older halogenated agents such as enflurane release potentially nephrotoxic concentrations of fluoride ions. This has not been found to be a problem with newer agents such as sevoflurane or isoflurane. Another concern relating to sevoflurane is the production of compound A by soda lime and other carbon dioxide absorbants. Compound A has been found to induce acute tubular necrosis in rats[49]. Recent work sheds doubt on the clinical significance of these findings. In the opinion of some authors, the FDA warning *'to minimize exposure to compound A, sevoflurane exposure should not exceed 2 MAC-hours at flow rates of 1 to 2 L/min'* should be reviewed[50].

Inhalational agents have been used to investigate the reno-protective effect of 'ischaemic preconditioning'. Short periods of ischaemia followed by reperfusion appear temporarily to increase resistance to further ischaemic damage. Preconditioning with 4% sevoflurane for 10 min at the beginning of cardiopulmonary bypass resulted in lower serum cystatin C concentrations (a marker of renal dysfunction) in a small, recent trial[51].

Inhalational agents cause peripheral vasodilatation and myocardial depression. Consequently, there is the need to maintain adequate renal blood flow and glomerular filtration rate (GFR)through the use of fluids and/or pharmacological agents. Fluid management is complicated by the stress response to surgery, with the increase in antidiuretic hormone (ADH) leading to impaired water and sodium excretion and increased potassium loss. Some authorities suggest that balanced salt solution should be used in preference to sodium chloride. Animal data show a reduction in GFR and renal blood flow when saline-based fluids are used, and large quantities of saline can lead to a hyperchloraemic acidosis[52].

The use of thoracic epidural anaesthesia and postoperative analgesia has been shown to reduce the incidence of ARF in patients undergoing coronary artery bypass graft surgery, possibly through improved haemodynamic stability and blunting of the stress response[53]. Clonidine may also exert a renoprotective effect[54].

Strategies for prevention of renal dysfunction, with the exception of adequate hydration, by and large have little evidence of clinical efficacy although they are widely used.

Mannitol is commonly used to promote urine production in high-risk patients as well as those undergoing renal transplantation. Although its use is associated with increased diuresis, an effect on preservation of renal function is less certain[55]. Loop diuretics such as frusemide are also used widely although current evidence suggests that they have little effect on mortality and may be nephrotoxic[56]. Solomon showed that hydration alone preserved renal function more effectively than either hydration with mannitol or treatment with loop diuretics in high-risk patients undergoing coronary angiography[57].

Although 'low-dose' dopamine ($0.5-3$ $\mu g.kg^{-1}.min^{-1}$) is widely used to enhance renal blood flow, recent meta-analyses have shown a lack of renal protection in both surgical and ITU patients[58]. Dopexamine may provide some protection to patients undergoing vascular but not cardiac surgery[59,60]. A more recent addition to this list is atrial natriuretic peptide (ANP). ANP improves renal perfusion in animal models, although to date, human studies are inconclusive[61]. The selective dopaminergic α_1-agonist fenoldopam has also failed to show protective effects in large randomized studies[62].

Patients with chronic renal failure (CRF) present to the anaesthetist for transplantation surgery, urological procedures, and surgery unrelated to the renal disease. The main challenges posed by these patients are the multi-system manifestations of CRF and the effect of CRF on the response to anaesthesia and surgery.

Cardiovascular disease is common and, in younger patients, can follow a rapidly progressive course. Cardiovascular mortality is increased 100-fold in this group, with implications for anaesthesia even for minor surgery[63]. A history of stroke, hypertension, or cardiac failure is associated with an increased risk of adverse perioperative cardiac events[64].

The aims of preoperative preparation are treatment of co-morbidity wherever possible and provision of a 'near normal physiological environment' prior to surgery. To this end, dialysis is carried out within 12–24 h of surgery to within 0.5 kg of ideal body weight[65].

Potential problems are subsequent hypovolaemia and hypokalaemia (although these patients show increased tolerance of swings in serum potassium concentration). Residual anticoagulation should be checked. Erythropoietin used to treat severe chronic anaemia may worsen hypertension and increase the risk of coagulation at vascular access sites[66].

Both regional and general anaesthesia have been used for renal transplantation. Vascular access may be difficult. The problem of prolonged surgery may be overcome using a combined spinal-epidural technique. Coagulation abnormalities may contraindicate this technique and up to 40% of cases require conversion to general anaesthesia. Fluid preloading should probably be avoided as it does not ensure haemodynamic stability and has been associated with the development of pulmonary oedema[65].

Intravenous general anaesthesia is associated with less postoperative nausea but shows no advantages when compared with inhalational techniques in terms of graft survival or overall mortality. The presence of autonomic neuropathy (particularly in diabetics) or uraemia can slow gastric emptying significantly and are indications for antacid premedication and rapid sequence induction. Abnormal respiratory function necessitates meticulous pre-oxygenation. Normothermia should be maintained to prevent vasoconstriction, facilitate fluid management, and decrease bleeding.

Drug handling is affected by chronic renal dysfunction. The duration of action of non-depolarizing neuromuscular blocking drugs can be unpredictable and should be monitored. Hofmann degradation of atracurium makes this an attractive option. Although the immunosuppressive regimens used to treat transplant patients often make antibiotic prophylaxis essential, antibiotics with nephrotoxic properties, e.g. gentamicin, should be avoided if possible. Steroid supplementation may be required.

Postoperative analgesia may be challenging. Non-steroidal anti-inflammatory analgesic drugs are contraindicated[67]. Accumulation of active metabolites of some opioids (e.g. morphine and pethidine) may prolong their effect and increase their side-effects. Patient-controlled intravenous fentanyl may be suitable after major surgery. There has been recent work on the use of buprenorphine, which is an opioid almost totally without renal metabolism[68].

Transplant patients have a 68% reduction in mortality compared with those on dialysis[69]. Post-transplant mortality is related to infection (especially early on), cardiovascular disease, and malignancy. Diabetic patients have a higher mortality from any cause than non-diabetics[70].

Cardiovascular disease accounts for 40–55% of deaths in transplant patients. Strict blood pressure control postoperatively has been shown to increase graft survival time although not overall cardiovascular mortality[71]. Some malignancies are more common in transplant patients than in the general population, and the increased incidence is thought to be due to immunosuppresive regimens. Antiviral therapy may be helpful in the prevention or treatment of virus-related tumours. Death from infection has fallen faster than mortality associated with other causes, in part due to patient selection, use of prophylaxis in high-risk cases, and early and aggressive treatment when infection is suspected[70].

References

1. Harness, J.K., Fung, L., Thompson, N.W., et al. (1986). Total thyroidectomy: complications and techniques. *World Journal of Surgery*, **10**, 781–6.
2. Foster, R.S. (1978). Morbidity and mortality after thyroidectomy. *Surgical Gynecology and Obstetrics*, **146**, 423–9.
3. Bouaggad, A., Nejmi, S.E., Bouderka, M.A., and Abbassi, O. (2004). Prediction of difficult tracheal intubation in thyroid surgery. *Anesthesia and Analgesia*, **99**, 603–6.
4. Hisham, A.N. and Aina, E.N. (2002). A reappraisal of thyroid surgery under local anaesthesia – back to the future? *Australian and New Zealand Journal of Surgery*, **72**, 287–9.

5. Maroof, M., Siddique, M., and Khan, R.M. (1992). Post-thyroidectomy vocal cord examination by fibreoscopy aided by the laryngeal mask airway. *Anaesthesia*, **47**, 445.

6. Farling, P.A. (2000). Thyroid disease. *British Journal of Anaesthesia*, **85**, 15–28.

7. www.endocrinesurgeon.co.uk(last accessed 17th December 2008).

8. Sheldon, D.G., Lee, F.T., Neil, N.J., and Ryan, J.A. (2002). Surgical treatment of hyperparathyroidism improves health related quality of life. *Archives of Surgery*, **137**, 1022–8.

9. Sunderland. (2001). Anaesthesia for amiodarone induced thyrotoxicosis: a case review. *Anesthesia and Intensive Care*, **29**, 24–9.

10. Lynn, J. and Studley, R.G.N. (1993). Surgical anatomy of the thyroid gland and the technique of thyroidectomy. In *Surgical endocrinology* (J. Lynn and S.R. Bloom eds.). Butterworth-Heinemann, Oxford.

11. Lundgren, E., Lind, L., Palmer, M. *et al.* (2001). Increased cardiovascular mortality and normalized serum calcium in patients with mild hypercalcaemia followed up for 25 years. *Surgery*, **130**, 978–85.

12. Mihai, R. and Farndon, J.K. (2000). Parathyroid disease and calcium metabolism. *British Journal of Anaesthesia*, **85**, 29–43.

13. Palazzo, F.F. and Sadler, G.P. (2004). Minimally invasive parathyroidectomy. *British Medical Journal*, **328**, 849–50.

14. Hughes, S. and Lynn, J. (1997). Surgical anatomy and surgery of the adrenal glands. In Surgical endocrinology (eds. J. Lynn and S.R.Bloom). Butterworth-Heinemann, Oxford.

15. Stoelting,R.K., Dierdorf, S.F., and McCammon, R.L. (1988). *Anaesthesia and Co-existing disease*, 2nd edition, Churchill Livingstone, New York.

16. Prys-Roberts, C. (2000). Phaeochromocytoma – recent progress in its management. *British Journal of Anaesthesia*, **85**, 44–57.

17. Bittar, D.A. (1982). Unsuspected phaeochromocytoma. *Canadian Anaesthetic Society Journal*, **29**, 183–6.

18. Prys-Roberts, C. and Fardon, J.R. (2001). Doxazosin versus phenoxybenzamine in the peri-operative management of patients with phaeochromocytoma. *British Journal of Surgery*, **88**, 1272.

19. James, M.F.M. (1989). Use of magnesium sulphate in the anaesthetic management of phaeochromocytoma; a review of 17 anaesthetics. *British Journal of Anaesthesia*, **62**, 616–23.

20. Kinney, M.A.O., Warner, M.E., vanHeerden, J.A., *et al.* (2000). Perianesthetic risks and outcomes of pheochromocytoma and paraganglioma resection. *Anesthesia and Analgesia*, **91**, 1118–23.

21. Rivers, E.P., Gaspari, M., Saad, G., *et al.* (2001). Adrenal insufficiency in high-risk surgical ICU patients. *Chest*, **119**, 889–96.

22. Smith, M. and Hirsch, N.P. (2000). Pituitary disease and anaesthesia. *British Journal of Anaesthesia*, **85**, 3–14.

23. Murrant, N.J. and Gatland, D.J. (1990). Respiratory problems in acromegaly. *Journal of Laryngology and Otology*,**104**, 52–55.

24. Schmitt, H., Buchfelder, M., Radespiel-Tröger, M., and Fahlbusch, R. (2000). Difficult intubation in acromegalic patients: incidence and predictability. *Anesthesiology*, **93**, 110–14.

25. Seidman, P.A., Kofke, W.A., Policare, R., and Young, M. (2000). Anaesthetic complications of acromegaly. *British Journal of Anaesthesia*, **84**, 179–82.

26. Diabetes in the UK 2004. http://www.diabetes.org.uk

27. McAnulty, G.R., Robertshaw, H.J., and Hall, G.M. (2000). Anaesthetic management of patients with diabetes mellitus. *British Journal of Anaesthesia*, **85**, 80–90.

28. Treiman, G.S., Treiman, R.L., Foran, R.F., *et al.* (1994). The influence of diabetes mellitus on the risk of abdominal aortic surgery. *American Journal of Surgery*, **60**, 436–40.

29. Manske, C.L., Wang, Y., Rector, T., *et al.* (1992). Coronary revascularisation in insulin-dependant diabetic patients with chronic renal failure. *Lancet*, **340**, 998–1002.

30. Watkins, P.J. (2003). Cardiovascular disease, hypertension and lipids. *British Medical Journal*, **326**, 874–6.

31. UK Prospective diabetes study group. (1998). Efficacy of atenolol and captopril in reducing macrovascular and microvascular complications in Type 2 diabetes UKPDS 39. *British Medical Journal*, **317**, 713–20.

32. Lewis, E.J., Hunsicker, L.G., Bain, R.P., and Rohde, R.D. (1993) for the Collaborative Study group: The effect of angiotensin-converting-enzyme inhibition on diabetic nephropathy. *New England Journal of Medicine*, **329**, 1456–62.

33. Furnary, A.P., Gao, G., Grunkemeier, G.L., *et al.* (2003). Continuous insulin infusion reduces mortality in patients with diabetes undergoing coronary artery bypass grafting. *Journal of Thoracic and Cardiovascular Surgery*, **125**, 1007–21.

34. Kindler, C.H., Seeberger, M.D., and Staender, S.E. (1998). Epidural abscess complicating epidural anesthesia and analgesia. An analysis of the literature. *Acta Anaesthesiologica Scandinavica*, **42**, 614–20.

35. Kahn, L. (1997). Neuropathies masquerading as an epidural complication. *Canadian Journal of Anaesthesia*, **44**, 313–6.

36. Klingstedt, C., Giesecke, K., Hamberger, B., and Jarnberg, P.O. (1987). High and low-dose fentanyl anaesthesia: circulatory and plasma catecholamine responses during cholecystectomy. *British Journal of Anaesthesia*, **59**, 184–8.

37. Sear, J.W. (2005). Kidney dysfunction in the postoperative period. *British Journal of Anaesthesia*, **95**, 20–32.

38. Kishen, R. (1999). Acute renal failure. In *Handbook of ICU therapy* (ed. I.McConachie), pp. 161–72. Greenwich Medical Media, London..

39. Liano, F. and Pascual, J. (1996). The Madrid acute renal failure study group. Epidemiology of acute renal failure: a prospective, multicentre, community-based study. *Kidney International*, **50**, 811–8.

40. Guerin, C., Girard, R., Selli, J.M., *et al.* (2000). Initial versus delayed acute renal failure in the intensive care unit. *American Journal of Respiratory and Critical Care Medicine*, **161**, 872–9.

41. Menash, P.L., Ross, S.A., and Gottleib, J.E. (1088). Acquired renal failure in critically ill patients. *Critical Care Medicine*, **16**, 1106–9.

42. McConachie, I. (2006). *Anaesthesia for the high risk patient*. Cambridge University Press, Cambridge, 179–97.

43. Levi, E.M., Viscoli, C.M., and Horwitz, R.I. (1996). The effect of acute renal failure on mortality: a cohort analysis. *Journal of the American Medical Association*, **275**, 1489–94.

44. Chertow, G.M., Levy, E.M., and Hammermeister, K.E. (1998). Independent association between ARF and mortality following cardiac surgery. *American Journal of Medicine*, **104**, 343–48.

45. Svensson, L.G., Coselli, J.S., Safi, H.J., *et al.* (1989). Appraisal of adjuncts to prevent acute renal failure after surgery on the thoracic or thoracoabdominal aorta. *Journal of Vascular Surgery*, **10**, 230–9.

46 Bertrand, M., Godet, G., Meersschaert, K. *et al.* (2001). Should angiotensin II antagonists be discontinued before surgery? *Anesthesia and Analgesia*, **92**, 26–30.

47. Griffin, M.R., Yared, A., and Ray, W.A. (2000). Nonsteroidal anti-inflammatory drugs and acute renal failure in elderly persons. *American Journal of Epidemiology*, **151**, 488–96.

48. Hynninen, M.S., Niemi, T.T., Poyhia, R., *et al.* (2006). N-acetylcysteine for the prevention of kidney injury in abdominal aortic surgery: a randomized, double-blind, placebo-controlled trial. *Anesthesia and Analgesia*, **102**, 1638–45.

49. Gonowski, C.T., Laster, M.J., Eger, E.I., *et al.* (1994). Toxicology of compound A in rats: effect of a 3-hour administration. *Anesthesiology*, **80**, 556–65.

50. Croinin, D.F. and Shorten, G.D. (2002). Anesthesia and renal disease. *Current Opinion in Anaesthesiology*, **15**, 359–63.

51. Julier, K., Da Silva, R., Garcia, C. *et al.* (2003). Preconditioning by sevoflurane decreases biochemical markers for myocardial and renal dysfunction in coronary artery bypass graft surgery: a double blind placebo-controlled multi-center study. *Anesthesiology*, **96**, 1315–27.

52. Scheingarter, S., Rehm, M., Sehmisch, C., Finsterer, U. (1999). Rapid saline infusion produces hyperchloraemic acidosis in patients undergoing gynaecologic surgery. *Anesthesiology*, **90**, 1265–70.

53. Scott, N.B., Turfrey, D.J., Ray, D.A.A., *et al.* (2001). A prospective randomized study of the potential benefits of thoracic epidural anesthesia and analgesia in patients undergoing coronary artery bypass grafting. *Anesthesia and Analgesia*, **93**, 528–35.

54. Kulka, P.J., Tryba, M., and Zenz, M. (1996). Preoperative alpha$_2$-adrenergic receptor agonists prevent the deterioration of renal function after cardiac surgery: results of a randomized controlled trial. *Critical Care Medicine*, **24**, 947–52.

55. Nicholson, M.L., Baker, D.M., Hopkinson, B.R., *et al.* (1996). Randomised controlled trial of the effect of mannitol on renal reperfusion injury during aortic aneurysm surgery. *British Journal of Surgery*, **83**, 1230–3.

56. Lassnigg, A., Donner, E., Grubhofer, G., *et al.* (2000). Lack of renoprotective effects of dopamine and furosemide during cardiac surgery. *Journal of the American Society of Nephrology*, **11**, 97–104.

57. Solomon, R., Werner, C., Mann, D., *et al.* (1994). Effects of saline, mannitol and furosemide to prevent acute decreases in renal function induced by radio contrast agents. *New England Journal of Medicine*, **331**, 1416–20.

58. Bellomo, R., Chapman, M., Finfer, S., *et al.* (2000). For ANZICS Clinical Trials group. Low-dose dopamine in patients with early renal dysfunction: a placebo-controlled randomised trial. *Lancet*, **356**, 2139–43.

59. Welch, M., Newstead, C.G., Smith, J.V., *et al.* (1995). Evaluation of dopexamine hydrochloride as a renoprotective agent during aortic surgery. *Annals of Vascular Surgery*, **9**, 488–92.

60. Allen, S.J., Penugonda, S.P., Baker, R.C., *et al.* (2003). Low dose dopexamine does not alter subclinical renal indices following cardiac surgery, *European Journal of Anaesthesiology*, **20**(S29), A28.

61. Kellum, J.A., Leblanc, M., Gibney, N., *et al.* (2005). Primary prevention of acute renal failure in the critically ill. *Current Opinion in Critical Care*, **11**, 537–41.

62. Bove, T., Landoni, G., Calabro, M.G. *et al.* (2005). Renoprotective action of fenoldopam in high-risk patients undergoing cardiac surgery. A prospective placebo controlled trial. *Circulation*, **110**, 3230–5.

63. Baigent, C., Burbury, K., and Wheeler, D. (2000). Premature cardiovascular disease in chronic renal failure. *Lancet*, **356**, 147–52.

64. Eagle, K.A., Berger, P.B., Calkins, H., *et al.* (2002). ACC/AHA guideline update for perioperative cardiovascular evaluation for non-cardiac surgery: a report of the American College of Cardiology/American Heart Association Task Force on practice guidelines. *Anesthesia and Analgesia*, **94**, 1052–64.

65. Rabey, P.G. (2001). Anaesthesia for renal transplantation. *British Journal of Anaesthesia CEPD Reviews*, **1**, 24–7.

66. Rang, S.T., West, N.L., Howard, J., Cousins, J.. (2006). Anaesthesia for chronic renal disease and renal transplantation. *EAU-EBU Update Series*, **30**, 1–11.

67. Clive, D.M. and Stoff, J.S. (1984). Renal syndromes associated with non-steroidal anti-inflammatory drugs. *New England Journal of Medicine*, **310**, 563–72.

68. Hand, C.W. (1990). Buprenorphine in patients with renal impairment: single and continuous dosing with special reference to metabolites. *British Journal of Anaesthesia*, **64**, 276–82.

69. Woolf, R.A., Ashby, V.B., Milford, E.L., *et al.* (1999). Comparison of mortality in all patients on dialysis, patients on dialysis awaiting transplantation, and recipients of first cadaver transplant. *New England Journal of Medicine*, **341**, 1725–30.

70. Briggs, J.D. (2001). Causes of death after renal transplantation. *Nephrology, Dialysis, Transplantation*, **16**, 1545–9.

71. Stewart, G.A., Tan, C.C., Rodger, R.S.C., *et al.* (1999). Graft and patient survival following renal transplantation: new targets for blood pressure control. In *Cardionephrology 5* (eds. TimioM, V. Wizeman, and S. Venanzi), pp. 357–61. Ediotoriale Bios, Cosenza..

Chapter 18

Injury during anaesthesia

Robert A McCahon & Jonathan G Hardman

This chapter will deal specifically with injury arising during anaesthesia as result of technical procedures, posture, or external, physical threat. Other forms of injury occur during anaesthesia (e.g. cerebrovascular events, myocardial infarction, and awareness) but these are covered separately. Nerve and spinal cord injuries arising during general or regional anaesthesia, while clearly qualifying as 'injury arising during anaesthesia', are dealt with in Chapter 15.

In the main, the chapter is organized by the physical location of the injury; these locations comprise: oral, laryngeal, tracheal, ocular, cutaneous, orthopaedic, muscular, and vascular. External ocular injury is discussed in this chapter, but postoperative visual loss is dealt with in Chapter 15.

Incidence

Injury during anaesthesia is very common. Removal of the patient's natural, protective mechanisms of pain perception and movement of the affected part causes the risk of superficial injury to be increased. The great majority of such injuries (e.g. cut lips, bruised limbs, pinched skin) are minor and recover rapidly and without the need for medical intervention[1]. The minor associated symptoms and the brief discomfort produced result in few accusations of blame and litigation. Substantial, life-altering injuries do occur. Occasionally, apparently minor injuries may lead to a chronic pain syndrome in the affected part, especially if neurological injury has occurred.

Oropharyngeal and dental injury

Injury to the mucosa of the oropharynx and to the teeth is common during general anaesthesia (5%)[2]. Unconscious patients inevitably require a degree of mechanical adjustment of the airway or insertion of devices to assure airway patency. These techniques each involve forces being exerted upon the delicate structures of the oropharynx. Clearly, the risk of injury increases with the use of increasing force. Greater force is required to assure the patency of a partially obstructed airway; in this context, lips may be trapped between teeth or between the facemask and the face, and lacerations and bruising may result. All such injuries are avoidable through attention to the correct placement of the patient's anatomy and the airway device.

Dental injury

When devices are placed within the pharynx, the risk of injury increases. However, the advantage of such devices almost always outweighs the extra risk of injury that they bring. Laryngoscopy using a rigid, handheld laryngoscope carries the risk of laceration of the lips, the oropharyngeal mucosa, and the uvula. Proper attention to detail can avoid these injuries. Dental injury is commonly associated with direct laryngoscopy (1%)[3–5]. The upper incisors are affected in 87% of cases[3]. The majority (98%) of dental injuries do not require surgical intervention[3], but crown fracture, dislocation, or dislodgement may require surgical management. Complaint and litigation are common following significant dental injury. Dental injuries are associated with difficulty in laryngoscopy; in particular, difficulty in visualizing the glottis may cause the anaesthetist to exert greater force or to use the upper incisors as a fulcrum to apply leverage to lift the epiglottis. However, the majority of dental injury is not associated with predicted difficult laryngoscopy[6] [Givol 2004]. Airway intervention may, of course, be life-saving, and dental injury is an occasional and inevitable consequence of desperate attempts to secure a dangerous airway. In this scenario, fault is mitigated, but the majority of dental injury arises from inadequate attention to proper technique in laryngoscopy. Dental injury occurs most commonly in patients aged 50–70 years[6], but it is not clear whether this reflects the more fragile state of older patients' dentition or the increased likelihood of difficult laryngoscopy. The use of dental protectors has been proposed for patients with fragile dentition or prominent incisors[7]. These may reduce the risk of dental injury, but frequently increase the difficulty of laryngoscopy and their usefulness remains unproven[8].

Dental injury has been reported during the removal of tracheal tubes and laryngeal masks[3]. During emergence from general anaesthesia, patients will often bite upon an intra-oral device, and forceful traction can avulse or fracture teeth. Even gentle traction may, feasibly, injure very fragile teeth during device removal, but substantial force is required to injure healthy teeth during airway device removal. The risk of dental injury during airway device removal may be reduced by inserting a bite-block prior to emergence or by postponing device removal until the patient is cooperative.

Oropharyngeal injury

The oropharyngeal mucosa may be injured through deployment of a rigid laryngoscope (resulting in laceration or bruising) or through ischaemia caused by prolonged compression by airway devices. Oropharyngeal laceration followed by positive pressure ventilation may result in surgical emphysema; such an outcome is rare. Uvular ischaemia and necrosis has been reported following placement of a tracheal tube[9] and the use of a Guedel airway. It is clear that any device which remains in the oropharynx should be justified against the potential risk it brings of mucosal ischaemia.

Sore throat following tracheal intubation or laryngeal mask placement is common. Its incidence is 45% when a tracheal tube is used, reducing to 18% when a laryngeal mask is used and to 3% when a facemask is used alone[10–13]. Laryngoscopy is responsible for some of the post-anaesthesia discomfort, but the indwelling airway device also accounts for some. Gentle laryngoscopy, use of the smallest appropriate airway device, and inflation of cuffs to minimum acceptable pressures reduces the risk of post-anaesthesia sore throat.

Laryngeal and tracheal injury

Postoperative vocal hoarseness has been reported in up to 50% of patients undergoing general anaesthesia[14]. It is usually self-limiting, but prolonged voice change has been reported, and may be due to more significant laryngeal injury[15].

Mucosa may be injured within the larynx and on the vocal cords. Such injury is more common with the use of tracheal tubes, and when these remain for prolonged periods (i.e. more than 24 h)[16]. Vocal cord and laryngeal ulceration and granulation are fairly common sequelae of mechanical ventilation via an orotracheal tube in the intensive care unit (ICU), but are rare following surgical anaesthesia. Mucosal injury is minimized by using the smallest appropriate device for the shortest time possible and by minimizing the pressure exerted on the mucosa by the inflatable cuff[16]. Cuff-induced mucosal injury is now much less common because of the introduction of high-volume low-pressure cuffs, which spread the area of cuff-mucosa contact considerably. Gradual cuff distension by the inward diffusion of nitrous oxide during anaesthesia may cause mucosal ischaemia, and this may be reduced by the inflation of the cuff using saline or a gas mixture containing nitrous oxide[14]. Cuff pressures larger than 15 mm Hg have been demonstrated to increase the risk of laryngeal injury, and the use of a manometer and/or methods to limit cuff-pressure is indicated if prolonged tracheal intubation is anticipated[17].

Laceration and penetration of the tracheal wall have been reported[18,19]. Such injuries have a potentially fatal outcome through the leakage of gas into the neck and mediastinum with compression of the great vessels and surgical emphysema. The application of excessive force via a tracheal tube, bougie, or stylet is usually to blame.

Injury to the arytenoid cartilages is uncommon but has been reported[20]. Dislocation or subluxation causes pain and a hoarse voice and may require surgical treatment.

The major risk factor for laryngeal and vocal cord injury is laryngo-tracheal instrumentation and intubation. It is likely that difficulty in laryngoscopy increases the risk of injury, but the majority (80%) of injuries are not associated with reported difficult intubation, and most (85%) occur following short-term tracheal intubation[19].

Oesophageal injury

The potentially fatal complication of oesophageal perforation is rare, but can occur following inadvertent instrumentation or intubation of the oesophagus during attempted endotracheal intubation[21].

Ocular injury

Perioperative eye injury is relatively rare, occurring during 0.1% of general anaesthetics. Such injuries account for around 2% of legal claims against anaesthetists[22]. The majority of injuries are minor, resulting in a few days' postoperative discomfort. However, blindness may follow apparently uneventful surgery and anaesthesia, and this may be utterly devastating for the patient; postoperative visual loss is discussed in Chapter 15.

Table 18.1 Incidence of oral, dental, pharyngeal, laryngeal, tracheal, and oesophageal injury during general anaesthesia

Injury	Incidence(%)	
All oral trauma	5–7	[Fung 2001 [5]]
Dental injury		
- Total	1	[Burton 1987 [4]]
- During laryngoscopy	0.5	[Warner 1999 [3]]
- Requiring surgical treatment	0.02	[Warner 1999 [2]]
Sore throat after general anaesthesia		[Higgins 2002 [10]]
- Total	12	
- Tracheal tube	45	
- Laryngeal mask	18	
- Facemask only	3	
Laryngeal injury		[Mencke 2003 [14]]
- Hoarse voice	50	
- Persistent hoarseness	1	

Corneal injury

Corneal injury accounts for two-thirds of intra-operative ocular injury[23]; this painful but usually self-limiting injury is caused usually by direct, physical trauma to the cornea, but may be caused by exposure keratopathy or chemical injury. The eyelids tend not to appose during general anaesthesia because of the reduction in the tonic contraction of the orbicularis oculi muscle. Placing tape or gel pads over the closed eyelids or applying lubricating ointment to the eyes reduces the risk of external objects abrading the cornea and of exposure keratopathy due to corneal drying, which results from the cessation of blinking. The reduction in tear formation and in tear-spreading through blinking make the cornea unusually sensitive to injury and contact with the cornea that appears trivial during anaesthesia may result in an exquisitely painful corneal abrasion postoperatively. Chemical injury to the cornea may occur following direct exposure of the cornea to cleaning solutions. Povidone–iodine 10% aqueous solution is considered not to cause corneal injury, but other skin preparations (e.g. chlorhexidine) may cause injury and should be avoided[22].

Cutaneous injury

Pressure on an area of skin reduces cutaneous perfusion; if this pressure is substantial and/or prolonged, then ischaemia and tissue necrosis may result[24]. Injury is most likely when pressure is exerted over bony prominences and in patients who are elderly, poorly nourished, immobile, incontinent, have chronic disease, or diminished

Table 18.2 Incidence of ocular injury during general anaesthesia

Injury	Incidence (%)	
All ocular injuries	0.17	[Cucchiara 1988 [25]]
	0.056	[Roth 1996 [23]]
Corneal abrasion	0.03–0.1	[Gild 1992 [26]]

conscious level. Pressure sores may occur in the postoperative period because of events that occurred during the intra-operative period, so it is essential to dissipate pressure over as large a surface area as possible when positioning the patient using appropriate padding; vulnerable areas should be checked and re-checked throughout surgery.

Thermal injury

Monopolar diathermy generates local temperatures of up to 1000°C using high-frequency alternating current. If the patient plate electrode is incorrectly placed then points of contact between metal and skin (e.g. ECG electrodes) can provide alternative return pathways and can result in serious burns. Incorrect placement of the patient plate electrode is the most common cause of accidental diathermy burns. Less commonly, careless surgical technique can cause local burns. Pools of spirit-based skin preparation fluids can heat up and ignite during monopolar or bipolar diathermy use.

Lasers can produce cutaneous, ocular, and mucosal burns. Currently, anaesthetists do not use lasers, and such accidental injury is usually through surgical mishap.

Chemical injury

Skin preparation solutions may cause cutaneous injury, especially when left in pools for prolonged periods or when they penetrate under a tourniquet. Such chemical cutaneous injury resembles thermal injury in appearance. Skin (and deeper tissues) may also be injured by injection of solutions subcutaneously through a misplaced intravenous cannula. Strongly acidic and strongly basic solutions have the greatest potential for tissue injury. Of the anaesthesia induction agents, thiopentone is the most dangerous in this regard, but even the apparently innocuous propofol has been reported to cause skin necrosis following inadvertent subcutaneous injection. Intra-arterial injury has even greater potential for injury, and this is discussed later in this chapter (see "Arterial injury").

Alopecia

Postoperative alopecia areata is a rare complication due to ischaemia induced by prolonged pressure on the scalp; it is associated with the use of head supports such as the head ring or jelly donut[27,28]. Additional risk factors are prolonged surgery, intra-operative hypotension, hypoxaemia, and anaemia. Intra-operative repositioning of the patient's head may reduce its incidence.

Muscular injury

Prolonged and substantial extrinsic compression or forced limb flexion may cause muscle ischaemia and necrosis. Myoglobinuria and hyperkalaemia can result. During prolonged surgery, sympathetic positioning and occasional checking and re-positioning seem likely to reduce the risk of this complication. Tourniquets may also cause muscle ischaemia and the duration of inflation and the inflation pressure determine the risk of injury. Inflation pressures should be 50–100 mmHg higher than systolic blood pressure for arms and legs, respectively, and inflation time should not exceed 2 h without a reperfusion window of at least 20 min in healthy patients[29,30]. Furthermore, the tourniquet should be applied to the proximal limb, avoiding bony prominences, and with adequate padding.

Compartment syndrome may follow prolonged muscular compression or significant trauma. Tourniquets and poor positioning may cause ischaemia with subsequent compartmental pressure increases and reduced compartmental perfusion. Compartment syndrome has been associated with prolonged lithotomy and Lloyd–Davies positioning[31–33].

Bone and joint injury

Operating tables with detachable sections or moveable parts bring the risk of trapping fingers (and other appendages) and subsequent crush injuries and/or amputation. Patients may fall from operating tables, with consequent fractures or intracranial injury. Care in positioning is of utmost importance, and extremes of operating table tilt (lateral and long-axis tilt) must be performed carefully and only when necessary.

It is a relatively common occurrence for an upper limb to swing free of its restraints while the patient is supine. This is particularly common during repositioning. Such accidental limb movement may result in shoulder injury through the forceful extension and abduction of the joint, limb injury through collision during its fall, or nerve injury (i.e. brachial plexus) through excessive stretch. Neck injury may also occur through uncontrolled movement of the head. The head is a heavy, spherical object that has a tendency to roll, especially in the anaesthetized patient. Patients with existing neck injury, nerve entrapment, cervical osteoarthritis, or rheumatoid arthritis should have their head positioned carefully, and preferably while awake, and this position should be maintained carefully throughout their unconsciousness.

Joints may be injured through prolonged positioning at the extreme of their range of movement. The lithotomy and knee-chest position carry particular risk of joint pain postoperatively.

Inhalational injury

The unconscious patient is supplied with a gas mixture via an airway device and a breathing system. Medical gases are stringently quality-controlled, but contaminants may enter the patient's airway via a number of routes. Regurgitation of gastric contents during general anaesthesia may lead to their inhalation and subsequent pulmonary injury. This is covered in detail in Chapter 10.

Water may accumulate in the breathing system; this often occurs in circle breathing systems when a low fresh gas flow rate is used, and exhaled water vapour condenses in the breathing system tubing. Such accumulated water may be tipped into the patient's airway if the tubing is moved. Inhalation may cause lung injury, haemolysis, and disturbance of gas exchange. Previously, inhaled gases were warmed and/or humidified occasionally using a hot water bath or nebulizer; these devices carried the risk of over-saturation of inhaled gases, with the risk for near-drowning.

The growing use of rebreathing (circle) breathing systems in recent years has brought many reductions in cost and in the risk of airway dehydration and cooling. However, there have been reports of carbon monoxide poisoning[34]. The carbon dioxide absorbant in circle systems may dry out, especially if fresh gas continues to enter the breathing system between operating lists[35,36]. When certain volatile anaesthetic agents react with the carbon dioxide absorbant, carbon monoxide may be produced. Desflurane and enflurane produce the most carbon monoxide; isoflurane produces less and sevoflurane and halothane produce very little or no carbon monoxide[36,37]. Of the carbon dioxide absorbants, Baralyme™ appears to produce greater quantities of carbon monoxide than does sodalime[35,36].

Several volatile anaesthetic agents may produce breakdown products within breathing systems. Some of these may be toxic in humans. The problem is most apparent during very low fresh gas flow into circle systems. This issue is covered in more detail in Chapter 21.

Vascular injury

Arteries may be injured through needling techniques, sustained external compression, or impact. By far the most common of these in anaesthesia practice is injury through needling, which may occur during attempted venous cannulation, regional anaesthesia, or intended arterial cannulation or blood sampling. Substantial haematomata may form following puncture, and rarely, distal perfusion may be adversely affected with subsequent ischaemia. False aneurysm formation is a risk, and surgical treatment may very rarely be required. More detailed discussion of the risks associated with vascular access is in Chapter 20.

It seems likely that the use of ultrasound guidance for needling techniques reduces the risk of inadvertent arterial or venous injury[38], although the evidence is minimal currently (partly through the novelty of the use of ultrasound, and partly through the difficulty in researching a rare complication).

The use of arterial tourniquets may (very rarely) injure arteries and may displace thrombi from vessel walls to generate emboli that most frequently travel to the lungs, causing pulmonary hypertension and disturbed gas exchange. Rarely, such pulmonary emboli may be fatal.

The accidental injection of drugs into arteries is usually harmless. Most drugs disperse very rapidly into the circulation, but some may provoke intense vasospasm or may deposit out of solution and block arterioles. The injection of thiopentone into an artery may cause intense vasospasm and has been reported to cause distal necrosis[39]. Intra-arterial vasoconstrictors, such as adrenaline and noradrenaline, may also produce distal ischaemia that may threaten tissue viability. Prevention of such complications requires proper labelling of vascular catheters so that venous and arterial lines are not confused and maintaining a degree of suspicion of arterial placement of a catheter, especially when located near the site of an artery (e.g. at the antecubital fossa, the groin or the front of the wrist).

Other organ injury

All organs are threatened during hypotension, hypoxia, anaemia, reduced cardiac output, impaired venous drainage, or extrinsic compression. Those organs with large basal metabolic rate and the incapacity for anaerobic metabolism are most at risk; these include the brain and heart, which are discussed in detail in Chapter 13 and Chapter 15. The liver and the kidneys may also be injured during anaesthesia. External compression of the liver, possibly associated with positioning, has been associated with postoperative liver dysfunction. The kidneys may be injured through medullary ischaemia, and the combination of dehydration, hypotension, and nephrotoxic drugs (e.g. non-steroidal anti-inflammatories, radio-contrast agents, or aminoglycoside antibiotics) generates a high risk of postoperative renal dysfunction.

References

1. Wu, C.L., Berenholtz, S.M., Pronovost, P.J., and Fleisher, L.A. (2002). Systematic review and analysis of postdischarge symptoms after outpatient surgery. *Anesthesiology*, **96**, 994–1003.

2. Jenkins, K. and Baker, A.B. (2003). Consent and anaesthetic risk. *Anaesthesia*, **58**, 962–84.

3. Warner, M.E., Benenfeld, S.M., Warner, M.A., Schroeder, D.R., Maxson, P.M. (1999). Perianesthetic dental injuries: frequency, outcomes, and risk factors. *Anesthesiology*, **90**, 1302–5.

4. Burton, J.F. and Baker, A.B. (1987). Dental damage during anaesthesia and surgery. *Anaesthesia and Intensive Care*, **15**, 262–8.

5. Fung, B.K. and Chan, M.Y. (2001). Incidence of oral tissue trauma after the administration of general anaesthesia. *Acta Anaesthesiologica Sinica*, **39**, 163–7.

6. Givol, N., Gershtansky, Y., Halamish-Shani, T., Taicher, S., Perel, A., and Segal, E. (2004). Perianesthetic dental injuries: analysis of incident reports. *Journal of Clinical Anesthesia*, **16**, 173–6.

7. Chadwick, R.G. and Lindsay, S.M. (1996). Dental injuries during general anaesthesia. *British Dental Journal*, **180**(7), 255–8.

8. Skeie, A. and Schwartz, O. (1999). Traumatic injuries of the teeth in connection with general anaesthesia and the effect of use of mouthguards. *Endodontics and Dental Traumatology* **15**, 33–6.

9. Harris, M.A. and Kumar, M. (1997). A rare complication of endotracheal intubation. *Lancet*, **350**, 1820–1.

10. Higgins, P.P., Chung, F., and Mezei, G. (2002). Postoperative sore throat after ambulatory surgery. *British Journal of Anaesthesia*, **88**, 582–4.

11. Dingley, J., Whitehead, M.J., and Wareham, J. (1994). A comparative study of the incidence of sore throat with the laryngeal mask airway. *Anaesthesia*, **49**, 251–4.

12. Taylor, T.H. (1992). Avoiding iatrogenic injuries in theatre. *British Medical Journal*, **305**, 595–6.

13. McHardy, F.E. and Chung, F. (1999). Postoperative sore throat: cause, prevention and treatment. *Anaesthesia*, **54**, 444–53.

14. Mencke, T., Echternach, M., Kleinschmidt, S., *et al.* (2003). Laryngeal morbidity and quality of tracheal intubation: A randomized controlled trial. *Anesthesiology*, **98**, 1049–56.

15. Maktabi, M.A., Smith, R.B., and Todd, M.M. (2003). Is routine endotracheal intubation as safe as we think or wish? *Anesthesiology*, **99**(2), 247–8.

16. Combes, X., Schauvliege, F., Peyrouset, O., *et al.* (2001). Intracuff pressure and tracheal morbidity: influence of filling with saline during nitrous oxide anesthesia. *Anesthesiology*, **95**, 1120–4.

17. Suzuki, N., Kooguchi, K., Mizobe, T., Hirose, M., Takano, Y., and Tanaka, Y. (1999). Postoperative hoarseness and sore throat after tracheal intubation: effect of a low intracuff pressure of endotracheal tube and the usefulness of cuff pressure indicator. *Masui*, **48**(10), 1091–5.

18. Törnvall, S.S., Jackson, K.H., and Enrique, T,O. (1971). Tracheal rupture, complication of cuffed endotracheal tube. *Chest*, **59**, 237–9.

19. Kambic, V. and Radsel, Z. (1978). Intubation lesions of the larynx. *British Journal of Anaesthesia*, **50**(6), 587–90.

20. Talmi, Y.P., Wolf, M., Bar-Ziv, J., *et al.*(1996). Postintubation arytenoid subluxation. *Annals of Otology, Rhinology,and Laryngology*, **105**(5), 384–90.

21. Hilmi, I.A., Sullivan, E., Quinlan, J., Shekar, S. (2003). Esophageal tear: an unusual complication after difficult endotracheal intubation. *Anesthesia and Analgesia*, **97**, 911–91.

22. White, E. (2004). Care of the eye during anaesthesia. *Anaesthesia and Intensive Care*, **5**, 302–3.

23. Roth, S., Thisted, R.A., Erickson, J.P., Black, S., and Schreider, B.D. (1996). Eye injuries after nonocular surgery. A study of 60,965 anesthetics from 1988 to 1992. *Anesthesiology*, **85**(5), 1020–7.

24. Knight, D.J.W. and Mahajan, R.P. (2004). *Continuing Education in Anaesthesia, Critical Care & Pain*, 4(5), 160–3.

25. Cucchiara, R.F. and Black, S. (1988). Corneal abrasion during anaesthesia and surgery. *Anesthesiology*, **69**, 978–9.

26. Gild, W.M., Posner, K.L., Caplan, R.A., and Cheney, F.W. (1992). Eye injuries associated with anaesthesia. A Closed Claims analysis. *Anesthesiology*, **76**, 204–8.

27. Wiles, J. and Hansen, R. (1985). Postoperative (pressure) alopecia. *Journal of the American Academy of Dermatology*, **12**,195–8.

28. Patel, K. and Henschel, E. (1980). Postoperative alopecia. *Anesthesia and Analgesia*, **59**, 311–3.

29. Pedowitz, R.A., Gershuni, D.H., Friden, J., Garfin, S.R., Rydevik, B.L., and Hargens, A.R. (1992). Effects of reperfusion intervals on skeletal muscle injury beneath and distal to a pneumatic tourniquet. *Journal of Hand Surgery*, **17**(2), 245–55.

30. Horlocker, T.T., Hebl, J.R., Gali, B., *et al.* (2006). Anesthetic, patient, and surgical risk factors for neurologic complications after prolonged total tourniquet time during total knee arthroplasty. *Anesthesia and Analgesia*, **102**(3), 950–5.

31. Halliwill, J.R., Hewitt, B.S., Joyner, M.J., and Warner, M.A. (1998). Effect of various lithotomy positions on lower extremity pressure. *Anesthesiology*, **89**, 1373–6.

32. Turnbull, D, and Mills, G.H. (2001). Compartment syndrome associated with the Lloyd Davies position. Three case reports and review of the literature. *Anaesthesia*, **56**, 980–7.

33. Warner, M.E., LaMaster, L.M., Thoeming, A.K., Shirk Marienau, M.E., and Warner, M.A. (2001). Compartment syndrome in surgical patients. *Anesthesiology*, **94**, 705–8.

34. Berry, P.D., Sessler, D.I., and Larson, M.D. (1999). Severe carbon monoxide poisoning during desflurane anesthesia. *Anesthesiology*, **90**, 613–6.

35. Davies, M.W. and Potter, F.A. (1996). Carbon monoxide, soda lime and volatile agents. *Anaesthesia*, **51**, 90.

36. Fang, Z.X., Eger, E.I., Laster, M.J., Chortkoff, B.S., Kandel, L., and Ionescu, P. (1995). Carbon monoxide production from degradation of desflurane, enflurane, isoflurane, halothane, and sevoflurane by soda lime and Baralyme. *Anesthesia and Analgesia*, **80**, 1187–93.

37. Frink, E.J. Jr, Nogami, W.M., Morgan, S.E., and Salmon, R.C. (1997). High carboxy hemoglobin concentrations occur in swine during desflurane anesthesia in the presence of partially dried carbon dioxide absorbents. *Anesthesiology*, **87**, 308–16.

38. Hopkins, P.M. (2007). Ultrasound guidance as a gold standard in regional anaesthesia. British Journal of Anaesthesia, **98**(3), 299–301.

39. Mazumder, J.K., Metcalf, I.R., and Holland, A.J. (1980). Inadvertent intra-arterial injection of thiopentone. *Canadian Anaesthesia Society Journal*, **27**(4), 395–8.

Chapter 19

Temperature

Simon P Holbrook & Philip M Hopkins

Humans are homeothermic, that is, in the face of considerable variation in the temperature of the environment, the core body temperature is kept comparatively constant. The enzyme reactions that preserve homeostasis operate most favourably when body temperature is maintained within a narrow range. Normal core body temperature follows a circadian pattern, varying by 0.5 to 0.7°C, being highest in the evening and lowest at approximately 06:00 h; the morning oral temperature averages at 36.7°C, but in 95% of young adults this value lies between 36.3 and 37.1°C. Therefore, core body temperature values outside this range may be normal. In addition, the luteal phase or latter half of the menstrual cycle is associated with an increase of 0.3 to 0.5°C in basal body temperature.

Maintenance of a normal body temperature depends on equilibrium between the production of heat and heat loss. Cell metabolism, muscular activity, and food ingestion are the major sources of heat. Heat is lost through the processes of radiation, conduction, convection, and evaporation. The control centre for temperature regulation is the hypothalamus, which integrates afferent information from peripheral and central thermoreceptors to primarily produce appropriate autonomic and behavioural responses. The principal effectors triggered by cold are vasoconstriction, particularly of arteriovenous shunts in fingers and toes, and shivering. Those triggered by heat are sweating and active cutaneous vasodilatation. These mechanisms maintain tight control of core body temperature around a set point, for example, 37°C. When heat loss exceeds heat production, body temperature falls: when the threshold temperature, say 36.8°C, is breached, vasoconstriction occurs; shivering may not commence though until 35.5°C is reached. The threshold for sweating may typically be 37.1°C. The difference between the thresholds for vasoconstriction and sweating is defined as the inter-threshold range and is approximately 0.2 to 0.4°C.

Disturbances of thermoregulation that may be encountered during anaesthesia may be categorized into hypothermia, fever (pyrexia), and hyperthermia. Most patients are rendered hypothermic during general anaesthesia, but fever and hyperthermia are seen less frequently and may be difficult to distinguish. On a physiological basis, hyperthermia is the outcome of heat production exceeding heat loss but with the set point remaining normal: the thresholds for sweating and cutaneous vasoconstriction also remain normal. Fever, however, results from endogenous pyrogens stimulating the hypothalamic control centre producing an increase in the set-point and the thresholds, although the inter-threshold range remains normal. We shall now consider these perturbations of thermoregulation in turn in the context of anaesthesia, exploring contributory factors and clinical consequences, incorporating the risks and benefits associated with temperature management.

Hypothermia

Definition

A precise definition of hypothermia states that it occurs when the core temperature is greater than one standard deviation below the mean, under resting conditions, in a thermoneutral environment[1]. The majority of the clinical literature would consider that mild hypothermia refers to a core temperature between 34 and 36°C.

Risk

Hypothermia is the most frequent perioperative thermal abnormality encountered[2]. During the operative period, a number of factors may contribute: uncovering of the patient to the ambient temperature of the operating theatre, aggravated by convective losses due to air turnover; a cold table and the use of cold antiseptic skin solutions; dry anaesthetic gases; body cavity exposure; and infusion of cold intravenous fluids. The root causes, though, are the effects of anaesthesia on human thermoregulation itself. Under normal conditions, the human body can be depicted as consisting of a core thermal compartment (consisting anatomically of the head and trunk) and a peripheral compartment; the temperature of the latter is typically 2 to 4°C less than the former, depending on the environment. Smaller gradients exist when the environment is warm or when there is cutaneous vasodilatation, and larger gradients in cold surroundings or when vasoconstriction confines heat to the core[3]. General anaesthesia inhibits arteriovenous shunt vasoconstriction and shivering, and to a lesser degree impedes sweating. The threshold for warmth response is raised, and the threshold for cold response lowered, thus broadening the inter-threshold range up to 10-fold[4]. The patient is rendered poikilothermic over a 4°C range of core body temperature; it exhibits variability directly dependent on the environmental temperature[1,5].

The initial vasodilatation occurring on induction of general anaesthesia produces redistribution of heat from the core to the peripheral compartment; core body temperature decreases 1°C during the first 30 min[6]. Heat is lost predominantly as the result of radiation and convection; evaporative losses depend on the nature of the surgery, and conductive losses are minimal. As time proceeds, redistribution diminishes but heat production also falls due to a reduced metabolic rate. Heat loss continues to exceed heat production at a slower rate for two to four hours, at which time a plateau may be reached when they become equal[3]. This may be attained more quickly with active warming measures. Active cutaneous vasoconstriction is not triggered until the core temperature falls to between 34 and 35°C or even lower[7–9]. This constrains metabolic heat to the core, preventing additional core hypothermia, but allows the peripheral tissues to continue to cool through reduced but continued cutaneous heat loss[10]. As the core body temperature plateau may take three to five hours to occur, it is rarely achieved during the course of most general anaesthetics[5].

Regional anaesthetic techniques commonly cause similar disturbances of thermoregulation; initial core hypothermia during epidural anaesthesia is primarily the result of heat redistribution from the core to the legs[11]. Sympathetic and motor nerve block prevents vasoconstriction and shivering distal to the level of the block. However, redistribution continues unabated even after the first hour. Shivering and vasoconstriction may occur in the upper body but are not enough to prevent core hypothermia; in addition the active cutaneous vasoconstriction that creates the plateau phase during general anaesthesia does not occur[3]. Central control of thermoregulation is also affected because of erroneous afferent signals from peripheral receptors in the blocked region: the thresholds for shivering and vasoconstriction are decreased and the inter threshold range increased three- to fourfold[5,12]. The major concerns are, principally, that patients often do not complain of coldness and the majority of anaesthetists do not monitor core temperature during neuraxial anaesthesia, only 33% routinely implementing temperature monitoring in one survey[13].

Case study 1

A 60 kg, 75-year-old lady presented for elective bilateral total knee replacement. She had a past medical history of osteoarthritis, hypertension, and mild chronic obstructive pulmonary disease. Preoperative haemoglobin concentration was 12.3 g/dl. She consented to a combined spinal and epidural technique for anaesthesia. A 16-gauge peripheral venous cannula was inserted. The regional anaesthetic procedure continued uneventfully and standard monitoring was implemented. A urethral urinary catheter was inserted for urine output monitoring and patient comfort. The surgery took nearly three hours to perform. An epidural infusion of 0.1% bupivacaine and 2 µg/ml fentanyl was commenced at 12 ml per h, one hour into the procedure. The patient remained haemodynamically stable and comfortable throughout, requiring no additional intravenous analgesia or sedation. Blankets and an intravenous fluid warmer (set at 42°C) were employed for thermal management. Three litres of crystalloid were infused in total. On arrival in the post operative care unit (PACU,) the patient was pain-free but shivering and complaining of feeling cold. Her core body temperature measured using a tympanic membrane probe was 35.1°C. Additional warming was provided with a forced-air warming blanket. She became asymptomatically hypotensive with a systolic blood pressure of 85mmHg and was oliguric. She temporarily responded to a 250-ml fluid challenge but her haemoglobin measured 6 g/dl. She received 3 units of packed red cells but ultimately spent 3 h in PACU, her discharge being delayed as a consequence of ongoing hypotension and hypothermia. She received additional blood transfusions during the postoperative period but otherwise made a successful recovery.

The case study highlights the need for temperature monitoring when using regional anaesthesia but also illustrates one group of patients at increased risk of developing perioperative hypothermia, the elderly, and one of the potential clinical consequences, increased blood loss.

Before we proceed to explore the benefits of maintaining perioperative normothermia, it must be noted that patients receiving combined general and neuraxial anaesthesia are the most likely to develop perioperative hypothermia. There is rapid heat loss because of redistribution; the threshold for vasoconstriction is reduced even further; shivering that may occur during neuraxial blockade is inhibited by general anaesthesia; and when the hypothalamus initiates the efferent signal to commence active vasoconstriction, to achieve the plateau phase, it is less successful because of sympathetic blockade in the legs[3]. In conclusion, these patients not only lose heat more rapidly but also suffer continuing heat loss, their core body temperature not achieving a plateau during lengthy procedures.

This emphasizes the need for vigilance and the institution of warming measures in all patients undergoing general and/or regional anaesthesia but most notably when in combination. In order to reinforce this, the clinical consequences of perioperative hypothermia will be explored.

Consequences

Awareness of the importance of tight thermoregulatory control to maintain human homeostasis leads to an appreciation that temperature perturbations will have a widespread effect on multiple systems. The physiological consequences are widely known and are described in Table 19.1. What is more important to the practising clinician is how avoidance of perioperative hypothermia may be of benefit to patient care. The results of prospective randomized trials are summarized in Table 19.2, and the clinical consequences will now be considered in turn.

Cardiovascular

The maintenance of perioperative normothermia in patients undergoing thoracic, vascular, or peripheral vascular surgery has been demonstrated to reduce significantly the incidence of ECG evidence of myocardial ischaemia and ventricular tachycardia[14]. Hypothermic patients also more frequently suffer morbid cardiac events postoperatively during the first 24 h, namely, unstable angina, cardiac arrest, and myocardial infarction. The avoidance of perioperative hypothermia reduces the probability of a morbid cardiac event in 55% of these patients. Also, in cardiac surgery patients, maintenance of normothermia has been shown to result in an increase in cardiac index and a decrease in systemic vascular resistance up to 4 h postoperatively; it also significantly lowers troponin-I levels at 24 h postoperatively[15].

A heightened adrenergic response, as opposed to increased metabolic demand and oxygen consumption, has been proposed as a mechanism for cardiac morbidity[14]. Perioperative hypothermia leads to a postoperative rise in mean norepinephrine levels, with a subsequent increase in the incidence of peripheral vasoconstriction and a higher systemic arterial pressure[16]. The mechanisms behind the harmful cardiovascular effects of hypothermia are not completely clear, but hypothermia also enhances the effects of volatile anaesthetic agents on baroreceptor function, depressing baroreceptor control of heart rate and prolonging its recovery[17]. The effects of perioperative hypothermia on baroreceptor function may explain the haemodynamic changes that occur.

Ultimately, in terms of cardiac risk, there is good evidence to support the maintenance of perioperative normothermia, especially in those patients with a background of, or at high risk of, cardiovascular disease.

Table 19.1 Physiological effects of hypothermia

System	Consequence
Respiratory	Left shift of oxygen haemoglobin dissociation curve; reduced oxygen delivery
	Increased tissue oxygen demand and consumption (especially if shivering) initially; reduces with worsening hypothermia
	Increased oxygen and carbon dioxide solubility; reduced PaO_2 and $PaCO_2$
	Depression of ventilatory drive as hypothermia worsens
Cardiovascular	Mild:
	Vasoconstriction producing increased systemic vascular resistance and mean arterial pressure
	Increased heart rate and cardiac output
	Moderate to severe
	Decreased cardiac contractility and thus output, hypotension, bradycardia
	Arrhythmias and conduction defects
	J waves at <30°C
	Ultimately ventricular fibrillation then asystole
Neurological	Confusion and thereafter reduced conscious level
	Prolonged awakening from general anaesthesia
Renal	Reduced glomerular filtration rate and renal blood flow: reduced renal function
	Polyuria due to reduced anti-diuretic hormone secretion and reduced renal tubular function leading to reduced sodium reabsorption and decreased plasma volume
Metabolic/ Endocrine	Reduced basal metabolic rate
	Insulin resistance and increased catecholamine response, and thus hyperglycaemia
	Reduced hepatic blood flow, metabolic, and excretory function
	Metabolic acidosis
Haematological	Coagulopathy (multifactorial) and platelet dysfunction
	Increased blood viscosity
Pharmacological	Prolonged drug action e.g. neuromuscular blocking agents
	Increased solubility of volatile anaesthetic agents resulting in prolonged induction and recovery but reduced requirement

Table 19.2 Clinical consequences of perioperative hypothermia

Consequence	Mean Δ T_{core} (°C)	Patient group	References
Increased incidence of postoperative:			
Ventricular tachycardia (8% vs. 2%); Morbid cardiac events (6% vs. 1%)	1.3	Abdominal, thoracic, vascular surgical patients with cardiac risk factors	[14]
Increased blood loss 184 ml (intraoperative)	0.5	Hip arthroplasty (spinal anaesthesia)	[21]
500 ml (intra- and postoperative)	1.5	Hip arthroplasty (general anaesthesia)	[19]
147 ml (intra- and postoperative)	0.5	Hip arthroplasty (combined spinal/ epidural anaesthesia)	[22]
Increased transfusion requirements	1.5	Hip arthroplasty (general anaesthesia)	[19]
Increased surgical wound infection			
19 vs. 6%	1.9	Colorectal surgery	[23]
14 vs. 5%	2.0ᵃ	Breast, varicose vein, or hernia surgery	[24]
Prolonged duration of action of neuromuscular blocking agents			
Vecuronium (mean = 34 min)	2.0	Elective surgery (non abdominal, non thoracic	[37]
Atracurium (mean = 24 min)	3.0	Healthy volunteers	[38]
Increased postoperative shivering 24% vs. 6%	1.3	Abdominal, thoracic, vascular surgical patients with cardiac risk factors	[14]
Increased postoperative oxygen consumption 269 vs. 141 ml min⁻¹ m⁻²	2.3	Elective abdominal surgery	[39]
Increased postoperative thermal discomfort	2.6	Elective colon surgery	[34]
Prolonged post anaesthetic recovery (mean = 40 min)	1.9	Elective abdominal e.g. colon resection	[40]
Prolonged duration of hospitalization (2.6 days)	1.9	Colorectal surgery	[23]
Increased protein catabolism	1.5	Hip arthroplasty	[36]

ᵃ Intervention was prewarming prior to surgery; none of the patients was warmed intraoperatively.

Haematological

The mechanism through which mild hypothermia produces a bleeding diathesis is probably multifactorial. It is thought to be the result of a failure in clot formation through platelet dysfunction and disruption to the coagulation pathway, as opposed to increased fibrinolysis[18]. The benefits of maintenance of normothermia in patients undergoing hip arthroplasty have been thoroughly investigated[19–22]. Three studies have illustrated that perioperative hypothermia significantly increased blood loss and one concluded a negative result. They exhibit heterogeneity in terms of anaesthetic technique employed and they highlight the difficulties of accurately assessing blood loss. They are all flawed to some extent, and it is difficult to extrapolate the results to other patient groups. However, the results do illustrate that the severity of hypothermia is a significant factor, with the largest difference in blood loss associated with the greatest disparity in core body temperature[19].

In conclusion, it would seem that maintaining normothermia is potentially a valuable and easily implemented approach to reducing operative blood loss and minimizing the need for transfusion.

Infectious

An important effect of perioperative hypothermia is an increased incidence of wound infection. Intraoperative core hypothermia in patients undergoing colorectal surgery results in a 13% absolute increase in the occurrence of surgical wound infection[23]. Wound healing is delayed, leading to a delay in suture removal and ultimately prolongation of the duration of hospitalization. Local or systemic preoperative warming of patients undergoing clean surgery (breast, varicose vein, or hernia) also reduces wound infection from 14 to 5%, resulting in a reduction in antibiotic usage[24].

Systemic cooling reduces subcutaneous oxygen tension, and wound infection rates are inversely proportional to subcutaneous oxygen tension[25]. Oxidative killing and phagocytosis by neutrophils has a linear relationship with core body temperature; intraoperative hypothermia causes a significant reduction in neutrophil function and thus resistance to infection[26]. Intraoperative core hypothermia also reduces lymphocyte activation and production of the anti-inflammatory interleukins 1β (IL1β) and 2 (IL2), potentially contributing to impaired immune defence, increased susceptibility to infection, and delayed wound healing[27]. Furthermore, human and animal studies have shown a relative blunting of the inflammatory response and a rise in the pro-inflammatory cytokine IL6 through maintenance of normothermia or correction of hypothermia[15,28].

Finally, whatever the processes behind hypothermia leading to an increase in surgical wound infection, there is currently no evidence to suggest that hypothermia increases the incidence of perioperative infections at other sites, for example, pneumonia[6].

Pharmacological

As mentioned previously, the enzyme systems that maintain homeostasis rely on precise thermoregulatory control to function optimally, and thus drug metabolism is dependent on body temperature. Volatile agent solubility is enhanced by hypothermia, which may subsequently delay recovery from general anaesthesia, and the minimum alveolar concentration (MAC) is reduced[18,29,30].

The effects of hypothermia on intravenous anaesthetic agents and opioids are probably of little clinical relevance, but hypothermia does prolong neuromuscular blockade. Furthermore, elimination of aminosteroid agents is reduced, compounding the pharmacodynamic effect.

Post-anaesthetic discomfort and recovery

Postoperative shivering is a frequent consequence of both general and regional anaesthesia and has been reported to occur in between 3.5% and 66% of patients[4,30–32]. Core hypothermia is significantly associated with an increase in the incidence of post-anaesthetic shivering (PAS)[14], but other factors contribute, including young age, prolonged surgery, and orthopaedic surgery. In addition to increasing patient discomfort, shivering also produces a two to threefold increase in oxygen consumption. The resultant hypoxaemia may cause myocardial ischaemia in elderly patients or those with cardiovascular risk factors. Fortunately, as a result of impaired thermoregulatory control, elderly patients are less likely to shiver, and hypoxia actually inhibits the shivering response[31,33].

Unsurprisingly, intraoperative hypothermia also increases the number of patients complaining of feeling uncomfortably cold postoperatively, and subsequently prolongs recovery[34]. Hypothermia has also been demonstrated to delay tracheal extubation[35]. Nevertheless, the consequences of hypothermia extend far from the operating room, delaying wound healing, prolonging return to a solid diet, and increasing the duration of hospital stay in colonic-surgery patients[23]. Hypothermia also increases protein breakdown and nitrogen loss, which may be attenuated through maintaining normothermia[36]. Protein wasting and coagulopathy secondary to hypothermia are both thought to play a role in delayed wound healing[18].

Modifying factors

Certain groups of patients require special consideration because of their increased risk of developing perioperative hypothermia, and in these instances, extra vigilance may be required to maintain normothermia. The most easily identifiable are those at the extremes of age and the critically ill. The latter group may incorporate numerous pathologies, including polytrauma patients, and those suffering from chronic debilitating illnesses, such as alcohol dependency. Other more specific groups prone to perioperative hypothermia include those with: acute alcohol intoxication and/or drug overdose (especially phenothiazines); loss of the protective skin barrier, such as severe burns or exfoliative conditions; endocrine disorders such as adrenocortical insufficiency and hypothyroidism; and lastly, autonomic neuropathies (associated, e.g., with spinal cord injuries and diabetes mellitus).

In contrast, obese patients are more likely to maintain their core body temperature as a result of less redistribution of heat under anaesthesia and reduced heat loss due to the insulating effect of body fat. They also have a higher vasoconstriction threshold. This restriction of heat to the core may actually lead to an increase in temperature, similar to the effect seen in paediatric patients with limb tourniquets[41] (see following paragraphs).

One final area to consider is those surgical specialties where hypothermia may be employed as a protective mechanism. The efficacy of induced hypothermia in clinical practice for neuroprotection is controversial: studies investigating its use in traumatic brain injury, stroke, surgery for intracranial aneurysm repair, and out-of-hospital cardiac arrest have met with mixed results[42–45]. These areas are not explored in any further detail here. However, hypothermia is used during cardiac surgery for protection against cardiac and cerebral ischaemia and this will be considered.

Extremes of age

Children and infants, but most notably preterm neonates, are prone to perioperative hypothermia. Redistribution of heat under general anaesthesia contributes less because of relatively small extremities, but their large surface area-to-volume ratio results in greater cutaneous loss of heat, especially from the head. Heat loss actually exceeds heat production after induction of general anaesthesia[46]. As a result of large radiant and convective heat losses, it is vital to maintain the ambient temperature (temperatures of 24 to 25°C or more may be used) and employ heat-conserving measures, especially in neonates where hypothermia may result in many of the consequences discussed earlier in addition to difficulty in weaning from ventilation[47]. Neonates do not shiver but produce heat through non-shivering thermogenesis, which continues up to the age of two years. The overall incidence of shivering is low and is associated with lower core body temperature, use of intravenous induction agents, age greater than six years, and longer duration of surgery[48]. Temperature monitoring should be employed as standard practice in paediatric patients, not only to avoid hypothermia but also to minimize the risk of over-warming (see following paragraphs).

Elderly patients (>60 years) experience more marked and prolonged perioperative hypothermia[49]. They have a lower basal metabolic rate, less subcutaneous tissue, and impaired thermoregulatory control: they are less likely to shiver and under general anaesthesia, the vasoconstriction threshold is significantly less[33]. The increased likelihood of comorbidities in these patients and the adverse outcomes linked to hypothermia demand that temperature monitoring and measures to maintain normothermia are more frequently utilized.

Sickle cell disease

In patients with sickle cell disease, hypothermia may precipitate a crisis, so cautious monitoring and good thermal management are essential components of anaesthesia.

Neuromuscular disorders

Patients with neuromuscular disease are not only susceptible to hypothermia but may also suffer harm as a result of it. Hypothermia may aggravate muscular weakness in myotonias and periodic paralyses, delaying recovery from general anaesthesia. In addition, the muscle damage associated with metabolic and mitochondrial myopathies may be exacerbated by hypothermia[50].

Coronary artery bypass surgery

Hypothermia is employed in cardiac surgery to minimize myocardial and neurological sequelae, despite a lack of good evidence to support it. A systematic review concluded that, despite the fact that hypothermia was associated with a reduced incidence of perioperative stroke, this was counterbalanced by a trend towards increased myocardial damage and perioperative mortality[51]. It was commented that there was also a lack of data regarding its benefits for the reduction of subtler neurological dysfunction, and a more recent prospective randomized trial demonstrated that hypothermic cardiopulmonary bypass (CPB) conferred no additional cerebral protection[52].

The main consideration in this group of patients is that the alterations in core body temperature occur much more rapidly and on a much greater scale. CPB permits the addition or removal of heat at astonishing rates. The most significant occurrence is the phenomenon known as 'afterdrop', which describes the rapid fall in core body temperature following the withdrawal of CPB, after initial rewarming of the patient using the bypass pump. Heat redistributes from the core to the peripheral tissues as a result of a substantial temperature gradient and subsequently results in postoperative hypothermia. This phenomenon may be likened to the redistribution of heat from the core to the periphery following induction of general anaesthesia. The magnitude of the afterdrop is dependent on the temperature at which CPB is conducted[53]. In addition to the consequences highlighted earlier, it has been shown that post-CPB patients who have a core temperature less than 36°C on admission to the ICU require more blood transfusion, require more prolonged mechanical ventilation, ICU and hospital stay, and have a greater mortality[54]. As a result, a variety methods of minimizing afterdrop have been explored[3].

Summary

The evidence demonstrating the consequences of perioperative hypothermia is summarized in Table 19.2. All these studies emphasize the clinical implications of intraoperative hypothermia and the gains to be reaped from maintaining normothermia. The consequences are far-reaching and the secondary economic costs must also be realized for any modern healthcare system. For an anaesthetist to be vigilant and endeavour to maintain normothermia during any major surgical procedure, the financial cost would seem minimal, especially when considering the gains in terms of patient outcome.

Fever

Definition

Fever is an abnormal rise in core body temperature due to stimulation of the thermoregulatory centre of the hypothalamus by endogenous pyrogens (e.g. IL2); the target set point and thresholds for sweating, vasoconstriction and shivering are raised but there is maintenance of the inter-threshold range.

Risk

Fever occurs infrequently during anaesthesia but may be observed during anaesthesia for septic surgical conditions. However, it is very common during the postoperative period as a component of the surgical stress response. It is argued that fever may be advantageous for host defence mechanisms; however, the physiological consequences (such as increased oxygen consumption) may be detrimental in some patients (e.g. those with significant cardiac or pulmonary disease)[55,56]. This is a controversial topic and will not be explored any further here.

The effects of general anaesthesia on thermoregulation have already been illustrated, predominantly the widening of the inter-threshold range. Intuitively, volatile anaesthetic agents, intravenous opioids and, probably, intravenous anaesthetics suppress fever, running the risk of concealing it intraoperatively, the first two groups doing so in a dose-dependent manner[57,58]. This has most clinical relevance for opioid use postoperatively and in critical care settings. It must always be remembered that inhibition of fever by opioids may mask evidence of an infection and therefore hinder patient care.

Modifying factors

Aortic endovascular stents

Aortic endovascular stenting is associated with a significant postoperative inflammatory response, incorporating rapidly spiking pyrexia and an increase in white cell count and acute phase proteins. This is abacteraemic but may result in problematic cardiovascular stress, triggering tachyarrhythmias and cardiac ischaemia. Invasive monitoring and postoperative vigilance in an appropriate setting are essential in these cases[59].

Epidural catheters

Epidural catheters are utilized frequently for surgical anaesthesia and the management of acute postoperative pain, and have a major role in obstetric analgesia and anaesthesia. Epidural catheters used for postoperative and labour analgesia have been shown to be associated with higher mean core body temperatures[60,61]. This may be a consequence of the fact that intravenous opioids, frequently employed as an alternative to epidural analgesia (local anaesthetic agent +/−opioid), inhibit fever[58].

Intrapartum pyrexia is significantly associated with younger maternal age; lower parity and gravity; greater duration of labour, and duration of ruptured membranes; and not only increased use of epidural analgesia, but also longer duration of epidural analgesia[62]. An inflammatory process has been implicated as intrapartum pyrexia is associated with raised IL6 levels; more importantly, serum IL6 levels are significantly higher in those with epidural analgesia, compared to those without[73]. Conversely, the increase in core body temperature during labour may be the result of passive hyperthermia: in the region blocked, sweating is diminished and thus heat loss is reduced, therefore when heat production increases during labour, hyperthermia may develop. Whatever the mechanism, maternal pyrexia occurring during epidural analgesia precipitates work-ups for neonatal sepsis, increases the use of neonatal anti-biotics and may account for higher rates of Caesarean section and assisted vaginal deliveries; however there is nothing to suggest a direct causal link between epidural catheter use and neonatal sepsis or adverse outcome[63,64].

Case study 2

A 70 kg, 28-year-old primigravida with type 1 diabetes presented at 37 weeks' gestation for induction of labour because of poor glycaemic control. Labour was slow to progress and required augmentation. An epidural catheter was sited at the L2/3 interspace on the delivery suite, prior to starting a syntocinon infusion. The obstetricians decided to proceed to delivery via Caesarean section 12 h later. Over the four hours prior to attending theatre, the patient had been pyrexial. Blood cultures had been taken and the white cell count was 8.0 x 10^9 /L. The midwives commented that epidural analgesia was 'patchy' and 20 ml of 1.5% lidocaine with 100 µg of fentanyl failed to produce adequate anaesthesia. A subarachnoid block was therefore performed. The operation and remainder of the anaesthetic management proceed-ed uneventfully. Cefuroxime 750 mg was administered prophylactically as per local practice. Epidural catheter removal was delayed until 36 h postpartum. On the 5th post operative day the patient developed dysuria, back pain, fever, and rigors. There was bruising, swelling, and erythema at the epidural site. Neurological examination was normal. Blood and urine sam-ples and a swab of the epidural site were taken for culture. Intravenous cefuroxime 750 mg eight-hourly was commenced. Two days later the patient developed bilateral leg paraesthesia and weakness; her back pain had worsened and she remained pyrexial. Neurological examina-tion confirmed the leg weakness; ankle jerks were absent and there was also loss of sensation to pinprick from L3 to S5 bilaterally. The white cell count was 20.1 × 10^9/L and C-reactive protein >250mg/L. Blood cultures grew staphylococcus aureus. An MRI scan revealed an epidural abscess and the patient was referred for neurosurgical intervention.

Spinal epidural abscess is rare but the total incidence has risen from 0.2–1.2 per 10 000 hospital admissions per year to 1.96 cases per 10 000 hospital admissions per year[65,66]. Whether this is the result of advancing technology and improved diagnostic tools or sim-ply the reflection of an ageing, more debilitated population is unclear. Spinal epidural abscess complicating the use of neuraxial blockade is even rarer and there is a broad range of reported incidences from retrospective data: published figures are from none of nearly 9000 procedures up to one in 800[67–72]. The quality and diversity of the evidence does not allow exact quantification of risk. An exhaustive review of the evidence is not provided here, but the risk factors associated with *all cause* spinal epidural abscess (i.e. not just those associated with central neuraxial blockade) will be discussed.

Various risk factors have been implicated for spinal epidural abscess. Diabetes mellitus is the most frequently associated comorbidity, followed by intravenous drug use, alcohol abuse, and immunocompromise (including chronic steroid use and human immunodeficiency virus infection)[73,74]. Concurrent infections feature highly, including skin, pulmonary, and urinary tract infections. Other associated factors are trauma (spinal and extra-spinal), degenerative spinal disorders, chronic renal impair-ment and, most relevant to anaesthetic practice, invasive procedures. However, epidural anaesthesia was only identified as a risk factor in 5% of cases, and spinal anaesthesia 1%, in one series[73].

Currently there is no strong evidence to suggest that the use of epidural analgesia and anaesthesia *per se* causes fever; however, it does not appear to suppress fever. A high core body temperature associated with the use of an epidural catheter may be true fever, akin to the surgical stress response, and it must be stressed that fever in this setting does not usually signify infection. Nevertheless, vigilance is paramount, especially in high-risk groups, as in rare circumstances, pyrexia may indicate the development of spinal epidural abscess.

Hyperthermia

Definition

Hyperthermia is defined as an abnormally high body temperature in the presence of a normal central thermoregulatory set-point. The implication is that heat gain cannot be compensated sufficiently by heat loss. In broad terms, hyperthermia can result from excessive heat production by the body, adverse environmental conditions (high environmental temperature, which is exacerbated by high humidity), or impairment of the normal mechanisms of heat loss.

Risk

Heat stroke describes severe hyperthermia at levels associated with tissue damage. This is often defined as a core temperature above an arbitrary value, such as 41°C. Classical heat stroke refers to heat stroke resulting from high environmental temperature and this is possible under anaesthesia with aggressive and prolonged active warming, especially in small children. Such an iatrogenic event is totally preventable by using temperature monitoring and no published reports of such cases are apparent in the literature.

Mild to moderate hyperthermia resulting from passive heat gain is likely to become more common with increasing efficiency of active warming devices[75]. Aside from iatrogenic classical heat stroke, other forms of life-threatening hyperthermia under anaesthesia are rare; an estimate of the overall incidence is less than 1:10 000 anaesthetics.

Consequences

The fate of cells exposed to thermal stress depends on the temperature and duration of exposure. At the molecular level, increasing temperature is related to increased translational, rotational, and vibratory motion of atoms and molecules. At temperatures less than 40°C, temperature-dependent changes in cellular processes result almost exclusively from this increased kinetic energy of molecules leading to increased rates of reactions of enzymatic processes or rates of interaction within cell signalling pathways. The overall effect of a change in temperature is not, however, always predictable with the cellular response being a composite of the temperature-dependence of many subcellular components. Below 40°C, hyperthermia does increase apoptosis and this is thought to result from increased transcription of factors in the apoptotic pathways. This is probably the mechanism for hyperthermia-induced sensitization of cells to other cytotoxic stressors such as ionizing radiation and cancer chemotherapeutic agents that is the basis for the use of therapeutic regional and whole-body hyperthermia in the treatment of cancer, especially in the advanced stages. However, the major consequences of moderate hyperthermia are related to the adaptive responses of increased blood flow to the skin (these can double the resting cardiac output, further increasing oxygen consumption) and salt and water depletion from sweating, which can amount to 2000 ml/h.

At temperatures greater than 40°C, the more sinister effect of protein denaturation occurs, in which there is unfolding of the tertiary protein structure with dysfunction and intracellular protein aggregation. The denaturation threshold varies between proteins and the specific proteins affected in thermal cytotoxicity have not been identified, but cellular respiration and signal transduction are predominantly affected with exposures above 41°C of relatively modest duration. Most cells are tolerant to denaturation of up to 5% of their protein content, but fewer than 5% of cells will survive 10% protein denaturation. Hyperthermia induces the expression of heat shock proteins, which are protective against metabolic and cytotoxic effects of subsequent heat exposure. Heat shock proteins have been implicated as important factors in heat acclimatization. The major protein so far identified, Hsp70 (a 70 kDa protein), prevents protein unfolding and aggregation.

Brain function is acutely sensitive to high temperature. Electroencephalographic changes are evident in conscious subjects at brain temperatures above 38°C and these may be accompanied by changes in behaviour, cognitive function, and mental fatigue. Clinical manifestations are more likely to become pronounced as temperatures exceed 41°C, with delirium, ataxia (cerebellar), and coma being common. Convulsions can occur but they are most common during cooling. Clinical features of altered brain function will obviously be masked during anaesthesia but may become apparent in the immediate postoperative period.

Sustained severe hyperthermia will, sooner or later, lead to the development of multi-organ failure. Hyperthermia causes an increase in vascular permeability and an increase in the expression of cell surface adhesion molecules. The result is endothelial interaction with activated leukocytes, stimulating production of inflammatory cytokines and procoagulant factors. Microvascular thrombosis and a consumptive coagulopathy are prominent features of severe hyperthermia. It has also been proposed that relative ischaemia of the gut from diversion of blood flow to the skin and vital organs may compound the cytokine response by permitting absorption of endotoxin through dysfunctional gut endothelium. The combination of a portal endotoxin load and visceral ischaemia may account for the significant incidence of liver failure (requiring transplantation in some cases) in heat stroke.

Hyperthermic disorders associated with excessive heat production are associated with rhabdomyolysis. The degree of rhabdomyolysis reflects the intensity and duration of muscle activity and not whether the activity is caused by a direct effect on muscle (e.g. in malignant hyperthermia, or by an indirect mechanism such as neuroleptic malignant syndrome). Muscle activity in the presence of hyperthermia is sinister because force generation (which is directly related to potassium and myoglobin release from muscle) is not only related to temperature but also becomes metabolically less efficient with increasing temperature, generating more heat and increasing oxygen consumption.

Modifying factors

Extremes of age

Just as the large body surface area relative to mass makes small children prone to lose heat under anaesthesia in a cold environment, it makes active warming more efficient. There is a real risk of hyperthermia developing if temperature monitoring is not used during active warming, especially in procedures lasting more than 45–60 min (see following paragraphs).

Elderly patients are not more likely to develop hyperthermia than healthy adults, but if it does occur they are less able to mount and sustain the cardiovascular responses required to prevent a progressive rise in temperature. The same obviously applies to younger people with limited cardiovascular reserve. Furthermore, the induced increase in myocardial work in combination with reduced systemic vascular resistance present conditions favouring myocardial ischaemia. These factors explain why the majority of classical heat stroke deaths during heat waves occur in the elderly.

Duration of anaesthesia

Even with the use of active warming measures, core temperature falls following induction of anaesthesia, as described in the section on hypothermia earlier, and eventually reaches a plateau. Active warming devices reduce the temperature drop and the time to reach the nadir, depending on their efficiency and the proportion of the patient's body surface exposed for the purposes of the surgery. The patient at this stage responds in a poikilothermic fashion and if heat delivery is greater than heat loss, the core temperature will start to rise at a reasonably fixed rate. This may be observed in warmed paediatric patients after 15 min, but in adults may not occur until 2 h or more of anaesthesia. If the positive thermal balance is maintained, the core temperature will continue to rise to hyperthermic levels. Cardiovascular and cutaneous responses to hyperthermia will reduce the tendency for the temperature to rise further depending on their efficiency. However, use of core temperature monitoring should, by this stage, have produced the appropriate reduction in active warming.

Limb tourniquets

Limb tourniquets aid conservation of core body temperature and thus hinder the development of hypothermia as minimal heat is exchanged between the isolated limb and the rest of the body[3]. The effect on heat distribution may be amplified in the absence of regional anaesthesia to the limb, when autonomic responses to the nociceptive stimulus of prolonged tourniquet application (>45 min) increase the metabolic rate. Core body temperature actually increases in children with the use of limb tourniquets[76]. In addition, heating measures utilized to maintain normothermia are more effective in children than adults. The risk of over-warming paediatric patients must be emphasized and reinforces the need for close temperature monitoring.

Malignant hyperthermia susceptibility

As malignant hyperthermia is a hyperthermic syndrome triggered solely by anaesthetic drugs, it will be discussed separately later in the chapter.

Muscular dystrophies and myotonias

Malignant hyperthermia-like crises have been described in progressive muscular dystrophies (Duchenne and Becker) and myotonic patients. Suxamethonium should always be avoided in these patients[29].

Neuroleptic malignant syndrome

This is an idiosyncratic reaction to dopamine-antagonist drugs, most commonly depot neuroleptic preparations. It has, however, been reported after use of metoclopramide, droperidol, and prochlorperazine—antiemetics used perioperatively. The incidence of neuroleptic malignant syndrome is reported as 0.07%–2.2% of psychiatric patients receiving neuroleptic medication[77]. The higher incidence may reflect less stringent diagnostic criteria. Cases have been reported in patients with Parkinson's disease following perioperative omission of dopamine agonist anti-Parkinsonian medication[78].

Neuroleptic malignant syndrome is characterized by hyperthermia, extrapyramidal rigidity, autonomic disturbances (especially diaphoresis), and rhabdomyolysis. The mortality is up to 30%[77].

Serotonin toxicity

This is a predictable, dose-dependent reaction to drugs that increase central intra-synaptic serotonin concentrations. It is characterized by hyperthermia, clonus, hyper-reflexia and, in the awake patient, agitation. Hyperthermia is secondary to increased autonomic nervous system output and neuromuscular activation. The severe, life-threatening form has only been described in patients receiving combinations of drugs that raise intra-synaptic serotonin by different mechanisms[79]. Invariably one of the drugs is a monoamine oxidase inhibitor (MOAI) and the other either a serotonin re-uptake inhibitor or a serotonin releaser (amphetamines and derivatives). Many opioid drugs prevent serotonin re-uptake and death from serotonin toxicity has been reported following administration of pethidine, tramadol, dextromethorphan, and possibly fentanyl to patients receiving MAOIs. No severe reactions have been reported in patients receiving MAOIs given morphine, codeine, or remifentanil[79].

Other drugs

A variety of other drugs have predictable effects to increase heat production or reduce heat loss; notably, sympathomimetics increase skeletal muscle metabolic activity, while anticholinergics reduce sweating.

Endocrine disorders

Thyrotoxicosis and phaeochromocytoma are associated with increased metabolic activity and therefore heat production. In an uncontrolled hyperthyroid patient anaesthesia can induce a 'thyroid storm' with features similar to malignant hyperthermia (see below).

Case study 3

A 63-year-old man was anaesthetized for a total hip replacement. He received thiopentone, fentanyl, and atracurium at induction followed by enflurane. After induction, he was given a further dose of fentanyl because his heart rate was 130 bpm and BP 210/120 mm Hg (pre-operative BP 160/90 mm Hg). His skin was noted to be hot with subsequent nasopharyngeal temperature reading 38.3°C. A provisional diagnosis of malignant hyperthermia was made and the 24 h postoperative creatine kinase concentration was 990 iu/L (normal <210 iu/L). Because of the prominent haemodynamic changes (marked increases in blood pressure are unusual in human malignant hyperthermia) we requested measurement of urinary catecholamine metabolites before accepting him for testing for malignant hyperthermia. Urinary catecholamines were markedly elevated and subsequent CT scan confirmed an adrenal tumour consistent with phaeochromocytoma.

Whole-body hyperthermia

Whole-body hyperthermia (WBH) is employed in the treatment of advanced malignancies. It encompasses the raising of the core body temperature to approximately 42°C for 60 min, or more, under general anaesthesia or sedation. This results in significant cardiovascular and respiratory stress, most notably: increases in the cardiac output, central venous pressure, oxygen consumption, and lactate level; and decreases in the mean arterial pressure, systemic vascular resistance, and PaO_2. These physiological changes may precipitate tachyarrhythmias or pulmonary oedema. Fluid management may be difficult as a result of high losses secondary to sweating and hyperglycaemia-induced diuresis. Other complications include renal toxicity, encephalopathy, and peripheral neuropathies due to positioning. The last may be prevented by regular limb mobilization. These may be challenging cases requiring meticulous selection and suitable vigilance whilst under anaesthesia[80].

Malignant Hyperthermia

Definition

Malignant hyperthermia (MH) is a pharmacogenetic disorder of skeletal muscle intracellular calcium homeostasis predisposing to a potentially life-threatening adverse reaction to potent inhalational anaesthetics and/or suxamethonium (succinylcholine). The name derives from the first cases described in the 1960s, which were characterized by a rapid rate of rise in body temperature, usually resulting in death.

Risk

Estimating the risk of MH is fraught with pitfalls. There is no risk to the individual known not to carry the genetic susceptibility and no risk to any patient who does not receive the triggering drugs. For most patients, however, their genetic susceptibility to MH is not known, while more than 90% of general anaesthetics include administration of a potent inhalational agent. Until recently, all estimates of risk were based on data from clinical reports and they varied from 1:1300[81] to 1:250 000[82] anaesthetics. The large incidence reported by Mauritz *et al.*[81] was from a small hospital in a secluded area of Austria where there may be a relatively small gene pool. More representative, perhaps, is their estimate of 1:23 600 based on results from Vienna. Ording's data[82] are based on a national survey in Denmark. The incidence of 1:250 000 relates to "fulminant" or severe cases, consisting of all the classical features of MH. However, this excludes those cases in which early signs of MH were detected and acted upon before the reaction became imminently life-threatening. When all cases of suspected MH were considered, Ording found the incidence to be 1:16 000 anaesthetics[82]. This is perhaps the more useful value as it is the clinical suspicion of MH that leads to a change in anaesthetic (and possibly surgical) management, transfer of the patient to a high-dependency or intensive care unit postoperatively, and the need for subsequent diagnostic testing.

A remarkably similar incidence (1:15 000) had, in fact, been estimated previously by Britt and Kalow working in Canada[83]. In the United Kingdom, we used the number of confirmed cases of MH in children to estimate the prevalence of MH susceptibility to be 1:8000[84], assuming the chance of an MH-susceptible child developing a reaction under anaesthesia to be 0.4 (MH patients have, on average, 2–3 uneventful anaesthetics prior to the diagnosis being made). Genetic risk may be even higher, however. In a study of French and Italian MH families in which a mutation associated with MH was known, Monnier et al.[85] detected a second mutation in a surprisingly large number of families, compatible with a prevalence of MH mutations of up to 1:2000. Similar analyses of UK MH families concur with these findings (unpublished).

Consequences

An MH reaction presents as a combination of cellular hypermetabolism, hyperthermia, muscle rigidity and rhabdomyolysis. The consequences depend on the severity of each of the components of the reaction. The consequences of hyperthermia have been described earlier, but even before the development of significant hyperthermia, a mixed respiratory/metabolic acidosis, hypoxaemia, and sympathetic stimulation can result from hypermetabolism. Muscle rigidity and rhabdomyolysis tend to be more profound when suxamethonium has been given. Seventy percent of patients with susceptibility to MH develop immediate rigidity of the jaw muscles after suxamethonium. This masseter muscle spasm can last for 5–15 min and make airway instrumentation impossible. Fortunately, oxygenation of the lungs is invariably feasible, and this may be because upper airway striated muscles retain their tone. Later, generalized muscle rigidity is an ominous sign as it is associated with compromised muscle blood supply (failure of the therapeutic agent dantrolene to reach its site of action) and failure of ATP production (ATP is required by the most important cellular calcium-sequestrating mechanisms). If the patient survives after late-onset muscle rigidity, fasciotomies may be required to treat compartment syndrome. Rhabdomyolysis poses the dual threat of hyperkalaemia (cardiac bradydysrhythmias) and myoglobin-induced acute renal failure. Some patients report recurrent episodes of muscle cramps and/or muscle weakness after an MH episode.

Even if the patient makes a complete recovery from the clinical episode, the suspected diagnosis has consequences. It may not have been possible for the planned surgery to be completed; the patient will have been admitted to a critical care unit for at least 24 h; the presumed clinical diagnosis should be confirmed. At present, the only definitive test for refuting a suspected clinical case involves *in vitro* pharmacological contracture studies on muscle biopsy specimens. As the specimens must be fresh, the patient is required to travel to the regional or national MH testing centre to undergo the biopsy, which leaves a 5- to10-cm scar. Until proven otherwise, patients with a suspected MH reaction should be counselled to inform all contactable blood relatives that MH susceptibility may be present within the family.

Modifying factors

Anaesthetic drugs

Even though all the potent inhalational anaesthetics can trigger MH within the first 5–15 min of administration, the onset can be delayed with the diethyl ether derivatives compared with halothane. Co-administration of suxamethonium tends to make reactions more florid. There is debate over the ability of suxamethonium alone to trigger the hypermetabolic/hyperthermic components of MH. Suxamethonium can, however, provoke life-threatening hyperkalaemia and/or myoglobinaemia sufficient to cause acute renal failure.

Case study 4

A 29-year-old man underwent colectomy because of inflammatory bowel disease. He received enflurane throughout the 2-h procedure, which was uneventful. Four hours postoperatively, he returned to theatre because of bleeding. On this occasion, rapid sequence induction, including suxamethonium, was followed by maintenance of anaesthesia with isoflurane. Within 15 min of induction of anaesthesia, he developed a rising end-tidal CO_2 and a tachycardia. He developed a maximum temperature of 39.7 °C at which point blood gases revealed a $PaCO_2$ of 9.1kPa and base excess of −12.1 mmol/L. He survived. It is not known why MH susceptible patients do not trigger on every exposure to triggering drugs.

Patient age, sex, and type of surgery

The age distribution of patients experiencing MH reactions is skewed, with the majority occurring in children over 5 years and young adults. Reactions occur in almost double the number of males compared to females. Neither of these observations has been explained satisfactorily in the context of a susceptibility trait that is inherited in an autosomal dominant fashion. There is also an association of MH with emergency, especially trauma, surgery. It has been suggested that high circulating catecholamine levels predispose to MH developing in a susceptible individual, and this explains the association with trauma surgery and the predominance of young males among MH reactors. There is no consensus on whether any of these associations are causal.

Temperature

Animal experiments have demonstrated that hypothermia can prevent triggering in MH susceptible pigs. Cases of MH have been reported in patients during rewarming after hypothermic cardiopulmonary bypass but not during the hypothermic phase.

Conditions associated with MH

Various musculoskeletal abnormalities, for example squints, scoliosis, talipes, have been linked to an increased incidence of MH but the evidence is unconvincing. These abnormalities may be found, however, in children with the rare core-type (central core disease, multi-minicore myopathy) congenital myopathies. The core myopathies are frequently associated with malignant hyperthermia susceptibility and result from mutations in the RYR1 gene, the gene most frequently implicated in MH.

References

1. Bligh, J. and Johnson, K.G. (1973). Glossary of terms for thermal physiology. *Journal of Applied Physiology*, **35**(6), 941–61.

2. Carli, F. and Macdonald, I.A. (1996). Perioperative inadvertent hypothermia: what do we need to prevent? *British Journal of Anaesthesia*, **76**(5), 601–3.

3. Sessler, D,I. (2000). Perioperative heat balance. *Anesthesiology*, **92**(2), 578–96.

4. Buggy, D.J. and Crossley, A.W.A. (2000). Thermoregulation, mild perioperative hypothermia and post anaesthetic shivering. *British Journal of Anaesthesia*, **84**(5), 615–28.

5. Sessler, D.I. (1997). Mild perioperative hypothermia. *New England Journal of Medicine*, **336**(24), 1730–7.

6. Leslie, K. and Sessler, D.I. (2003). Perioperative hypothermia in the high risk surgical patient. *Best Practice & Research Clinical Anaesthesiology*, **17**(4), 485–98.

7. Annadata, R.S., Sessler, D.I., Tayafeh, F., Kurz, A., and Dechert, M. (1995). Desflurane slightly increase the sweating threshold, but produces marked nonlinear decreases in the vasoconstriction and shivering thresholds. *Anesthesiology*, **83**(6), 1205–11.

8. Xiong, J., Kurz, A., Sessler, D.I., *et al.* (1996). Isoflurane produces marked and nonlinear decreases in the vasoconstriction and shivering thresholds. *Anesthesiology*, **85**(2), 240–5.

9. Matsukawa, T., Kurz, A., Sessler, D.I., Bjorksten, A.R., Merrifield, B., Cheng, C. (1995). Propofol linearly reduces the vasoconstriction and shivering thresholds. *Anesthesiology*, **82**(5), 1169–80.

10. Kurz, A., Sessler, D.I., Christensen, R., and Dechert, M. (1995). Heat balance and distribution during the core temperature plateau in anesthetized humans. *Anesthesiology*, **83**(3), 491–9.

11. Matsukawa, T.M.D, Sessler, D.I.M.D., Christensen, R.B.A., Ozaki, M.M.D., and Schroeder, M.B.A. (1995). Heat flow and distribution during epidural anesthesia. *Anesthesiology*, **83**(5), 961–7.

12. Kurz, A.M.D., Sessler, D.I.M.D., Schroeder, M.B.A., and Kurz, M.M.D. (1993). Thermoregulatory response thresholds during spinal anesthesia. *Anesthesia and Analgesia*, **77**(4), 721–6.

13. Frank, M., Nguyen, J.M., Garcia, C., and Barnes, R.A. (1999). Temperature monitoring practices during regional anaesthesia. *Anesthesia and Analgesia*, **88**, 373–7.

14. Frank, S.M., Fleisher, L.A., Breslow, M.J., *et al.* (1997). Perioperative maintenance of normothermia reduces the incidence of morbid cardiac events. A randomized clinical trial. *Journal of the American Medical Association*, **277**(14), 1127–34.

15. Nesher, N., Uretzky, G., Insler, S., *et al.* (2005). Thermo-wrap technology preserves normothermia better than routine thermal care in patients undergoing off-pump coronary artery bypass and is associated with lower immune response and lesser myocardial damage. *Journal of Thoracic and Cardiovascular Surgery*, **129**(6), 1370–7.

16. Frank, S.M.M.D., Higgins, M.S.M.D., Breslow, M.J.M.D., *et al.* (1995). The catecholamine, cortisol, and hemodynamic responses to mild perioperative hypothermia: a randomized clinical trial. *Anesthesiology*, **82**(1), 83–93.

17. Tanaka, M., Nagasaki, G., and Nishikawa, T. (2001). Moderate hypothermia depresses arterial baroreflex control of heart rate during, and delays its recovery after, general anaesthesia in humans. *Anesthesiology*, **95**(1), 51–5.

18. Doufas, G. (2003). Consequences of inadvertent perioperative hypothermia. *Best Practice & Research Clinical Anaesthesiology*, **17**(4), 535–49.

19. Schmied, H., Kurz, A., Sessler, D.I., Kozek, S., and Reiter, A. (1996). Mild hypothermia increases blood loss during total hip arthroplasty. *Lancet*, **347**, 289–92.

20. Johannson, T., Lisander, B., and Ivarsson, I. (1999). Mild hypothermia does not increase blood loss during total hip arthroplasty. *Acta Anaesthesiologica Scandinavica*, **43**, 1005–10.

21. Widman, J., Hammarqvist, F., and Sellden, E. (2002). Amino acid infusion induces thermogenesis and reduces blood loss during hip arthroplasty under spinal anaesthesia. *Anesthesia and Analgesia*, **95**,1757–62.

22. Winkler, M., Akca, O., Birkenberg, B., *et al.* (2000). Aggressive warming reduces blood loss during hip arthroplasty. *Anesthesia and Analgesia*, **91**, 978–84.

23. Kurz, A., Sessler, D.I., and Lenhardt, R. (1996). Perioperative normothermia to reduce the incidence of surgical wound infection and shorten hospitalization. *New England Journal of Medicine*, **334**(19),1209–15.

24. Melling, A.C., Baqar, A., Scott, E.M., and Leaper, D.J. (2001). Effects of preoperative warming on the incidence of wound infection after clean surgery: a randomised controlled trial. *Lancet*, **358**, 876–80.

25. Hopf, H.W.M.D, Hunt, T.K.M.D, West, J.M.D.N.S., *et al.* (1997). Wound tissue oxygen tension predicts the risk of wound infection in surgical patients. *Archives of Surgery*, **132**(9), 997–1004.

26. Wenisch, C.M.D., Narzt, E.M.D., Sessler, D.I.M.D., *et al.* (1996). Mild intraoperative hypothermia reduces production of reactive oxygen intermediates by polymorphonuclear leukocytes. *Anesthesia and Analgesia*, **82**(4), 810–6.

27. Beilin, B.M.D., Shavit, Y.P., Razumovsky, J.M.D., Wolloch, Y.M.D., Zeidel, A.M.D., and Bessler, H.P. (1998). Effects of mild perioperative hypothermia on cellular immune responses. *Anesthesiology*, **89**(5),1133–40.

28. Xiao, H.M.D. and Remick, D.G.M.D. (2005). Correction of perioperative hypothermia decreases experimental sepsis mortality by modulating the inflammatory response. *Critical Care Medicine*, **33**(1),161–7.

29. Liu, M.M.D., Hu, X.M.D., and Liu, J.M.D. (2001). The effect of hypothermia on isoflurane MAC in children. *Anesthesiology*, **94**(3), 429–32.

30. Complications and treatment of mild hypothermia. (2001). *Anesthesiology*, **95**(2),531–43.

31. De Witte, J. and Sessler, D.I. (2002). Perioperative shivering. *Anesthesiology*, **96**, 467–84.

32. Akin, A., Esmaoglu, A., and Boyaci, B. (2005). Postoperative shivering in children and causative factors. *Paediatric Anaesthesia*, **15**, 1089–93.

33. Ozaki, M.M.D., Sessler, D.I.M.D., Matsukawa, T.M.D., *et al.* (1997). The threshold for thermoregulatory vasoconstriction during nitrous oxide/sevoflurane anesthesia is reduced in the elderly. *Anesthesia and Analgesia*, **84**(5), 1029–33.

34. Kurz, A., Sessler, D.I., Narzt, E., *et al.* (1995). Postoperative hemodynamic and thermoregulatory consequences of intraoperative core hypothermia. *Journal of Clinical Anesthesia*, **7**, 359–66.

35. Fleisher, L.A.M.D., Metzger, S.E.M.D., Lam, J.B.S., and Harris. (1998). Perioperative cost-finding analysis of the routine use of intraoperative forced-air warming during general anesthesia. *Anesthesiology*, **88**(5), 1357–64.

36. Carli, F., Emery, P.W., and Freemantle, C.A.J. (1989). Effect of perioperative normothermia on postoperative protein metabolism in elderly patients undergoing hip arthroplasty. *British Journal of Anaesthesia*, **63**, 276–82.

37. Heier, T., Caldwell, J.E., Sessler, D.I., and Miller, R.D. (1991). Mild intraoperative hypothermia increases duration of action and spontaneous recovery of vecuronium blockade during nitrous oxide-isoflurane anesthesia in humans. *Anesthesiology*, **74**(5), 815–9.

38. Leslie, K.M.B.B.S.F., Sessler, D.I.M.D., Bjorksten, A.R.P., and Moayeri, A.B.A. (1995). Mild hypothermia alters propofol pharmacokinetics and increases the duration of action of atracurium. *Anesthesia and Analgesia*, **80**(5), 1007–14.

39. Just, B., Delva, E., Camus, Y., *et al.* (1992). Oxygen uptake during recovery following naloxone. *Anesthesiology*, **76**, 60–4.

40. Lenhardt, R., Marker, E., and Goll, V. (1997). Mild intraoperative hypothermia prolongs postanesthetic recovery. *Anesthesiology*, **87**(6), 1318 –23.

41. Kasai, T., Hirose, M., Matsukawa, T., Takamata, A., and Tanaka, Y. (2003). The vasoconstriction threshold is increased in obese patients during general anaesthesia. *Acta Anaesthesiologica Scandinavica*, **47**(5), 588–92.

42. Nolan, J.P., Morley, P.T., Hoek, T.L.V., and Hickey, R.W. (2003). Therapeutic hypothermia after cardiac arrest.: An advisory statement by the Advanced Life Support Task Force of the International Liaison Committee on Resuscitation. *Resuscitation*, **57**(3), 231–5.

43. Todd, M.M., Hindman, B.J., Clarke, W.R., and Torner, J.C. (2005) The Intraoperative Hypothermia for Aneurysm Surgery Trial (IHAST) investigators. mild intraoperative hypothermia during surgery for intracranial aneurysm. *New England Journal of Medicine*, **352**(2), 135–45.

44. Fritz, H.G. and Bauer, R. (2004). Secondary injuries in brain trauma: effects of hypothermia. *journal of neurosurgical anesthesiology*, **16**(1), 43–52.

45. Luscombe, M. and Andrzejowski, J.C.(2006). Clinical applications of induced hypothermia. *Continuing Education in Anaesthesia Critical Care and Pain*, **6**(1), 23–7.

46. Antonnen, H., Puhakka, K., Niskanen, J., and Ryhanen, P. (1995). Cutaneous heat loss in children during anaesthesia. *British Journal of Anaesthesia*, **74**(3), 306–310.

47. Millar, C. (2005). Principles of anaesthesia for term neonates. *Anaesthesia in Intensive Care*, **6**(3), 92–6.

48. Akin, A., Esmaoglu, A., and Boyaci, A. (2005). Postoperative shivering in children and causative factors.

49. Vaughan, M.S., Vaughan, R.W., and Cork, R.C. (1981). Postoperative hypothermia in adults: relationship of age, anesthesia, and shivering to rewarming. *Anesthesia and Analgesia*, **60**(10), 746–51.

50. Klingler, W., Lehmann-Horn, F., and Jurkat-Rott, K. (2005). Complications of anaesthesia in neuromuscular disorders. *Neuromuscular Disorders*, **15**(3), 195–206.

51. Rees, K., Beranek-Stanley, M., Burke, M., and Ebrahim, S. (2001). Hypothermia to reduce neurological damage following coronary artery bypass surgery. *Cochrane Database of Systematic Reviews*, **1**, CD002138.

52. Grigore, A.M., Mathew, J., Grocott, H.P., *et al.* (2001). Prospective randomized trial of normothermic versus hypothermic cardiopulmonary bypass on cognitive function after coronary artery bypass graft surgery. *Anesthesiology*, **95**(5), 1110–9.

53. Rajek, A., Lenhardt, R., Sessler, D.I., *et al.* (1998). Tissue heat content and distribution during and after cardiopulmonary bypass at 31°C and 27°C. *Anesthesiology*, **88**(6), 1511–8.

54. Insler, S.R., O'Connor, M.S., Leventhal, M.J., Nelson, D.R., and Starr, N.J. (2000). Association between postoperative hypothermia and adverse outcome after coronary artery bypass surgery. *The Annals of Thoracic Surgery*, **70**(1), 175–81.

55. Negishi, C. and Lenhardt, R. (2003). Fever during anaesthesia. *Best Practice and Research, Clinical Anaesthesiology*, **17**(4), 499–517.

56. Jampel, H., Duff, G., Gershon, R., Atkins, E., and Durum, S. (1983). Fever and immunoregulation. III. Hyperthermia augments the primary in vitro humoral immune response. *Journal of Experimental Medicine*, **157**(4), 1229–38.

57. Lenhardt, R., Negishi, C., Sessler, D.I., *et al.* (1999). The effect of pyrogen administration on sweating and vasoconstriction thresholds during desflurane anesthesia. *Anesthesiology*, **90**(6), 1587–95.

58. Negishi, C., Lenhardt, R., Ozaki, M., *et al.* (2001). Opioids inhibit febrile responses in humans, whereas epidural analgesia does not: an explanation for hyperthermia during epidural analgesia. *Anesthesiology*, **94**(2), 218–22.

59. Eberle, B., Weiler, N., Duber, C., *et al.* (1996). Anesthesia in endovascular treatment of aortic aneurysm. Results and perioperative risks. *Anaesthesist*, **45**(10), 931–40.

60. Lieberman, E. and O'Donoghue, C. (2002). Unintended effects of epidural analgesia during labor: A systematic review. *American Journal of Obstetrics and Gynecology*, **186**(5, Supplement 1), S31–S68.

61. Bredtmann, R. D., Herden, H. N., Teichmann, W., Moecke, H. P., Kniesel, B., Baetgen, R., and Tecklenburg, A. (1990). Epidural analgesia in colonic surgery: Results of a randomized prospective study. *British Journal of Surgery*, **77**(6), 638–42.

62. Smulian, J.C., Bhandari, V., Vintzileos, A.M., *et al.* (2003). Intrapartum fever at term: Serum and histologic markers of inflammation. *American Journal of Obstetrics and Gynecology*, **188**(1), 269–74.

63. Lieberman, E., Lang, J.M., Frigoletto, Jr., F., Richardson, D.K., Ringer, S.A., and Cohen, A. (1997). Epidural analgesia, intrapartum fever, and neonatal sepsis evaluation. *Pediatrics*, **99**(3), 415–9.

64. Lieberman, E., Cohen, A., Lang, J., Frigoletto, F., and Goetzl, L. (1999). Maternal intrapartum temperature elevation as a risk factor for Cesarean delivery and assisted vaginal delivery. *American Journal of Public Health*, **89**(4), 506.

65. Baker, A.S., Ojemann, R.G., Swartz, M.N., and Richardson, E.P., Jr. (1975). Spinal epidural abscess. *New England Journal of Medicine*, **293**(10), 463–8.

66. Hlavin, M.L., Kaminski, H.J., Ross, J.S., and Ganz, E. (1990). Spinal epidural abscess: a ten-year perspective. *Neurosurgery*, **27**(2), 177–84.

67. Gosavi, C., Bland, D., Poddar, R., Horst, C., and Roberts, C.J. (2004). Epidural abscess complicating insertion of epidural catheters. *British Journal of Anaesthesia*, **92**(2), 294–5.

68. Phillips, J.M.G., Stedeford, J.C., Hartsilver, E., and Roberts, C. (2002). Epidural abscess complicating insertion of epidural catheters. British Journal of Anaesthesia, **89**(5), 778–82.

69. Royakkers, A.A.N.M., Willigers, H., van der Ven, A.J., Wilmink, J., Durieux, M., and van Kleef, M. (2002). Catheter-related epidural abscesses - Don't wait for neurological deficits. *Acta Anaesthesiologica Scandinavica*, **46**(5),611–5.

70. Dahlgren, N. and Tornebrandt, K. (1995). Neurological complications after anaesthesia. A follow-up of 18,000 spinal and epidural anaesthetics performed over three years.*Acta Anaesthesiologica Scandinavica*, **39**(7), 872–80.

71. Kindler, C., Seeberger, M., Siegemund, M., and Schneider, M. (1996). Extradural abscess complicating lumbar extradural anaesthesia and analgesia in an obstetric patient. *Acta Anaesthesiologica Scandinavica*, **40**(7), 858–61.

72. Wang, L.P., Hauerberg, J., and Schmidt, J.F. (1999). Incidence of spinal epidural abscess after epidural analgesia: a national 1-year survey. *Anesthesiology*, **91**(6), 1928–36.

73. Reihsaus, E., Waldbaur, H., and Seeling, W. (2000). Spinal epidural abscess: a meta-analysis of 915 patients. *Neurosurgical Review*, **23**(4), 175–204.

74. Tang, H-J., Lin, H-J., Liu, Y-C., and Li, C-M. (2002). Spinal epidural abscess–experience with 46 patients and evaluation of prognostic factors. *journal of infection*, **45**(2), 76–81.

75. Cassey, J.G., Armstrong, P.J., Smith, G.E., Farrell, P.T. (2006). The safety and effectiveness of a modified convection heating system for children during anesthesia. *Pediatric Anesthesia*, **16**(6), 654–62.

76. Bloch, E.C., Ginsberg, B., Binner, R.A.J., and Sessler, D.I. (1992). Limb tourniquets and central temperature in anesthetized children. *Anesthesia and Analgesia*, **74**(4), 486–9.

77. Adnet, P.J., Reyford, H., and Krivosic-Horber, R.M. (1996). Neuroleptic malignant syndrome. In *Hyperthermic and Hypermetabolic Disorders* (eds. P.M. Hopkins and F.R. Ellis), pp. 223–38. Cambridge University Press.

78. Stotz, M., Thummler, D., Schurch, M., Renggli, J.C., Urwyler, A., and Pargger, H. (2004). Fulminant neuroleptic malignant sydrome after perioperative withdrawal of antiParkinsonian medication. *British Journal of Anaesthesia*, **93**, 868–71.

79. Gillman, P.K.(2005). Monoamine oxidase inhibitors, opioid analgesics and serotonin toxicity. *British Journal of Anaesthesia*, **95**, 434–41.

80. Kerner, T., Hildebrandt, B., Ahlers, O., *et al.* (2003). Anaesthesiological experiences with whole body hyperthermia. *International Journal of Hyperthermia*, **19**(1), 1–12.

81. Mauritz, W., Sporn, P., and Steinbereithner, K. (1986). Malignant hyperthermia in Austria I: epidemiology and clinical aspects. *Anaesthesist*, **35**, 639–50.

82. Ording, H. (1985). Incidence of malignant hyperthemia in Denmark. *Anesthesia and Analgesia*, **64**, 700–4.

83. Britt, B.A. and Kalow, W. (1970). Malignant hyperthermia: a statistical review. *Canadian Anaesthetists Society Journal*, **17**, 293–315.

84. Hopkins, P.M. and Ellis, F.R. (1995). Inherited disease affecting anaesthesia. In *A Practice of Anaesthesia* (eds. T.E.J. Healy and P.J. Cohen), pp. 938–52. Edward Arnold, London.

85. Monnier, N., Krivosic-Horber, R., Payen, J-F., *et al.* (2002). Presence of two different genetic traits in malignant hyperthermia families: implication for genetic analysis, diagnosis, and incidence of malignant hyperthermia susceptibility. *Anesthesiology*, **97**(5), 1067–74.

Chapter 20

Equipment

Iain K Moppett

The equipment used by anaesthetists is largely for the benefit of the patient. The anaesthetic machine is explicitly designed to deliver a known, safe mixture of medical gases and vapours to the patient. Breathing systems and ventilators allow the anaesthetist to maintain or provide safe and efficient ventilation of the patient's lungs. Monitoring devices exist to warn the anaesthetist of actual or impending problems. Furthermore, equipment manufacturers have generally been responsive to theoretical problems, near misses, and episodes of patient harm, introducing safety features to minimize risk to the patient. Generally, the benefit of using modern anaesthetic equipment far exceeds the risks attached to it, but patients may sometimes suffer harm because of the equipment used by anaesthetists. In some instances, patients may also possibly suffer harm due to equipment that was not used. This chapter explores the risks associated with anaesthetic equipment, and the benefits associated with their use. Injuries specific to the airway and respiration are discussed in detail in Chapter 12.

Overall risks due to equipment

Only a small fraction of equipment errors and failures are reported. Most information is presented as single case reports detailing problems with a single piece of equipment. The manufacturers' published response to these tends to be defensive[1], but where manufacturing or design faults are identified, this does lead to change. The fact that case reports are published is indirect evidence of the rarity of the problem. One large, prospective, audit of over 83 000 anaesthetics in the late 1990s[2] identified equipment problems in 157 (0.19%); general anaesthesia had a higher rate (0.23%) and regional anaesthesia lower (0.05%), presumably reflecting the amount of equipment used for the different techniques. Around 70% of problems were trivial, 25% of intermediate severity, and 2.5% (4 out of 157) were serious. In this series, no patients died or suffered long-term morbidity. For comparison, in the same patient series, around 1% of anaesthetics were associated with intraoperative problems; equipment problems, therefore, accounted for around 20% of all problems. An earlier qualitative interview study[3] found a slightly smaller ratio of equipment failure to human error (4%).

There have been sporadic reports of death and serious permanent morbidity due solely to equipment disasters such as cross-over of nitrous oxide and oxygen supplies[4] and blockage of breathing circuits[5]. Most of these are probably preventable with appropriate checking of equipment as stipulated by the various national bodies and manufacturers.

Anaesthetic machine

Benefits

The modern anaesthetic machine is a highly engineered piece of equipment, which has numerous safety features designed to minimize the risk to the patient. When used by competent, vigilant individuals, it provides a controlled system for delivering oxygen and inhaled anaesthetic drugs to the patient. It has three main drawbacks: (1) large capital cost means that machines may not be available in every area where anaesthesia may be carried out; (2) ongoing maintenance needs may, if not met, result in faulty equipment; and (3) the machines are generally bulky and essentially not portable, meaning that patients are often disconnected and reconnected either for intra-hospital transfer or between anaesthetic room and operating room.

Risks

The prospective audit cited above[2] found that one-third of equipment problems were related to the anaesthetic machine. Similarly, the earlier study[3] found that the most frequently reported problems were breathing circuit disconnections, gas-flow control errors, and loss of gas supply. The American Closed Claims project[6] reported 72 of 3791 claims as associated with gas delivery equipment; This may represent an over-estimate of relative frequency of problems because the outcomes from the events were poor, with death or permanent brain damage in 55%. Only a quarter were due to unanticipated failure of equipment; the remainder were due to 'misuse'. Overall, one-third of gas delivery claims were due to misconnections and disconnections; 4 out of 5 of these were judged 'preventable' with appropriate monitoring (predominantly pulse oximetry and capnography). A literature review from 1993 concluded that 33–66% of all anaesthetic-related incidents involved hypoxic gas mixtures, gas flow, circuit, tracheal tube, airway and ventilation problems, and these accounted for most cases of brain damage dealt with by insurance companies[7]. The majority of these problems are detectable early in their course by appropriate monitoring.

Scavenging equipment

Benefits of scavenging

Scavenging of anaesthetic gases is of no direct benefit to the patient but is of benefit to theatre staff. Legal requirements exist pertaining to maximum permissible environmental concentrations of volatile anaesthetic agents and scavenging is required to achieve these.

Risks of scavenging equipment

Modern scavenging equipment is designed with air breaks to reduce the risk of excessive negative pressure being applied to the breathing circuits. In the light of previous adverse events, scavenging equipment can no longer be connected to pressure-relief valves. However, case reports have been published where faulty, obstructed, and unchecked scavenging systems have led to potential or actual patient harm[8–12].

It is not possible to estimate the frequency of these events, but given the paucity of reports, serious adverse events are probably rare.

Monitoring equipment

Benefits of monitoring

Monitoring in anaesthesia has developed over time, in parallel with greater physiological understanding and advances in technology. Standards of practice have been set by most national anaesthetic bodies, though for many of these, the evidence in favour of monitoring is not of particularly high quality. The Australian Incident, Monitoring Study (AIMS)[13], reporting on the first 2000 submitted incidents found that just over half the incidents were detected by monitoring, a figure which would have been higher (but not 100%) if the available monitoring had been used and alarms set appropriately. Monitors are, therefore, a useful adjunct to the most fundamental monitor—the presence of a trained anaesthetist.

Pulse oximetry

Pulse oximetry is generally held to be a part of minimum monitoring standards for anaesthesia, sedation, and intensive care[14,15]. The AIMS study[10] found that of the incidents detected by monitors, 27% were detected first by the pulse oximeter. A theoretical analysis by the AIMS investigators suggested that around 80% of incidents could be detected using pulse oximetry alone.

Pulse oximetry has been associated with injury, though rarely. One study[16] of 125 patients undergoing prolonged monitoring (more than 2 days) in intensive care found temporary skin necrosis occurred in 6 patients, despite changing the probe site every 2–3 h. There was an association of injury with vasopressor use, though this may have been linked to severity of illness. Other case reports have described sensory loss in the finger[17–19] and burns[20] associated with normal use of finger clip pulse oximeters. It is recommended that probe position should be changed very 2–3 h to reduce the risk of complications, although this is no direct evidence to support the practice.

Expired gas capnography

Measurement of the inspired and expired concentrations of carbon dioxide has been viewed as a minimum standard of anaesthetic monitoring for many years[14,15]. Capnography provides a diagnostic test for placement of breathing tubes and connection of breathing systems. Data from the AIMS study found that 24% of monitor-detected incidents were identified first through capnography, which would have risen to around 30%, had it been used. The American Closed Claims Study suggested that the combination of pulse oximetry and capnography could prevent around 80% of equipment-related claims[6]. To date, there have been no reports of direct injury caused by capnography. Quantitative and qualitative interpretation of the capnograph trace is a matter of clinical judgement, for which there are few direct studies associating end-tidal carbon dioxide levels with good or bad outcome. Data from patients with traumatic brain injury suggest that prolonged, severe hypocapnia is detrimental, and hypercapnia is associated with increased rates of cardiac dysrhythmmia in the presence of halothane.

Volatile agent monitoring

Continuous monitoring of inspired and expired anaesthetic agent concentrations is a minimum standard for anaesthesia involving inhaled agents. Lack of such monitoring increases the risk of inadequate dosing (leading to cardiovascular instability or awareness) or over-dosing (leading to increased cardiorespiratory depression). Whether the addition of monitors of anaesthetic depth (e.g. BIS®, auditory evoked potentials) is necessary for every patient is still a subject of debate (see Chapter 11).

Inspired oxygen monitoring

Monitoring the fraction of oxygen in the gases delivered to and inhaled by the patient is a minimum standard for all anaesthesia[15,16]. Failure to monitor this adequately (either due to lack of monitoring, or ignoring/disabling alarms) has led to deaths and permanent brain damage. The AIMS study found that the oxygen analyser was a relatively infrequent 'first detector' with only 4% of monitor-detected incidents (though it was somewhat underused). However, given the gravity of delivering hypoxic gas mixtures to patients, other than in extreme circumstances, it is difficult to envisage a situation where anaesthesia should be induced without such monitoring.

Blood pressure monitoring

The AAGBI recommendations[14] for blood pressure monitoring are that it should be recorded at least every five minutes, and more frequently if clinically necessary. This is based largely on custom and practice rather than any evidence demonstrating that 5 min is an optimal interval. Modern, automated, non-invasive blood pressure measurement is generally reliable enough for most patients, provided manufacturers' guidelines are followed. Injury following prolonged use of automated cuffs has been reported, though rarely. Nerve injury to both radial[21,22] and ulnar nerves has been described[23]. Compartment syndrome has been reported associated with machine malfunction[24], rapid cycling[25], tight cuff application, and marked elbow flexion[26]. Other reported complications include petechiae, bruising, and phlebitis[21]. The incidence of these complications is unknown. The ASA task force on prevention of perioperative peripheral neuropathies[27] consensus conclusion was that 'properly functioning automated blood pressure cuffs on the upper arms do not affect the risk of upper extremity neuropathies.'

Clinicians may elect to monitor arterial pressure invasively, either to avoid the risk associated with prolonged and frequent non-invasive monitoring, to allow more rapid assessment of blood pressure changes, or to allow frequent arterial blood sampling. Cannulation of the peripheral arteries is associated with various rare complications. One study has collated the various reports of complications of arterial cannulation from 1978–2001[28]. The most common reported complication is temporary occlusion of the radial artery which occurs in approximately 20% of cannulations. Permanent occlusion is rare with 3 reported cases out of 4200. Allen's test (of dependency upon radial arterial perfusion of the hand) does not appear to be a useful predictor of ischaemic problems[29]. Local infection occurs in around 0.7%, while sepsis is reported for around 0.1%. Haematoma (variously defined) occurs in around 15%. Pseudoaneurysm,

Table 20.1 Complication rates for arterial cannulation in anaesthesia and intensive care[23]

	Permanent ischaemic damage	Temporary occlusion	Sepsis	Local infection	Pseudo-aneurysm	Haematoma	Bleeding
Radial	0.09	19.7	0.13	0.72	0.09	14.4	0.52
	(4/4217)	(831/4217)	(8/6245)	(45/6245)	(14/15,623)	(418/2903)	(2/375)
Femoral	0.18	1.45	0.44	0.78	0.3	6.1	1.58
	(3/1664)	(10/688)	(13/2923)	(5/642)	(6/2100)	(28/461)	(5/316)
Axillary	0.2	1.18	0.51	2.24	0.1	2.28	1.41
	(2/989)	(11/930)	(5/989)	(16/713)	(1/1000)	(17/744)	(10/711)

Source: Modified from Sy, W.P. (1981). Ulnar nerve palsy possibly related to use of automatically cycled blood pressure cuff. *Anesthesia and Analgesia*, **60**, 687–8. With permission.

Note: Incidence (%) (cases/number of cannulations)

which is a risk factor for subsequent infection or rupture, is reported with an incidence of around 0.1%. Complications for femoral and axillary artery cannulation are similar, though temporary occlusion appears to be less common (Table 20.1). Risk factors for complications are not clear, though temporary occlusion appears to be more likely if the cannula is relatively large compared to the vessel and if cannulation is prolonged. Infection is more common if cannulae are left *in situ* for more than 96 h. A more recent study from a single centre[30] found lower complication rates (0.0067% (15/22 292) overall); the 2 patients with permanent damage had multiple co-morbidities. Fatal[31] and non-fatal[32] retrograde cerebral embolism from giving sets that have not been flushed free of air have been reported, as has nerve injury[33].

Central venous access

Central venous access may be required for the administration of drugs, for difficult or long-term venous access and for monitoring of central venous pressure. However, central venous access is associated with significant risk of injury; it follows that clinicians should be satisfied that the potential benefits outweigh the risks. Some drugs can only be given safely into central veins, in which case the indication for central access may be clear. Similarly, difficult or long-term access may only be achieved via a central route. The evidence for central venous pressure (CVP) monitoring is much less robust. Numerous studies have failed to demonstrate good predictive value for CVP as a marker of fluid responsiveness. Other techniques with better sensitivity for estimates of cardiac output, such as transoesophageal Doppler, transoesophageal echocardiography, and peripheral pulse variation with the respiratory cycle have better sensitivity[34]. The use of CVP monitoring has been associated with improved outcome in some clinical studies[35] particularly those assessing the effects of goal-directed therapy[36]. Alternative methods, such as transoesphageal Doppler, which do not carry the same traumatic and infection risks have also been shown to improve outcomes[37,38].

The benefits of central venous catheters (CVC) must be weighed against the risks associated with their insertion and use. Every nearby anatomical structure has been reported as damaged temporarily or permanently by attempts at central line insertion[39]: pleura and lung; associated arteries—carotid, vertebral, cervical, thyroidal, subclavian, and femoral; nerves—vagus[40], phrenic[41] sympathetic trunk, brachial plexus[42], femoral; heart and pericardium; thoracic duct; trachea; oesophagus. Resultant complications include: pneumothorax; haemothorax; chylothorax; cardiac tamponade; cardiac dysrhythmmia; embolism of air into both the venous system and (carotid) arterial supply to the brain; airway obstruction; mediastinitis; arteriovenous fistula; Horner's syndrome[43]; chronic pain syndrome. Pneumothorax accounts for around a quarter of all reported complications of CVC insertion[44] and is reported to occur with a frequency of around 5%[45] though this may be reduced in the hands of experienced operators[31]. Long-term complications include thrombus formation, vessel occlusion and erosion and infection.

One recent prospective study of nearly 1800 CVC insertion attempts by experienced operators has described the mechanical complications of insertion in an ICU population[46]. Overall failure rate was 2.8% at the initial site. Arterial puncture occurred in 3%, with arterial cannulation in 0.2%. In this series pneumothorax occurred in 0.6%, and overall, 6.7% of catheters were malpositioned.

Various trials have investigated the use of 2-D ultrasound to reduce complication rates. A meta-analysis of 18 trials[47] found a relative risk reduction for failed catheter placement, complications, and first attempt failure for internal jugular placement (Table 20.2). A systematic review from 2002 concluded that internal jugular line insertion is associated with more arterial punctures but less catheter misplacement than subclavian insertion. Haemo- and pneumothorax rates are similar between the two sites[48]. A more recent prospective and non-randomized study did not find

Table 20.2 Relative risk associated with landmark versus 2-D ultrasound technique for central venous access

Adults	Relative risk (95% CI)	
	Internal jugular	Subclavian
Failed catheter placement	0.14	0.14
	(0.06–0.33)	(0.04–0.57)
Complication with placement	0.43	0.1
	(0.22–0.87)	(0.01–0.71)
Failure on first attempt	0.59	—
	(0.39–0.88)	
Infants	—	—
Failed catheter placement	0.15	—
	(0.03–0.64)	
Complication with placement	0.27	—
	(0.08-0.91)	

Note: Relative risk <1 favours ultrasound guidance. CI = confidence interval.

a statistically significant difference in arterial puncture rate between internal jugular and subclavian, though the trend was also for higher arterial puncture rates with internal jugular approaches (4 vs. 2%)[31].

Catheter-associated infection is difficult to diagnose with certainty, leading to variation in reported rates of infection. Overall infection rates are around 5%[49]. Factors associated with increased rates of infection include: multi-lumen versus single lumen CVC (OR: 2.58)[49], not using maximal sterile precautions during insertion (OR: 3.3)[50], and emergency insertion (OR: 6.2)[51]. Femoral lines have traditionally been believed to present a greater infection risk but studies suggest that if strict sterile precautions are observed, the risks are similar for all three main sites[51,52].

Catheter-related thrombosis rates are affected by the interaction between catheter design, duration of placement, and patient characteristics. Reported rates of thrombosis vary widely between 2% and 67%, with an overall incidence of imaged (Doppler ultrasound or venography) thrombosis around 30%[53]. Clinically-manifested thrombosis is reported at 0–12%. These data include oncology, cardiology, haematology, and ICU patients. If solely ICU patients are included (which reflects the majority of CVCs inserted by anaesthetists) then diagnosed DVT occurs in around 30% of patients, whilst clinically manifest thrombosis occurs in around 0.5%. Femoral catheters may pose a greater risk than sublcalvian or internal jugular catheters[54]. The incidence of thrombosis is higher in patients with cancer, previous thromboembolism, and with CVC-associated infection[54,55]. One study found an approximately 15% rate of pulmonary embolism in patients with upper extremity CVC-associated DVT, of whom 2 of 13 died due to pulmonary embolism[56]. There are no convincing trial data to support the use of prophylactic treatment to prevent clinically manifest CVC-associated thrombosis[53].

Electrical risks

Electric-powered equipment is invaluable for modern anaesthetic and surgical practice. In the AIMS database, adverse events due to electricity were rare, with an incidence similar to ocular damage[57]. Safety standards, such as IEC 60601 apply to the manufacture of electrical equipment. Provided proper maintenance is carried out and use of equipment is in accordance with manufacturers' guidance, electrical events are rare.

Rapid infusion devices

Rapid infusion of intravenous fluids can be life-saving, and several devices exist to achieve this, some of which have in-built warming processes as well. All of these devices carry a risk of air embolus due to air entrainment, and various case reports have been published with fatal and non-fatal outcomes from such events[58]. Although the devices contain air-elimination devices, these cannot be guaranteed to prevent air embolism, and user vigilance is still an absolute requirement[59]. Medical device alerts have also been issued[60] concerning these devices with manufacturers providing more guidance on avoidance of injury. Hyperkalaemia of sufficient magnitude to cause ECG changes and cardiac arrest has been associated with the administration of bank blood via rapid infusion devices[61,62] and traditional pressure bags[62].

Miscellaneous risks

Almost every piece of equipment used by anaesthetists has been associated with an adverse event. Devices designed to function as open-ended cylinders (breathing systems, face masks, intravenous and epidural catheters and needles) have all been blocked due to manufacturing defects, accidental blockage, and possibly malice. Similarly, equipment designed not to have holes, can have holes in the wrong place, again due to design, manufacturing, storage, or usage faults. The checking processes promulgated by national associations such as AAGBI and equipment manufacturers should make these rare.

References

1. Moppett, I. and Spendlove, J. (2004). Manufacturers' response to criticism. *Anaesthesia*, **59**, 1143.
2. Fasting, S. and Gisvold, S.E. (2002). Equipment problems during anaesthesia – are they a quality problem? *British Journal of Anaesthesia*, **89**, 825–31.
3. Cooper, J.B., Newbower, R.S., and Kitz, R.J. (1984). An analysis of major errors and equipment failures in anesthesia management: considerations for prevention and detection. *Anesthesiology*, **60**, 34–42.
4. Herff, H., Paal, P., von Goedecke, A., Lindner, K.H., Keller, C., and Wenze, V. (2007). Fatal errors in nitrous oxide delivery *Anaesthesia*, **62**, 1202–6.
5. Carter, J.A. (2004). Checking anaesthetic equipment and the Expert Group on Blocked Anaesthetic Tubing (EGBAT). *Anaesthesia*, **59**, 105–7.
6. Caplan, R.A., Vistica, M.F., Posner, K.L., and Cheney, F.W. (1997). Adverse anesthetic outcomes arising from gas delivery equipment: A Closed Claims analysis. *Anesthesiology*, **87**, 741–8.
7. Runciman, W.B. (1993). Risk assessment in the formulation of anaesthesia safety standards. *European Journal of Anaesthesiology*, **Suppl 7**, 26–32.
8. Gray, W.M. (1985). Scavenging equipment. *British Journal of Anaesthesia*, **57**, 685–95.
9. Mantia, A.M. (1982). Gas scavenging systems. *Anesthesia and Analgesia*, **61**, 162–4
10. Tavakoli, M. and Habeeb, A. (1978). Two hazards of gas scavenging. *Anesthesia and Analgesia*, **57**, 286–7.
11. Carvalho, B. (1999). Hidden hazards of scavenging. *British Journal of Anaesthesia*, **83**, 532–3.
12. Farquhar-Thomson, D.R. and Goddard, J.M. (1996). The hazards of anaesthetic gas scavenging systems. *Anaesthesia*, **51**, 860–2.
13. Webb, R.K., van der Walt, J.H., Runciman, W.B., *et al.* (1993). The Australian Incident Monitoring Study. Which monitor? An analysis of 2000 incident reports. *Anaesthesia and Intensive Care*, **21**, 52942.
14. Recommendations for standards of monitoring during anaesthesia and recovery, 4th edition. (2007). Association of Anaesthetists of Great Britain and Ireland. London.
15. American Society of Anesthesiologists: Standards for Basic Anesthetic Monitoring. (2003). http://www.asahq.org/publicationsAndServices/standards/02.pdf#2. (last accessed 13th January 2009)
16. Wille, J., Braams, R., van Haren, W.H., and van der Werken, C. (2000). Pulse oximeter-induced digital injury: frequency rate and possible causative factors. *Critical Care Medicine*, **28**, 3555–7.

17. Gates, R.E., Kinsella, S.B., Moorthy, S.S. (1995). Sensory loss of the distal phalanx and pulse oximeter probe. *Anesthesia and Analgesia*, **80**, 855.

18. Clark, M. and Lavies, N.G. (1997). Sensory loss of the distal phalanx caused by pulse oximeter probe.*Anaesthesia*, **52**, 508–9.

19. Donahue, P.J. and Emery, S. (1995). Digital sensory loss without pulse oximeter malfunction. *Anesthesia and Analgesia*, **81**, 1312.

20. Baruchin, A.M., Nahlieli, O., Neder, A., and Shapira, Y. (1993). Finger injury from a pulse oximeter sensor during orthognathic surgery, *Annals of the Meditterranean Burns Club*, 6.

21. Lin, C-C., Bruno Jawan, B., de Villa, M.V.H., Chen, F-C., and Liu, P-P. (2001). Blood pressure cuff compression injury of the radial nerve. *Journal of Clinical Anesthesia*, **13**, 306–8.

22. Schaer, H.M. and Tschirren, B. (1982). Radial nerve paresis following automatic measurement of blood pressure. A case report. *Anaesthesist*, **31**, 151–2.

23. Sy, W.P. (1981). Ulnar nerve palsy possibly related to use of automatically cycled blood pressure cuff. *Anesthesia and Analgesia*, **60**, 687–8.

24. Yamada, M., Tsuda, K.N., Yamada, M., Nagai, S., Tadokoro, M., and Ishibe, Y. (1997). A case of crush syndrome resulting from continuous compression of the upper arm by automatically cycled blood pressure cuff. *Masui*, **46**, 119.

25. Vidal, P., Sykes, P.J., O'Shaughnessy, M., and Craddock, K. (1993). Compartment syndrome after use of an automatic arterial pressure monitoring device [published erratum appears in Br J Anaesth 1994; 72:738J]. *British Journal of Anaesthesia*, **71**, 902–4.

26. Sutin, K.M., Longaker, M.T., Wahlander, S., Kasabian, A.K., and Capan, L.M. (1996). Acute biceps compartment syndrome associated with the use of a noninvasive blood pressure monitor. *Anesthesia and Analgesia*, **83**, 1345–6.

27. ASA Task Force on prevention of peri-operative peripheral neuropathies. (2000). Practice advisory for prevention of peri-operative peripheral neuropathies. *Anesthesiology*, **92**, 1168–82.

28. Scheer, B.V., Perel, A., and Pfeiffer, U.J. (2002). Clinical review: Complications and risk factors of peripheral arterial catheters used for haemodynamic monitoring in anaesthesia and intensive care medicine. *Critical Care*, **6**, 198–204.

29. Slogoff, S., Keats, A.S., and Arlund, C. (1983). On the safety of radial artery cannulation. *Anesthesiology*, **59**, 42–7.

30. Rao, V.K., Hilmi, I., Damian, D., Salmon, A., and Galhotra, S.X. (2007). Etiology, Incidence and outcome of arterial injury following intraoperative arterial canulation. *Anesthesiology*, **107**, A1982.

31. Chang, C., Dughi, J., Shitabata, P., Johnson, G., Coel, M., and McNamara, J. (1988). Air embolism and the radial arterial line. *Critical Care Medicine*, **16**, 141–3.

32. Chilvers, M.B. (1999). Cerebral air embolism following a small volume of air inadvertently injected via a peripheral arterial cannula. The Internet Journal of Anesthesiology Vol3N1: http://www.ispub.com/journals/IJA/Vol3N1/air.htm; Published January 1, 1999; Last Updated January 1, 1999.

33. Wallach, S.G. (2004). Cannulation injury of the radial artery: diagnosis and treatment algorithm. *American Journal of Critical Care*, **13**, 315–9.

34. Michard, F., Teboul, J.L. (2002). Predicting fluid responsiveness in ICU patients. A critical analysis of the evidence. *Chest*, **121**, 2000–8.

35. Venn, R., Steeele, A., Richardson, P., Poloniecki, J., Grounds, M., and Newman, P. (2002). Randomized controlled trial to investigate influence of the fluid challenge on duration of hospital stay and perioperative morbidity in patients with hip fractures. *British Journal of Anaesthesia*, **88**, 65–71.

36. Rivers, E., Nguyen, B., Havstad, S. *et al.* (2001). Early goal directed therapy in the treatment of severe sepsis and septic shock. *New England Journal of Medicine*, **345**, 1368–77.

37. Sinclair, S., James, S., and Singer, M.(1997). Intraoperative intravascular volume optimisation and length of hospital stay after repair of proximal femoral fracture: randomised controlled trial. *British Medical Journal*, **315**, 909–12.

38. Abbas, S.M. and Hill, A.G. (2008). Systematic review of the literature for the use of oesophageal Doppler monitor for fluid replacement in major abdominal surgery. *Anaesthesia*, **63**, 44–51.

39. Boon, J.M., van Schoor, A.N., Abrahams, P.H., Meiring, J.H., and Welch, T. (2008). Central venous catheterization—an anatomical review of a clinical skill, Part 2: Internal Jugular Vein via the Supraclavicular Approach. *Clinical Anatomy*, **21**, 15–22.

40. Moosman, D.A. (1973). The anatomy of infraclavicular subclavian vein catheterization and its complications. *Surgical Gynecology and Obstetrics*, **136**, 71–4.

41. Vest, J.V., Pereira, M.B., and Senior, R.M. (1980). Phrenic nerve injury associated with venipuncture of the internal jugular vein. *Chest*, **78**, 777–9.

42. Thomas, S., Bhandarai, V. (2004). Nerve plexus injury with internal jugular cannulation. *Indian Journal of Anaesthesia*, **48**, 228–30.

43. Parikh, R.K. (1972). Horners syndrome - A complication of percutaneous catheterization of internal jugular vein. *Anaesthesia*, **27**, 327–9.

44. Seneff, M.G. (1987). Central venous catheterization: A comprehensive review. *Journal of Intensive Care Medicine*, **2**, 2218–23.

45. Sznajder, J.I., Zveibil, F.R., and Bitterman, H. (1986). Central vein catheterization. Failure and complication rates by three percutaneous approaches. *Archives of Internal Medicine*, **146**, 259–61.

46. Schummer, W., Schummer, C., Rose, N., Niesen, W-D., and Sakka, S.G. (2007). Mechanical complications and malpositions of central venous cannulations by experienced operators: A prospective study of 1794 catheterizations in critically ill patients. *Intensive Care Medicine*, **33**, 1055–9.

47. Hind, D., Calvert, N., McWilliams, R., *et al.* (2003). Ultrasonic locating devices for central venous cannulation: meta-analysis. *British Medical Journal*, **327**, 361–7.

48. Ruesch, S., Walder, B., and Tramer, M.R. (2002). Complications of central venous catheters: Internal jugular versus subclavian access-A systematic review. *Critical Care Medicine*, **30**, 454–60.

49. Zurcher, M., Tramer, M.R., and Walder, B. (2004). Colonization and bloodstream infection with single- versus multi-lumen central venous catheters: a quantitative systematic review. *Anesthesia and Analgesia*, **99**, 177–82.

50. Raad, II., Hohn, D.C., Gilbreath, B.J., *et al.* (1994). Prevention of central venous catheter-related infections by using maximal sterile barrier precautions during insertion. *Infection Control and Hospital Epidemiology*, **15**, 231–8.

51. Goetz, A.M,,Wagener, M.M., Miller, J.M., and Muder, R.R. (1998). Risk of infection due to central venous catheters: effect of site of placement and catheter type. *Infection Control and Hospital Epidemiology*, **19**, 842–5.

52. Deshpande, K.S., Hatem, C., Ulrich, H.L., *et al.* (2005). The incidence of infectious complications of central venous catheters at the subclavian, internal jugular, and femoral sites in an intensive care unit population. *Critical Care Medicine*, **33**, 13–20.

53. van Rooden, C.J., Tesselaar, M.E.T., Osanto, S., Rosendaal, F.R., and Huisman, M.V. (2005). Deep vein thrombosis associated with central venous catheters – a review. *Journal of Thrombosis and Haemostasis,* **3**, 2409–19.

54. Trottier, S.J., Veremakis, C., O'Brien, J., and Auer, A,I. (1995). Femoral deep vein thrombosis associated with central venous catheterization: results from a prospective, randomized trial. *Critical Care Medicine,* **23**, 52–9.

55. Timsit, J.F., Farkas, J.C., Boyer, J.M., *et al.* (1998). Central vein catheter-related thrombosis in intensive care patients: incidence, risks factors, and relationship with catheter-related sepsis. *Chest,* **114**, 207–13.

56. Monreal, M., Raventos, A., Lerma, R., *et al.* (1994). Pulmonary embolism in patients with upper extremity DVT associated to venous central lines – a prospective study. *Thrombosis and Haemostasis,* **72**, 548–50.

57. Singleton, R.J., Ludbrook, G.L., Webb, R.K., and Fox, M.A. (1993). The Australian Incident Monitoring Study. Physical injuries and environmental safety in anaesthesia: an analysis of 2000 incident reports. *Anaesthesia and Intensive Care,* **21**, 659–63.

58. Novitsky, Y.W., Mostafa, G., Sing, R.F., Lipford, E., and Heniford, B.T. (2006). Fatal cardiac embolism. *Injury,* **37**, 78–80.

59. Schnoor, J., Macko, S., Weber, I., and Rossaint, R. (2004). The air elimination capabilities of pressure infusion devices and fluid-warmers. *Anaesthesia,* **59**, 817–21.

60. Medical device alert MDA/2007/099 MHRA London 2008.

61. Carvalho, B.and Quiney, N.F. (1999). 'Near-miss' hyperkalaemic cardiac arrest associated with rapid blood transfusion. *Anaesthesia,* **54**, 1094–6.

62. Smith, H.M., Farrow, S.J., Ackerman, J.D., Stubbs, J.R., and Sprung, J. (2008). Cardiac arrests associated with hyperkalemia during red blood cell transfusion: a case series. *Anesthesia and Analgesia,* **106**, 1062–9.

Chapter 21

Drug reactions and drug errors

Ronnie J Glavin

As anaesthetists, we rely on drugs for our professional practice. We use drugs to interfere with the normal physiological controls of our patients to allow them to undergo diagnostic or therapeutic surgical procedures. We need to have an understanding of the nature and extent of adverse reactions to those drugs, not only so that we can disclose such facts to the patient before anaesthesia, but also so that we can engage in a meaningful dialogue with those patients. Quoting frequencies and incidences is only the first stage in a process of helping a patient make sense of the possible implications for the journey through the perioperative period. The aim of this chapter is to equip the anaesthetist with the necessary information to enable such a process to take place.

The first section provides a framework into which different kinds of adverse reaction can be placed. The second section deals with those reactions that are immunologically based; although not very frequent, their potential severity makes them of particular relevance. The third section describes some of the more important possible adverse reactions associated with each of the major classes of drugs which anaesthetists use. The fourth section discusses drug error, as this is not only an unfortunately common source of adverse reaction but has gone beyond the previous confines of the medical literature into the popular press. The final section contains a very short review of possible future directions, especially in the field of pharmacogenetics.

Definitions and framework

The World Health Organisation (WHO) definition of an adverse drug reaction is 'a response to a drug that is noxious and unintended and occurs at doses normally used in man for the prophylaxis, diagnosis and therapy of disease, or for the modification of physiological function'[1].

One of the difficulties of this definition relates to the use of the word noxious, because it does not quantify the extent of the harm or injury caused. Within the context of drug reporting this is important because, if minor unwanted effects are included, surveillance systems would be less effective in drawing attention to the more serious unwanted effects. This definition also includes neither contaminants nor drug errors. Edwards and Aronson[2] have therefore proposed the following definition of an adverse drug reaction: 'An appreciably harmful or unpleasant reaction, resulting from an intervention related to the use of a medicinal product which predicts hazard from future administration and warrants prevention or specific treatment, or alteration of the dosage regimen, or withdrawal of the product'.

The term 'adverse effect' is used when talking about responses from the individual drug perspective, whereas the term 'adverse reaction' is used when referring to the patient perspective. An 'adverse event' is an adverse outcome that occurs while the patient is taking a drug, but is not necessarily attributable to that drug. The term 'medicinal product' can go beyond the WHO definition of a drug because exposure to products, which contain substances such as latex can result in severe adverse reactions, such as anaphylaxis, for which the earlier definition would be appropriate.

The current classification of adverse drug reactions lists six categories, which are labelled A–F (see Table 21.1)[2].

Adverse event by classification of event

Augmented or dose-related

Anaesthetists titrate drugs against clinical effect and so are continuously monitoring their pharmacological actions. The inter-individual variation in response to drugs requires that close attention be paid to the effects of a drug, reducing the likelihood that a patient receives too much or too little. However, drug errors can result in significant overdosing of drug (e.g. a vaporizer allowed to deliver a high concentration, a syringe of local anaesthetic drug administered intravenously instead of via the epidural route, etc.). This aspect will be dealt with in greater detail in the section on drug error.

Bizarre or non-dose related

Included in this category are idiosyncratic responses such as anaphylactic reactions, which are discussed in Section 2.

Chronic or dose-related and time-related

Unlike many other physicians, anaesthetists usually administer drugs to patients over a very short period of time and do not usually prescribe prolonged courses of drugs (with the exception of those working in the field of chronic pain). However, maintenance

Table 21.1 Classification of adverse drug reactions, with some examples

Type of reaction	Mnemonic	Example
A: Dose-related	Augmented	Respiratory depression from a relative overdose of opioid drug
B: Non-dose-related	Bizarre	Anaphylactic shock
C: Dose-related and time-related	Chronic	Methoxyflurane-induced renal failure
D: Time-related	Delayed	Teratogenesis with thalidomide
E: Withdrawal	End of use	Hypothalamic pituitary adrenal suppression with prolonged course of corticosteroid drugs
F: Unexpected failure of a therapy	Failure	Awareness under anaesthesia related to drug error

of anaesthesia or sedation in the intensive care setting may result in a relatively prolonged, continuous exposure to inhalational agents or intravenous drugs.
A number of examples are discussed in later sections.

Delayed or time-related

Reactions in this category usually refer to carcinogenic or teratogenic effects of drugs.
The possible impact of anaesthetic drugs on pregnancy is reviewed later.

End-of-use or withdrawal

These effects are more usually associated with longer-term prescription of drugs. They
may present management challenges for the anaesthetist (e.g. patients on long-term
high-dose steroid therapy, or patients who have abused intravenous drugs) but will
not be discussed in any detail in this chapter.

Failure or unexpected failure of therapy

In cases of long-term drug administration, this reaction is seen when a drug that
has been working effectively ceases to do so. This is often due to an interaction with
another drug or to a new co-existing disease. For example, an oral contraceptive
may fail because of an interaction with antibiotics or because of a decrease in
absorption associated with diarrhoea and vomiting from an acute viral infection.
The most serious failure in anaesthetic practice is awareness under anaesthesia.
This is dealt with in Chapter 11. Drug errors may, of course, contribute to failure
of therapy and will be discussed in that Section of this chapter.

Major immunological adverse reactions

Sitter[3] quotes an incidence of anaphylaxis (IgE-mediated reaction) as high as 1 in
1000 anaesthetics. He also quotes an incidence of histamine-related reactions as high
1 in 10; these reactions include anaphylactoid reactions, i.e. reactions in which
the clinical appearance of the patient may resemble that associated with a reaction
mediated by IgE but in which an immunological mechanism cannot be demonstrated.
Mertes[4] quotes an incidence of anaphylactic/anaphylactoid reactions of 1:13 000 in
France in 1996, while Fisher[5] quotes a range of 1:10 000 to 1:20 000 in Australia.

Part of the difficulty in establishing the true incidence is due to uncertainty about the
accuracy of the diagnosis and the exhaustiveness of investigations. The clinical reaction
must be recognized for the diagnosis to be made, and this may be difficult in a draped
anaesthetized patient whose condition may be unstable due to the challenges of surgery.
It is also difficult to obtain denominator data, i.e. the number of patients exposed to the
possible risk in the population from which reactions are reported. Even if the number of
patients who were anaesthetized is known, there may be insufficient information about
how many were exposed to different classes of drugs.

The common presenting symptoms from a survey of units dealing with referrals
following suspected anaphylaxis in France from January 1997 to December 1998 are
shown in Table 21.2[6].

The reactions vary in intensity (Table 21.3) but even when appropriately treated, death
may result, with quoted mortality rates ranging of 3.5%[7] to 4.0%[8]. An additional 2%

Table 21.2 Most common clinical features of anaphylaxis under anaesthesia reported from a 2-year survey of French referral units[6]

Clinical feature	Percentage of patients in which signs appeared (%)
Cardiovascular symptoms	73.6
Cutaneous symptoms	69.6
Bronchospasm	44.2

of patients experience significant brain damage[8]. Reactions to antibiotics can occur following the removal of a tourniquet during orthopaedic surgery[9]. Common initial symptoms that have been documented include pulselessness, difficulty in inflation of the lungs, and reduced oxygen saturation[4]. A sudden decrease in end-tidal carbon dioxide tension may be the first sign of an anaphylactic reaction; if such a decrease occurs during anaesthesia, as opposed to immediately after induction, then a reaction to latex or to an intravenous colloid should be considered.

A detailed description of the mechanism of anaphylaxis is beyond the remit of this chapter. The reader who wishes a more detailed description should refer to the paper by Hepner[10]. The key feature of anaphylaxis is an immunological reaction to an antigen. In the case of drug-induced anaphylaxis, the antigen is often a carrier protein and either the drug or a product of drug metabolism. Subsequent exposure to the antigen may produce a more severe reaction. With neuromuscular blocking drugs, the main antigenic determinants are substituted ammonium ions[11]. This explains the cross-reactivity commonly found when anaphylaxis related to a neuromuscular blocker is investigated. Flexible molecules such as succinlycholine can stimulate sensitized basophils much more easily than rigid molecules such as pancuronium. Cross-reactivity also occurs between latex and various fruits, including avocado, banana, kiwi, and papaya.

The agents responsible for most of the anaphylactic reactions under anaesthesia are muscle relaxants, with induction agents, antimicrobials, latex and blood volume

Table 21.3. Grade of severity of anaphylactic reactions referred to specialist units in France during a survey in 1997 and 1998[6]

Grade	Signs	Incidence
1	Cutaneous signs, generalized erythema, urticaria, angio-oedema	10.1%
2	Measurable but not life-threatening symptomsCutaneous signs, tachycardia, hypotension, respiratory disturbance, cough, difficult to inflate lungs	22.9%
3	Life-threatening symptomsCollapse, tachycardia or bradycardia, arrhythmias, bronchospasm	62.6%
4	Cardiac and or respiratory arrest	4.4%
5	Death	0

Source: From Laxenaire, M-C. and Mertes, P.M. (2001). Anaphylaxis during anaesthesia. Results of a two-year survey in France. *British Journal of Anaesthesia*, **87**, 549–59. With permission.

Table 21.4 Agents responsible for anaphylactic reactions from a 2-year French survey[6]

Drug	Percentage(%)
Neuromuscular blocking drug	69
Latex	12
Antibiotics	8
Others	2.9
Colloids	2.7
Opioids	1.4

Source: From Laxenaire, M-C. and Mertes, P.M. (2001). Anaphylaxis during anaesthesia. Results of a two-year survey in France. *British Journal of Anaesthesia*, **87**, 549–59. With permission.

replacement solutions, comprising the majority of the remainder[6]. Table 21.4 shows the relative percentages of agents found in Mertes' study[4].

Agents responsible for anaphylaxis

Neuromuscular blocking drugs

The estimated incidence of anaphylactic reactions to muscle relaxants is 1:6500 anaesthetics in which these drugs are employed[10]. Table 21.5 shows the frequencies associated with the use of individual muscle relaxants.

An added danger with muscle relaxants is cross-reactivity. Patients who have had an anaphylactic reaction to one muscle relaxant may react subsequently to any future exposure to a different muscle relaxant.

Latex

The prevalence of latex sensitization varies with the population studied, ranging from 1%[12] to 6.6%[13] and reaching an incidence as high as 15.8% in anaesthetic staff[14]. This sensitivity does not mean that an anaphylactic reaction will occur.

In France, the incidence of allergy to latex increased from 0.5% before 1980 to 19% in 1994[4]. However, the 1997–1998 survey[6] revealed that the incidence had decreased

Table 21.5 Neuromuscular blocking drugs responsible for anaphylactic reactions from a 2-year French survey[6]

Drug	Percentage (%)
Rocuronium	29
Suxamethonium	23
Atracurium	21
Vecuronium	18
Pancuronium	16
Mivacurium	2.7
Cisatracurium	0.3

to 12.1%, suggesting that an increasing awareness of the risk of latex sensitization, and actions taken to reduce exposure of susceptible patients to latex by conducting surgery in a latex-free environment, were beginning to have an effect.

Hypnotic drugs

The estimated incidence of reactions due to thiopentone is 1:30 000, compared to 1:60 000 for propofol[10]. Current evidence suggests that patients who are allergic to egg are no more likely than other patients to suffer an anaphylactic reaction to propofol[10]. Etomidate appears to be the most immunologically safe intravenous anaesthetic drug. There have also been very few reactions reported with the use of ketamine.

Opioid drugs

Reactions to opioids are quoted as being infrequent[10] although the 1997–1998 French survey reported seven cases[6].

Local anaesthetic drugs

Although many patients claim to have had an adverse reaction to a local anaesthetic drug, it is estimated that less than 1% of all reactions have an allergic mechanism[4]. In a series of 208 patients over a 20-year period, Fisher and Bowey[15] found that four patients had an immediate allergic reaction and that another four patients experiencing delayed allergic reactions. Although allergy is more likely to be due to ester local anaesthetic drugs, reactions to amide drugs have also been reported. Some of these reactions may have been due to the preservatives in commercial preparations[16].

Colloid solutions

The range of reactions due to synthetic colloids appears to vary from 0.033% to 0.22%[17]. Reactions to urea-linked gelatin appear to be more frequent than those associated with modified gelatins[18]. Comparative figures for dextrans are 0.27%, albumin 0.009%, and hydroxyethyl starch 0.058%[17].

Other drugs

Antibiotics account for between 2% and 8% of all allergic reactions associated with anaesthesia[6,19]. Cephalosporins account for most in Australia, with penicillin leading the list in France. Protamine has also been incriminated[4] but no figures are quoted.

Screening for anaphylaxis

The enquiring patient may ask whether he or she could or should be screened for allergy. Whitby[20] has proposed criteria that should be used to determine whether screening confers a benefit or not. On the basis of these criteria, Fisher concludes that screening cannot currently be justified and is unlikely to be justified in the future[5].

Risk factors

There are two relevant groups: those with a history of drug allergy and, to a lesser extent, those with a history suggestive of latex sensitivity.

History of drug allergy

Any unexplained life-threatening reaction during a previous anaesthetic must be considered as a possible allergic reaction; if so, re-exposure to the drug or agent is likely to result in a reaction which is at least as severe[21]. The dangers of possible cross-reactions mean that avoiding only the drugs used on the previous occasion may not be sufficient, and so the patient's allergic status should be determined[22]. This is true particularly when a reaction to a neuromuscular blocking drug is suspected. The high incidence of cross-reactions mandates testing for allergy to a number of muscle relaxants before subsequent administration, including testing of drugs that were not available at the time of the possible reaction[23].

Latex allergy

Fisher[5] suggests that there is a strong case for delaying surgery where possible to determine if latex sensitivity is present in spina bifida patients, patients with fruit allergy, and health workers with contact glove allergy. Others have suggested that anaphylaxis to latex in spina bifida patients may be reduced by managing them in latex-free environments from birth[24]. If testing is not possible, it may be prudent to treat these three groups of patients in a latex-free environment.

Pretreatment

There is no evidence that pre-treatment with histamine H_1 or H_2 blockers, or corticosteroids, makes any difference to the likelihood or severity of an acute anaphylactic reaction[4].

Prevention of second or subsequent anaphylactic reactions

A patient who has been investigated appropriately after a suspected anaphylactic reaction should be in possession of relevant information[5]. A Medic-Alert™ bracelet or similar should be worn by the patient, which should contain three pieces of information:

a) Anaphylaxis to Drug X

b) The name of a safe alternative (this should be identifiable from skin testing performed after the reaction)

c) See letter

21.1 Incidence of anaphylaxis associated with the perioperative period

Estimated incidence of Anaphylaxis in the perioperative period ranges from 1 in 1000 to 1 in 20 000.

In the UK, extrapolated figures suggest that the number of reactions associated with anaesthesia is 500 per year.

Mortality, despite appropriate instigation of appropriate therapy, is 4% with a further 2% of patients sustaining severe brain damage.

The letter should be carried by the patient at all times and should detail what happened (the clinical events), the drugs that were used, the results of investigations, and any recommendations. The letter should be modified by the anaesthetist responsible for each subsequent anaesthetic.

Elective patients who have not been investigated should be referred as a matter of urgency. Patients who require emergency surgery should be anaesthetized using a technique that avoids as many potential allergens as possible (e.g. regional technique, or avoid neuromuscular blocking drugs if general anaesthesia is necessary)[25].

Further details of investigations and techniques are beyond the remit of this chapter and the reader is referred to the guidelines on the management of anaphylaxis by the Association of Anaesthetists of Great Britain and Ireland[25a].

Reactions to commonly used anaesthetic drugs

Space does not allow a comprehensive review of all aspects of the drugs commonly used by anaesthetists. The anaesthetist is expected to be familiar with the common pharmacological effects of the drugs that they use, including those effects that are dose-related, such as cardiovascular depression from the intravenous induction agents or inhalational anaesthetics. This section describes adverse reactions, which are not immunological in origin. The intention is to equip the anaesthetist with facts that will be useful in the dialogue with the patient. Common adverse effects will not be discussed in detail although they may be important in such a dialogue; for example, a patient who is already afraid of needles and is then warned of pain on injection from the use of propofol or etomidate may wish to discuss alternatives to intravenous induction of anaesthesia.

Intravenous induction agents

Ketamine and emergence reactions

Emergence reactions associated with the use of ketamine are characterized by vivid dreaming, often associated with excitement, confusion and fear, or a sense of floating out of one's body[26]. The reported incidences range from as low as 3–5% to as high as 100%, but the majority of the evidence suggests that 10–30% of adult patients who receive the drug as the sole or major component of the anaesthetic technique will suffer an emergence reaction[27]. Children appear to be less susceptible than adults[28]. Benzodiazepines appear to most effective in attenuating emergence reactions[27].

Etomidate and adrenal suppression

Etomidate has been shown to interfere with the synthesis of cortisol and so can bring about adrenocortical suppression[29]. This has raised the question of the significance of any adrenocortical suppression following a single dose of etomidate in relation to the overall response to stress associated with major surgery. Reves et al.[30] concluded that there are three facts which suggest that adrenocortical suppression after an induction dose of etomidate is not clinically significant.

1. There are no known reports of any negative clinical outcome associated with induction of anaesthesia using etomidate, despite millions of uses.

2. After induction of anaesthesia using etomidate, the serum cortisol concentration usually remains in the low normal range, and the adrenocortical suppression is a relatively short-lived phenomenon.

3. High-stress surgery can overcome the temporary adrenocortical suppression caused by etomidate.

Propofol infusion syndrome

This rare, but potentially lethal, syndrome is associated with infusions of propofol. Clinical features include cardiomyopathy with acute cardiac failure, metabolic acidosis, skeletal myopathy, hyperkalaemia, hepatomegaly, and lipaemia[31]. Although first described in children, it has been also observed in critically ill adults[32]. An infusion of at least 5 mg kg^{-1} h^{-1} for 48 h or longer appears to be required to generate the syndrome.

Inhalational agents

Hepatotoxicity

The two mechanisms responsible are intrinsic (or dose-related) and idiosyncratic[33]. Intrinsic reactions are dose-dependent and were seen with older agents such as chloroform. Idiosyncratic reactions are caused by products of metabolism of the inhalational agent combining with a protein to form an allergenic complex that provokes a hypersensitivity reaction on subsequent exposure to the drug. Several hundred cases of hepatotoxicity have been attributed to halothane and approximately 50 cases to enflurane[34] but hepatotoxicity appears to be rare in patients who have received isoflurane[35] or desflurane[36]. This pattern reflects the extent of oxidative metabolism of the drugs (halothane 20%, enflurane 2.5%, isoflurane 0.2%, and desflurane 0.01%)[37]. Sevoflurane has been associated with small increases in the serum concentration of liver transaminases but no cases of unequivocal hepatotoxicity have been recorded[38].

Cross-sensitivity may be a feature of fluorinated inhaled anaesthetics and therefore such agents should be avoided if patients give a history of postoperative unexplained hepatotoxicity[39].

Nephrotoxicity

Nephrotoxicity of inhaled anaesthetics has been attributed to fluoride ions generated by metabolism of fluorinated drugs. Serum concentrations of fluoride greater than 50 µmol L^{-1}, below which no renal damage occurs[40], have been reported after prolonged administration of methoxyflurane. These concentrations have not been reported with the use of enflurane, isoflurane or desflurane. After prolonged administration of sevoflurane, the serum concentration of fluoride can increase to more than 50 µmol L^{-1} but decreases much more rapidly than occurred following the use of methoxyflurane[41]. There is no convincing evidence that the use of sevoflurane is associated with nephrotoxicity. It appears to be a combination of peak concentration of serum fluoride and the duration of high concentration (area under the curve) that determines whether renal damage is likely to occur.

Sevoflurane and compound A

The dehydrofluorination of sevoflurane to form compound A is initiated by soda lime abstraction of a proton from the isopropyl group of sevoflurane. This has been shown to cause renal failure in rats when they inhale 25 and 50 parts per million of Compound A for 3 h[42]. It appears to be the total exposure that matters rather than the peak concentration. The safe concentration for compound A in humans is not known. This raises theoretical concerns about using sevoflurane in circle systems with a low fresh gas flow rate for patients with known renal disease.

Haematopoietic and neurological system effects

Nitrous oxide (N_2O) can cause oxidation of the cobalt ion in vitamin B_{12}. Marked megaloblastic changes are seen after 24 h of breathing N_2O at a concentration of 50%[43]. Bone marrow damage may occur even earlier in seriously ill patients[44]. However, subacute combined degeneration of the cord requires much longer exposure (months rather than days) and is only seen in individuals who abuse N_2O on a long-term basis. Experimental data suggest that there is a threshold concentration of 1,000 parts per million for N_2O; below this level, it has no biochemical effect[45].

Malignant hyperthermia

The quoted incidence is 1 in 15 000 anaesthetic procedures but it may be as low as 1 in 50 000 anaesthetic procedures in adults. The mortality rate is higher than 60% in untreated patients[46], but is less than 10% in those appropriately treated.

Anaesthesia and pregnancy

The evidence is that women who undergo surgery during pregnancy for non-obstetric conditions appear have an increased risk of premature birth and some suggestion that general anaesthesia is associated with lower birth weight than regional techniques, though the confounding effect of surgical pathology cannot be excluded[47].

Neuromuscular blocking drugs

Although many adverse effects attributable to the use of muscle relaxant drugs have been described[46], those which are most relevant for disclosure to the patient, and which may be relevant for further discussion between anaesthetist and patient, are myalgia and prolonged neuromuscular block caused by atypical pseudocholinsterase (butyrylcholinesterase), both of which are related to the use of succinylcholine. Malignant hyperthermia may also be attributable to the use of succinylcholine, and has been discussed earlier.

Myalgia

A meta-analysis of 52 randomized trials[48] found that the incidence of fasciculations associated with the use of succinylcholine was 95% and that the incidence of myalgia at 24 h was 50%. The authors were unable to find a clear relationship between fasciculation and myalgia. The best methods of preventing myalgia were administration of a non-steroidal anti-inflammatory drug (number needed to treat 2.5) or rocuronium or lignocaine (number needed to treat 3). Interestingly, they found a lower incidence

Table 21.6 Clinically relevant abnormal variants of butyrylcholinesterase (plasma cholinesterase)

Genotype	Incidence	Effect on duration of succinlycholine
Atypical		
Heterozygous	1 in 25 patients	Prolonged by 30–50%
Homozygous	1 in 3000 patients	Marked prolongation (4 h)
Silent		
Homozygous	1 in 167 000 patients	Extreme prolongation: many hours

of myalgia following administration of succinylcholine 1.5 mg kg^{-1} (44.6%) than after a dose of succinylcholine 1mg kg^{-1} (62.8%)[48].

Atypical butyrylcholinesterase (plasma cholinesterase)

The short duration of action of succinylcholine is due to its rapid hydrolysation by the enzyme butyrylcholinesterase (also known as plasma cholinesterase or pseudo-cholinesterase). In addition to the usual variant (U) of this enzyme, there are several others, which are less effective in the breakdown of succinylcholine, including atypical (A) and silent (S). Their clinical relevance is shown in Table 21.6[46].

Drug errors

Definitions

Human error is defined as the failure of a planned action to be completed as intended (an error of execution) or the use of a wrong plan to achieve an aim (error of planning)[49].

Brennan[50] defined an adverse event in this context as 'an injury caused by medical management rather than the underlying condition of the patient'. An adverse event attributable to error is a 'preventable adverse event'. Adverse drug events are defined as injuries resulting from medical intervention related to a drug[51].

Extent of the problem

The problem at inpatient level

The scale of drug use in health care is such that, even if the percentage experiencing adverse drug events is small, a large number of patients may be harmed. In England, general practitioners prescribe 660 million drugs annually[52].

21.2 Drug errors in anaesthesia

1 error every 133 anaesthetics
1 intravenous drug bolus error in every 200 anaesthetics

Table 21.7 Categories of drug error from a study of 36 health care facilities in the United States[54]

Error	Frequency (%)
Wrong time	43
Omission	30
Wrong dose	17
Unauthorised drug	4

Source: From Barker, K.N., Flynn, E.A., Pepper, G.A., *et al.* (2002). Medication errors observed in 36 health care facilities. *Archives of Internal Medicine*, **162**, 1897–903. With permission.

An analysis of 289 411 medication orders written during one year in a tertiary-care centre teaching hospital revealed that the overall error rate was 3.33 errors for each 1000 orders written[53]. The rate of significant errors was estimated to be 1.81 per 1000 orders. A study of direct observation on adult wards in 36 healthcare institutions reported a 19% frequency of drug administration errors, of which 17% were dose errors[54].

A review of US death certificates, on which death attributable to medication error is a category, showed a 2.57-fold increase in medication errors as the cause of death from 2876 deaths in 1983 to 7931 in 1993[55]. Outpatients deaths due to medication error rose by a factor of 8.48 during that period, compared with a 2.4-fold increase in inpatient deaths. Children are at particular risk of medication errors, primarily because of incorrect dosages[56]. The potential for medication-related error increases as the average number of drugs administered increases. These figures are likely to be an underestimate because not all drug errors are noticed, let alone documented or reported. Classen.[57] identified 731 adverse drug errors in 648 patients but only 92 of these were reported by healthcare providers; the remaining 631 were detected from automated signals.

The problem in anaesthesia

Webster and colleagues[58] provided an estimate of anaesthetic medication error in two New Zealand hospitals. They asked anaesthetists to complete a study form, indicating whether or not a drug administration error had taken place. This helped provide both a high return rate and denominator data. They obtained data for 8000 anaesthetics and found an administration error rate of 7.5 per 1000 anaesthetics, with a 'near miss' rate of 3.7 per 1000 anaesthetics. These translate as one error in every 133 anaesthetics, with one in every 200 involving intravenous administration of a drug bolus. The most frequent errors were dose errors (20%) and drug substitutions (20%). Most (63%) involved intravenous boluses, 20% involved infusions, and 15% related to inhalational agents. This study yielded a higher incidence of drug error than previous studies, which had shown medication error rates of 0.12 to 1.5 per 1000 anaesthetics[59,60]. However, these studies had used the number of anaesthetics administered as the denominator rather than a deliberate classification of each anaesthetic as having an error or not.

Table 21.8 Categories of anaesthetic drug error from a study of data from the Australian Incident Monitoring Study[63]

Errors	Frequency (Total = 896)
Syringe swap	155 (34%)
Ampoule labelling	125 (28%)
Equipment error	234 (26%)
Route of administration error	126 (14%)
Communication error	35 (4%)

Source: From Abeysekera, A., Bergman, I.J., Kluger, M.T., *et al.* (2005). Drug error in anaesthetic practice: a review of 896 reports from the Australian Incident Monitoring Study database. *Anaesthesia*, **60**, 220–7. With permission.

These figures appear to put anaesthesia in a good light compared to the figures for medication errors in inpatient wards. However, the observational studies used to obtain the data for ward studies are much more sensitive than reporting systems, such as those used in the anaesthetic studies. It is therefore difficult to make direct comparisons between ward data and anaesthetic data, using figures from studies carried out to date. One study from the United Kingdom reported 4 'drug-related events' in 130 h of direct observation of anaesthetists at work. Few of the patients in the Webster dataset experienced adverse events. There was no death or permanent disability but there was one case of awareness.

It is not surprising that drug errors occur. One study estimated that each anaesthetic drug administration can be associated with up to 40 component steps[62]. Anaesthetists seldom check drugs with a second individual and, even if they wished to do so, the resources, in the form of other personnel, may not be available. This is true particularly in a crisis, when anaesthetic assistants may have been delegated other tasks to perform.

Abeysekera[63] reviewed 896 reports of drug error in the Australian Incident Monitoring Study (AIMS). They define a drug error, for the purposes of this study, as 'a failure to give the drug or dose of drug that was intended'. They also used the category 'pre-error', which they defined as 'an incident that may have led to a drug error, but in which no drug was given'. They reviewed incidents reported between 1988 and December 2001. They found 896 incidents from 8088 reports. Over half (54%) were associated with emergency procedures, 40% with elective surgery and 6% not specified.

Approximately half of the incidents (452) involved syringe or drug preparation errors. These include syringe swaps, wrong ampoule or labelling errors, and pharmaceutical preparation errors. Syringe swaps accounted for 37% of these errors, with the most common being fentanyl intended but suxamethonium given ($n = 16$). Equipment errors due to misuse or malfunction accounted for 234 (26%) of incidents. Intravenous devices (94/234) and vaporizers (118/234) accounted for the clear majority of problems.

Communication errors were defined as occurring when the narrative suggested that miscommunication between anaesthetic staff and others (such as surgeons or recovery room staff) was the primary cause of failure to give the drug. There were 35 reports of communication error (4%), which included giving the same drug twice ($n = 10$) or failure to give a drug ($n = 5$).

Route of administration errors occurred in 126 (14%) of the reports. The most common errors were inadvertent arterial injection, subcutaneous injection due to a 'tissued' intravenous catheter, and inadvertent intravenous injection when performing epidural or peripheral nerve block.

The most common errors under the category of 'Others' were 'drug being given despite allergy or contra-indication' ($n = 17$) and 'overdose due to entire ampoule being given in one dose' ($n = 12$). It is interesting, but not surprising, that over half of these errors occurred during emergency procedures. The average anaesthetist in Australasia probably gives in excess of 250 000 drug administrations in a professional lifetime, a figure that is unlikely to be radically different from that in UK practice. An error rate of 1 in 133[58] anaesthetics would result in around 1880 errors solely from drug administration.

The psychology of error

The enquiring patient may ask what the individual anaesthetist is doing to prevent or reduce the number and type of errors. To answer this question requires a brief account of the psychology of human error. Reason[49] classifies errors into two categories: active and latent. Active errors may be divided into slips or lapses, and mistakes. A slip or lapse occurs when we are in a familiar environment engaged in routine activity but either fail to do something (a lapse) or do the wrong thing (a slip). Many of these errors are associated with distractions or fatigue. Mistakes occur when something different from routine happens. Normally, we resort to one of a set of precompiled responses that we have learned or acquired. If an inappropriate rule is applied, then this is labelled a 'rule-based mistake'. If we do not have a precompiled response for the situation, then we have to invent a solution. If that solution is inappropriate, then it is labelled a 'knowledge-based mistake'. Examples are given in Box 21.3.

Latent errors are compared to resident pathogens—they are continually present but do not normally cause any problems. However, under certain conditions, they can make a bad situation worse. Latent errors are usually referred to as system failures because they arise from some deficit in the system. An example is given in Box 21.4.

As the example in Box 21.4 illustrates, a serious adverse outcome usually requires a combination of active errors and latent errors. On most occasions when an active error occurs, layers of defence, such as protocols, bring the error to the notice of the anaesthetist or another member of the team before an adverse outcome results. If these defences are eroded (e.g. lack of protocols), or gaps appear (e.g. lack of a specialist nurse on the non-specialist ward), then the active error is more likely to bring about an adverse outcome. When addressing the cause of errors, both the active components and the latent errors must be addressed.

Possible countermeasures against error

The patient, having asked about drug errors, may then ask about the countermeasures that the individual anaesthetist regularly undertakes and about the systems in place in the hospital or department to learn from errors and near misses.

21.3 Different categories of active error with some illustrative examples

Slip

While drawing up my emergency drugs, the anaesthetic assistant asked me if I wanted any controlled drugs for the first patient. I replied fentanyl and promptly put a fentanyl label on to my atropine syringe. Cause—distraction during a task.

Lapse

I had just taken the patient into theatre from the anaesthetic room. The phone rang; the staff in the ward were querying my preoperative instructions for the next patient on the list. I had connected the patient to the breathing system but had not switched the ventilator on. It was only when I had dealt with the phone call that I noticed the lack of a CO_2 trace and then switched on the ventilator. Cause—distraction at a crucial time in a sequence of events.

Mistake (rule-based)

While working with a more junior trainee during a vascular list, the surgeon asked if we could 'reverse the patient'. My more junior colleague then administered intravenous neostigmine and glycopyrrolate. The surgeon had intended that we give protamine to antagonize the heparin that had been given intravenously one hour earlier.

Cause—my more junior colleague had applied the correct rule for 'reverse neuromuscular blockade' but an inappropriate one for 'antagonize heparin'. Right rule, wrong circumstances.

Mistake (knowledge-based)

This example is taken from experience at a simulation centre. As part of a course in dealing with unexpected anaesthetic emergencies, there is a scenario in which the catheter mount is partly obstructed. This brings about an increase in airway pressure and a decrease in oxygen saturation. The patient is a young male with a history of mild asthma who is undergoing an emergency appendicectomy. One trainee, not having a 'rule' to deal with this situation decided to treat the patient as having an acute episode of bronchospasm. He administered intravenous salbutamol. When there was no improvement in the airway pressure, he changed the vaporizer from isoflurane to halothane and then gave this hypoxic and hypercapnic patient an intravenous bolus of aminophylline, resulting in ventricular tachycardia.

Humans find it difficult to work things out from first principles during times of stress. When people are faced with a situation that is different from normal and associated with deterioration in the patient's condition, a normal response is to revert to a rule with which they are familiar that matches some of the features of the condition. Once committed to this course of action, it becomes increasingly difficult to abandon it. This is known as a fixation error. In this example, the trainee did not have a rule for 'unexpected rise in airway pressure' and so reverted to the rule for treating bronchospasm (which was the only condition he had experienced in which unexpected airway pressure appeared). The fixation error brought about an even worse deterioration in the condition of the patient in the scenario.

21.4 A case report illustrating a lethal combination of active and latent errors

This example is taken from the Department of Health publication—*An organization with a Memory*[64]. A child who was a patient in a District General Hospital was due to receive chemotherapy under general anaesthesia at a specialist centre. The child was allowed to eat and drink before leaving the District General Hospital. There then followed a series of events that concluded with the child receiving intrathecal vincristine with fatal consequences.

The case report demonstrates how a combination of active errors on the part of different health care providers combined with deficiencies in the system resulted in a tragic outcome.

Some of the events are listed in the following table:

Event	Type of Error
Child is allowed to eat and drink	Active error (mistake, rule-based)
No beds are available in the oncology ward	Latent error: the specialist knowledge in the oncology ward would be more likely to correct some of the subsequent errors
Patient's notes not available to ward staff on admission	Latent error: more difficult to correct subsequent active errors
No specialist oncology nurse available on ward to administer intravenous vincristine	Latent error: lack of specialist staff
Vincristine and methotrexate were transported together	Active error: mistake, rule-based (protocol violation)
Ward staff informed that both drugs were to go to theatre	Active error: mistake, rule-based (protocol violation)
	Latent error: specialist staff would have known that both drugs should not have gone to theatre so no defence present to counteract the active error

The Department of Health report[52] contains recommendations that attempt to address both active and system errors (see Table 21.9). Merry and colleagues[65] have published evidence-based recommendations to address some of the active error and latent error sources.

More work is currently being undertaken in the field of human factors, which is an iterative process. As the anaesthetic community becomes better acquainted with the vocabulary and terminology of active and latent errors, it should be possible to better reflect on critical incidents and submit more informed and detailed incident reports.

The future

A challenge faced by all anaesthetists is the ability to manage the inter-individual differences between patients. Predicting a patient's response to a particular drug has

Table 21.9 Recommendations to reduce risk of drug error in anaesthesia

1.	Anaesthetists should be aware of the risks of drug errors and ensure that checking procedures are in place. Errors often occur in situations of haste, distraction or fatigue.
2.	Lighting of the operating room environment is critical for safety. In situations of reduced lighting, specific arrangements should be made for checking anaesthetic drugs.
3.	Drug storage arrangements should be consistent in all anaesthetic care delivery units.
4.	Ampoules should be read and re-read before drugs are drawn up into a syringe. Errors are unlikely to be detected once the syringe is prepared.
5.	Ideally, drugs are prepared by the person who will administer them, immediately before use.
6.	Syringes should be labelled with the name and concentration.
7.	Syringes intended for an emergency should be stored away from the immediate work area.
8.	The international colour-coded syringe labelling system should be used.
9.	Consider using pre-filled syringes for emergency drugs that are prepared by the pharmacy unit to assure the quality of contents and accurate handling.
10.	Pharmacists should regularly visit operating theatres and anaesthetic rooms to ensure safe drug use.
11.	When drug manufacturer, packaging or formulations change, theatre staff should be alerted before the drug becomes routinely available in the operating theatre.

Source: From Orser, B.A. and Byrick, R. (2004). Anesthesia-related medication error: time to take action. *Canadian Journal of Anesthesia*, **51**, 756–60. With permission.

Modified by Orser from Department of Health. (2004). *Building a safer NHS for patients: improving medication safety* (ed. Jim Smith). A report by the Chief Pharmaceutical Officer. DH Publications, London.

long been a goal of clinicians[67]. Pharmacogenetics is well known to anaesthetists because of their understanding of malignant hyperpyrexia and atypical plasma cholinesterase. However, other causes of inter-individual variability in response to anaesthetic drugs are less clear[67,68].

References

1. WHO. International drug monitoring: the role of national centres. Technical Report Series WHO 1972, no 498.

2. Edwards, I.R. and Aronson, J.K. (2000). Adverse drug reactions: Definitions, diagnosis, and management. *Lancet*, **356**,1255–9.

3. Sitter, H., Torossian, A., Duda, D., and Sattler, J. (2004). Classification of perioperative histamine-related reactions. *Inflammation Research*, **Supplement 2**, S164–S168.

4. Mertes, P.M. and Laxenaire, M-C. (2002). Allergic reactions occurring during anaesthesia. *European Journal of Anaesthesiology*, **19**, 240–62.

5. Fisher, M.M. and Doig, G.S. (2004). Prevention of anaphylactic reactions to anaesthetic drugs. *Drug Safety*, **27**, 393–410.

6. Laxenaire, M-C. and Mertes, P.M. (2001). Anaphylaxis during anaesthesia. Results of a two-year survey in France. *British Journal of Anaesthesia*, **87**, 549–59.

7. Currie, M., Webb, R.K., Williamson, J.A., Russell, W.J., and Mackay, P. (1993). The Australian Incident Monitoring Study. Clinical Anaphylaxis: an analysis of 2000 incident reports. *Anaesthesia in Intensive Care*, **21**, 621–5.

8. Fisher, M.M. and Baldo, B.A. (1993). The incidence and clinical features of anaphylactic reactions during anaesthesia in Australia. *Annales Francaises D' anesthesie Et De Reanimation*, **12**, 97–104.

9. Laxenaire, M-C., Mouton, C., Frederic, A., Viry-Babel, F., and Bouchon, Y. (1996). Anaphylactic shock after tourniquet removal in orthopedic surgery. *Annales Francaises D' anesthesie Et De Reanimation*, **15**, 179–84.

10. Hepner, D.L. and Castells, M.C. (2003). Anaphylaxis during the perioperative period. *Anesthesia and Analgesia*, 97, 1381–95.

11. Baldo, B.A. and Fisher, M.M. (1983). Substituted ammonium ions as allergenic determinants in drug allergy. *Nature*. **306**, 262–4.

12. Turjanmaa, K. and Reunala, T. (1990). Incidence of positive prick test to rubber protein. *Contact Dermatitis*, **23**, 279.

13. AORN latex guideline. (1999). In *Standards, recommended practices and Guidelines*, 93–108. Association of Operating Room Nurses, Inc., Denver.

14. Konrad, C., Fieber, T., Gerber, H., Schuepfer, G., and Muellner, G. (1997). The prevalence of latex sensitivity among anesthesiology staff. *Anesthesia and Analgesia*, **84**, 629–33.

15. Fisher, M.M. and Bowey, C.J. (1997). Alleged allergy to local anaesthetics. *Anaesthesia in Intensive Care*, **25**, 611–4.

16. Dooms-Goossens, A., de Alam, A.G., Degreef, H., and Kochuyt, A. (1989). Local anaesthetic intolerance due to metabisulfite. *Contact Dermatitis*, **20**, 124–6.

17. Ring, J. and Messmer, K. (1977). Incidence and severity of anaphylactoid reactions to colloid volume substitutes. *Lancet*, **1**, 466–9.

18. Laxenaire, M.C., Charpentie,r C., and Feldman, L. (1994). Anaphylactoid reactions to colloid plasma substitutes: incidence, risk factors, mechanisms. A French multicenter prospective study. *Annales Francaises D' anesthesie Et De Reanimation*, **13**, 301–10.

19. Fisher, M.M. and Baldo, B.A. (1998). Mast cell tryptase in anaesthetic anaphylactoid reactions. *British Journal of Anaesthesia*, **80**, 26–9.

20. Whitby, L.G. (1974). Definitions and criteria: screening for disease. *Lancet*, **ii**, 3–5.

21. Fisher, M. and Baldo, B.A. (1994). Anaphylaxis during anaesthesia: current aspects of diagnosis and prevention. *European Journal of Anaesthesiology*, **11**, 263–84.

22. Laroche, D., Bricard, H., and Laxenaire, M.C. (1998). Allergo-anesthesia consultation: not enough patients are tested after an anaphylactoid anaesthetic incident. *Annales Francaises D' anesthesie Et De Reanimation*, **17**, 89–90.

23. Fisher, M.M., Merefield, D., and Baldo, B. (1999). Failure to prevent an anaphylactic reaction to a second neuromuscular blocking drug during anaesthesia. *British Journal of Anaesthesia*, **82**, 770–3.

24. Nieto, A., Mazon, A., Pamies, R., *et al.* (2002). Efficacy of latex avoidance for primary prevention of latex sensitisation in children with spina bifida. *Journal of Pediatrics*, **140**, 370–2.

25. Association of Anaesthetists of Great Britain and Ireland. (2003). *Suspected anaphylactic reactions associated with anaesthesia* (revised 3rd edition). Association of Anaesthetists of Great Britain and Ireland and British Society for Allergy and Clinical Immunology, London.

25a. Association of Anaesthetists of Great Britain and Ireland. Allergies and anaphylaxis. http://www.aagbi.org/anaphylaxisdatabase.htm (last accessed 2nd December, 2008).

26. Garfield, J.M., Garfield, F.B., Stone, J.G., Hopkins, D., and Johns, L.A. (1972). A comparison of psychologic responses to ketamine and thiopental-nitrous oxide-halothane anaesthesia. *Anesthesiology*, **36**, 329–38.

27. White, P.F., Way, W.L., and Trevor, A.J. (1982). Ketamine – its pharmacology and therapeutic uses. *Anesthesiology*, **56**, 119–36.

28. Sussman, D.R. (1974). A comparative evaluation of ketamine anaesthesia in children and adults. *Anesthesiology*, **40**, 459–64.

29. Lamberts, S.W., Bons, E.G., Bruining, H.A., and de Jong, F.H. (1987). Differential effects of the imidazole derivatives etomidate, ketoconazole and miconazole and of metyrapone on the secretion of cortisol and its precursors by human adrenocortical cells. *Journal of Pharmacology and Expermental Therapeutics*, **240**, 259–64.

30. Reves, J.G., Glass, P.S.A., Lubarsky, S.A., and McEvoy, M.D. (2005). Intravenous nonopioid anesthetics. In *Miller's Anesthesia* (ed. R.D. Miller), pp. 317–78, 6th edition. Elsevier, Philadelphia..

31. Hanna, J.P. and Ramundo, M.L. (1998). Rhabdomyolysis and hypoxia associated with prolonged propofol infusion in children. *Neurology*, **50**, 301–3.

32. Funston, J.S. and Prough, D.S. (2004). Two reports of propofol anesthesia associated with metabolic acidosis in adults. *Anesthesiology*, **101**, 6–8.

33. Pohl, L.R., Satoh, H., Christ, D.D., and Kenna, J.G. (1988). The immunologic and metabolic basis of drug hypersensitivities. *Annual Review of Pharmacology and Toxicology*, **28**, 367–87.

34. Lewis, J.H., Zimmerman, H.J., Ishak, K.G., and Mullick, F.G. (1983). Enflurane hepatotoxicity: a clinicopathologic study of 24 cases. *Annals of Internal Medicine*, **98**, 984–92.

35. Sinha, A., Clatch, R.J., Stuck, G., Blumenthal, S.A., and Patel, S.A. (1996). Isoflurane hepatotoxicity: a case report and review of the literature. *American Journal of Gastroenterology*, **91**, 2406–9

36. Martin, J.L., Plevack, D.J., Charlton, M., *et al.* (1995). Hepatotoxicity after desflurane anesthesia. Anesthesiology, **83**, 1125–9.

37. Njoku, D., Laster, M.J., Gong, D.H., Eger, E.I., Reed, G.F., and Martin, J.L. (1997). Biotransformation of halothane, enflurane, isoflurane, and desflurane to trifluoroacetylated liver proteins: Association between protein acylation and hepatic injury. *Anesthesia and Analgesia*, **84**, 173–8.

38. Ray, D.C., Bomont, R., Mizushima, A., Kugimiya, T., Forbes Howie, A., and Beckett, G.J. (1996). Effect of sevoflurane anaesthesia on plasma concentrations of glutathione S-transferase. *British Journal of Anaesthesia*, **77**, 404–7.

39. Martin, J.L. and Njoku, D.B. (2005). Metabolism and toxicity of modern inhaled anesthetics. In *Miller's Anesthesia* (ed. R.D. Miller), pp. 231–72, 6th edition. Elsevier, Philadelphia.

40. Mazze, R.I., Cousins, M.J., and Jackson, S.H. (1971). Renal dysfunction associated with methoxyflurane anaesthesia. A randomised prospective clinical evaluation. *Journal of the American Medical Association*, **216**, 278–88.

41. Kobayashi, Y., Ochiai, R., Takeda, J., Sekiguchi, H., and Fukushima, K. (1992). Serum and urinary inorganic fluoride concentrations after prolonged inhalation of sevoflurane in humans. *Anesthesia and Analgesia*, **74**, 753–7.

42. Gonsowski, C.T., Laster, M.J., Eger, E.I., Ferrell, L.D., and Kerschmann, R.L. (1994). Toxicity of compound A in rats. Effect of a 3-hour administration. *Anesthesiology*, **80**, 556–65.

43. O'Sullivan, H., Jennings, F., Ward, K., McCann, S., Scott, J.M., and Weir, D.G. (1981). Human bone marrow biochemical function and megaloblastic hematopoiesis after nitrous oxide anaesthesia. *Anesthesiology*, **55**, 645–9.

44. Amos, R.J., Amess, J.A., Hinds, C.J., and Mollin, D.L. (1982). Incidence and pathogenesis of acute megaloblastic bone-marrow change in patients receiving intensive care. *Lancet*, **2**, 835–8.

45. National Institute for Occupational Safety and Health (NIOSH). (1977). Criteria for a recommended standard for occupation exposure to waste anesthetic gases and vapors. pp. 77–140. NIOSH Publications, Washington D.C.

46. Naguib, M. and Magboul, M.M.A. (1998). Adverse effects of neuromuscular blockers and their antagonists. *Drug Safety*, **18**, 99–116.

47. Jenkins, T.M., Mackey, S.F., Benzoni,E.M., Tolosa, J.E., and Sciscione, A.C. (2003). Non-obstetric surgery during gestation: Risk factors for lower birthweight. The *Australian and New Zealand Journal of Obstetrics and Gynaecology*, **43**, 27–31.

48. Schreiber, J-U., Lysakowski, C., Fuchs-Buder, T., and Tramèr, M.R. (2005). Prevention of succinylcholine-induced fasciculation and myalgia: a meta-analysis of randomized trials. *Anesthesiology*, **103**, 877–84.

49. Reason, J. (1990). *Human Error*, Cambridge University Press, Cambridge, UK.

50. Brennan, T.A., Leape, L.L., Laird, N.M., *et al.* (1991). Incidence of adverse events and negligence in hospitalized patients. Result of the Harvard Medical Practice study. *New England Journal of Medicine*, **324**, 370–6.

51. Bates, D.W., Boyle, D.L., Vander vliet, M.B., Schneider, J., and Leape, L. (1995). Relationship between medication errors and adverse drug events. *Journal of General Internal Medicine*, **10**, 199–205.

52. Department of Health. (2004). *Building a safer NHS for patients: improving medication safety* (ed. Jim Smith). A report by the Chief Pharmaceutical Officer. DH Publications, London.

53. Lesar, T.S., Briceland, L., and Stein, D.S. (1997). Factors related to errors in medication prescribing. *Journal of the American Medical Association*, **277**, 312–7.

54. Barker, K.N., Flynn, E.A., Pepper, G.A., Bates, D.W., and Mikeal, R.L. (2002). Medication errors observed in 36 health care facilities. *Archives of Internal Medicine*, **162**, 1897–903.

55. Phillips, D.P., Christenfeld, N., and Glynn, L.M. (1998). Increase in US medication-error deaths between 1983 and 1993. *Lancet*, **351**, 643–44.

56. Koren, G. and Haslam, R.H. (1994). Pediatric medication errors: predicting and preventing tenfold disasters. *Journal of Clinical Pharmacology*, **34**, 1043–5.

57. Classen, D.C., Pestonik, S.L., Evans, R.S., and Burke, J.P. (1991). Computerised surveillance of adverse drug events in hospital patients. *Journal of the American Medical Association*, **266**, 2847–51.

58. Webster, C.S., Merry, A.F., Larsson, L., McGrath, K.A., and Weller, J. (2001). The frequency and nature of drug administration error during anaesthesia. *Anaesthesia in Intensive Care*, **29**, 494–500.

59. Craig, J. and Wilson, M.E. (1981). A survey of anaesthetic misadventures. *Anaesthesia*, **36**, 933–6.

60. Chopra, V., Bovill, J.G., and Spierdijk, J. (1990). Accidents, near accidents and complications during anaesthesia. A retrospective analysis of a 10-year period in a teaching hospital. *Anaesthesia*, **45**, 3–6.

61. Smith, A.F., Goodwin, D., Mort, M., and Pope, C. (2005). Categorisation and significance of non-conformities in anaesthetic practice: pointers from the Lancaster expertise study. *British Journal of Anaesthesia*, **94**, 405.

62. Fraind, D.B., Slagle, J.M., Tubbesing, V.A., Hughes, S.A., and Weinger, M.B. (2002). Reengineering intravenous drug and fluid administration processes in the operating room. Step one: task analysis of existing processes. *Anesthesiology*, **97**, 139–47.

63. Abeysekera, A., Bergman, I.J., Kluger, M.T., and Short, T.G. (2005). Drug error in anaesthetic practice: a review of 896 reports from the Australian Incident Monitoring Study database. *Anaesthesia*, **60**, 220–7.

64. Department of Health. (2000). *An organization with a memory*. A report by the Chief Medical Officer. (ed. Liam Donaldson) DH Publications, London.

65. Jensen, L.S., Merry, A.F., Webster, C.S., Weller, J., and Larsson, L. (2004). Evidence-based strategies for preventing drug administration errors during anaesthesia. *Anaesthesia*, **59**, 493–504.

66. Orser, B.A. and Byrick, R. (2004). Anesthesia-related medication error: time to take action. *Canadian Journal of Anesthesia*, **51**, 756–60.

67. Palmer, S.N., Giesecke, N.M., Body, S.C., Shrnan, S.K., Fox, A.A., and Collard, C.D. (2005). Pharmacogenetics of anesthetic and analgesic agents. *Anesthesiology*, **102**, 663–71.

68. Meyer, U.A. (2000). Pharmacogenetics and adverse drug reactions. *Lancet*, **356**, 1667–71.

Section 4

Personal perspectives

Chapter 22

Consent in anaesthesia

Bertie Leigh

Respect for the autonomy of the patient in the eyes of the law has increased, is increasing, and ought to be diminished. This chapter will examine the truth of this proposition, describe the mischief to which it gives rise, and identify steps that anaesthetists can take to protect themselves until the fashion changes.

It is almost 100 years since Cardozo J said:

> Every human being of adult years and sound mind has a right to determine what shall be done with his own body; and a surgeon who performs an operation without his patient's consent commits an assault, for which he is liable in damages[1].

This remark is now regarded as an axiom, having been cited with approval by the House of Lords on at least two occasions. The proposition is not in any way surprising, reflecting as it does the ancient principle in English Common Law that any intentional touching of a person is unlawful and amounts to the tort of battery unless it is justified by consent or some other lawful authority. In practice, this means that doctors operate on patients only when they consent or when they are incapable of consent. What is much newer, and has developed only during the last 50 years, is the idea that the doctor seeking the consent of a patient owes a duty to act as a reasonable doctor would act in advising of the risks involved. *Bolam*[2] was itself a case of consent, but the first case (*Chatterton*) concerned solely with the issue of what precisely a doctor has to do in order to avoid a finding of negligence was decided in 1981[3]. During the last 25 years, the law has become progressively more rigorous, and as I shall argue, the assumptions that prevail in the court now correspond less closely to the assumptions that prevail among staff and patients in the hospital. The danger is that this represents a loss of balance. At the time of the *Chatterton* case, medical ethics were much influenced by the view that there were four ethical propositions that had to be kept in balance. The most important was beneficence—the obligation to act in the patient's best interests; the second was non-maleficence—do no harm; the third was the obligation to act justly; and the fourth was an obligation to respect the patient's autonomy. Over the last 25 years, the last of these has grown like a cuckoo's egg until it threatens the health of the other inhabitants of the nest.

Because respecting autonomy is undoubtedly a good thing, it may, and certainly appears by the House of Lords, to be regarded as unobjectionable. However, a glance at the history of the Animal Rights campaign demonstrates that it is certainly possible to have too much of a good thing. At the time of Schloendorff's case[1], the partners in my firm were much preoccupied with the cruelty involved in vivisection on dogs.

Coleridge v Baylis (1903) was a *cause célèbre* tried by the Lord Chief Justice with a jury. It is easy to understand the feelings of the anti-vivisectionists of a century ago who were motivated by feelings of kindness and benevolence towards animals. Today, animal experiments are performed under quite different circumstances, and the animals are treated with more respect than vermin are in most of their other interactions with human society. Yet such is the intolerance of the activists that despite this improvement, they have adopted measures pioneered by political terrorists. They have sought, by threats and blackmail, to prevent third parties supplying innocuous services to people who are peripherally concerned with medical research. This represents a loss of the ability to balance the desirable objective of medical progress against another desirable objective for the avoidance of animal suffering. As a result of this loss of balance, people who set out with laudable intentions may find themselves acting in a fashion regarded by civil society and the law as evil.

The case of *Chester v Afshar*[4] shows how the law is also capable of losing its balance. I must declare an interest because my firm acted for Mr Afshar, but I do not believe this has much affected my view. The story is a familiar one. Miss Chester was a sophisticated journalist who went to see Mr Afshar, a surgeon, one Friday afternoon because she had a very unpleasant pain emanating from her back. She carried a referral letter saying that she was reluctant to undergo surgery. She had already undergone a series of medical treatments including injections over a period of six years, which had failed to relieve her pain. Her latest exacerbation was due to a prolapsed disc, which the experts agreed would be at least as hazardous to treat conservatively as it would be to treat surgically. Mr Afshar gave her what was found to be admirable advice about the diagnosis and prognosis and, as a result, she was persuaded to abandon her previous reluctance and to undergo a three level micro-discectomy on the following Monday.

Mr Afshar made no notes of the advice that he gave but insisted that he had given the conventional advice that this sort of surgery is associated with a 1% risk of permanent damage. The discussion between them lasted some 30 min. Miss Chester said that he told her only that he had never crippled anyone yet, which he agreed would not have on its own discharged his duty to warn. Unpersuaded by the proposition that Mr Afshar would be unlikely to abandon his standard pattern of advice so completely, or that Miss Chester would be unlikely to change her mind without asking more direct questions about the risks involved, the Judge preferred her memory of the conversation so that breach of duty was established.

The defence did not argue that a respectable body of opinion would not mention the risk. This demonstrates that, in the 20 years since we were preoccupied with the case of *Sidaway*[5], there has been a greater change in attitudes to consent than there has been progress towards greater safety in spinal surgery. Mrs Sidaway's operation was a far more ambitious and hazardous procedure than Miss Chester's. Mrs Sidaway underwent a C4 laminectomy and a facetectomy of the disc space between C4 and C5; she had previously undergone a C5/6 discectomy and fusion and suffered from a congenital fusion of C2 and C3 with a central canal stenosis at C5 and C6. In short, hers was a re-operation on a cervical spine which was congenitally abnormal. The progress in the arts of diagnostic imaging, surgery and anaesthesia between 1974 and 1994 must have reduced the real risks to Miss Chester considerably further. Yet 20 years of social progress meant that the respectable body of opinion which would have failed to mention the far lower risks involved in her surgery had vanished by 1994. The law had not changed, inasmuch as the obligation was still to mention those risks that a reasonable body of opinion would have mentioned. Because the *Bolam* test means that the law holds up a mirror to professional practice, the obligation on the doctor is quite different. Just as the anti-vivisectionists are less tolerant of less animal suffering, patients are, at least in the eyes of the law after a complication, insistent upon being told of much less likely hazards after much safer surgery.

It was thus common ground by the time the case came to appeal that whether Mr Afshar or the Almighty was responsible in law for Miss Chester's misfortune depended upon whether his failure to mention the risk had caused her harm. One might suppose that this was a simple issue of whether she would have had the operation if he had warned her of the risk. She said she did not know the answer to this question. She said she would have sought a second opinion. The evidence was that that second opinion would have come from Professor Crockard, who gave evidence that he would have advised that conservative treatment would be significantly more hazardous than surgery.

The Court of Appeal was persuaded by an Australian decision, *Chappel v Hart*[6], in which it was said that in such circumstances, the doctor would be liable. The facts were slightly different, however, because Mrs Chappel said that she would have made sure that she underwent the operation only in the hands of the foremost expert in Australia, which was not Miss Chester's case. What weighed with the Court of Appeal was the fact that, by the end of the operation on the Monday, Miss Chester had certainly been the victim of misfortune and had sustained her lesion. If she had delayed the operation, say until the Wednesday, when she would have obtained a second opinion, the chances that she would have experienced the misfortune on that day would have been 1%. Thus the chances were 99:1 that her misfortune had happened because, as a result of relying on Mr Afshar's advice, she had undergone the operation on the Monday. This argument always suffered from the weakness that it would have applied equally if the operation had been delayed only by a couple of hours. It was dismantled in the House of Lords by Lord Hoffman who likened it to the proposition that a man debating whether to try his luck in a casino would, on learning that the chances of No 7 coming up at roulette were 1 in 37, would decide to come back next week or go to a different casino.

The majority of the House of Lords saw what to most people looks like a question of fact—did Mr Afshar's breach of duty cause Miss Chester to undergo an operation—as being more usefully decided as a question of public policy. It should be better answered by asking whether, all things considered, the defendant *should* be held liable for the harm that ensued. They took cognizance of the imbalance of power between doctor and patient. They followed Professor Honoré, an Oxford academic, and decided the case on two simple propositions, both of which are so exaggerated as to be as misleading as the Animal Rights Activists' concern for animal welfare. They are:

1 That Miss Chester's right to autonomy is of profound importance and must be respected by the medical profession and the law; and

2 If the surgeon who fails to mention the risk is not put in the position of the insurer of that risk, the duty identified in Proposition 1 will be emptied of its content.

Remarkably, some of their Lordships felt that Miss Chester should not be penalized for her honesty in saying that she did not know whether she would have gone ahead with the procedure.

Let us examine the two propositions in turn. I suggest that one relevant question in respect of the first is whether it is a true reflection of the attitudes of a significant body of people who undergo medical treatment. When Miss Chester was forced to seek the advice of Mr Afshar, was she seeking an opportunity to exercise her right to autonomy, or a remedy for a disabling and very unpleasant condition? If it be the latter, is it very likely that the former would be uppermost in her mind, or is the reality that most patients pay as little attention to the risks of surgery as they do to the details printed in 6-point typeface on the reverse of a car hire insurance contracts?

Numerous studies have sought to ascertain what patients actually remember at an interval after being counselled for surgery. Thirty-two such studies were reviewed by Lemaire[7]. These questioned patients as to what they remembered at intervals varying between one day and nine months after they gave consent to surgery, which had proved uncomplicated. The studies varied in design and setting, so that it is not surprising that the results are similarly varied, but the overall direction is consistent. Inquiries on the same day that the information was given showed an 18–81% recall of significant details. After one week, between 25 and 58% of the information was recalled; after six weeks, the percentage recall was 40–48%, and after six months, the percentage of information recalled varied between 10 and 29%. In some studies, a significant proportion of patients failed to recall any of the major items about which they had been informed, particularly those related to risks and complications. These were patients who were not engaged in litigation and had no possible motive for dissimulating, but in one study, 16 of 20 patients wrongly denied that major risks had been discussed with them.

This is not exactly surprising. When we consult doctors, we do not go to exercise a dog named our Autonomy, we go to get better. The doctor may say 'I cannot decide for you' or offer options for our tentative consideration in an ostensibly undirective fashion. But however it is put, most people respond by asking what the doctor advises or what the doctor would do if he or she had the same problem. Most of us want the doctor's advice, not his or her doubts. When we hire a car on holiday, few people turn the form over and attempt to read the small print on the back of the agreement. Some of us, especially lawyers, feel that we should, but in almost every case, we do not bother, trusting the hire company to have written a reasonable agreement, and the law to ensure that it will not be enforced to our detriment if it is unreasonable.

Nor is it entirely surprising that the majority of the House of Lords should have forgotten this. They are only human and no more likely to remember their few altercations with surgeons than the rest of society. That said, Lemaire did find good evidence that the ability to understand information is related to age and education: most studies reported that a lower education level was associated with a negative influence on comprehension and memory. Recall of information was also negatively influenced by older age.

Lemaire himself suggested that this impugned the patients' capacity to consent. This does not seem right. Many of us have to be prompted by the waiter before we remember what we ordered in a restaurant, and few of us could reel off the dishes we did not order—which is a closer analogy to the risks we decide not to deter us from having a procedure. Yet, no one suggests that deficiency should deprive us of the right to choose. Nevertheless, it does suggest that Professor Honoré and the House of Lords put substantially more importance on the patient's right to be informed of every risk than patients do themselves. As a result, the behaviour of both doctors and patients is being distorted to fit a model designed by the Judiciary: 'I do not care what you want to do, Mrs Sidaway: we must now have a discussion which is designed to command the approval of three members of the House of Lords and I will refuse to operate on you unless you pay attention.'

The second premise of the decision in Afshar is not central to this argument, but I suggest that it is no more robust than the first. The duties on doctors do not depend for their force on any obligation on those who indemnify the doctors to compensate the patient if things go wrong. The obligation to counsel appropriately is no different from any other duty in this respect. It is enforced through a multiplicity of pressures, including the requirements of the GMC and the clinical governance arrangements of employers. Most formative is probably the pressure from peers: this is communicated by the Association of Anaesthetists of Great Britain and Ireland and the Royal College of Anaesthetists by trainers and through the host of writings and lectures that contribute to continuing medical education. The revolution in attitudes as to what should be said in the 20 years between *Sidaway* and *Afshar* has not been in response to any specific decision of the GMC or the courts.

It would be wrong to suppose that the rule in *Afshar* appears to have significant implications for other professionals. By an extraordinary coincidence, less than one month after the judgement for Miss Chester, her barrister, Miss Jacqueline Perry, appealed to the Lords herself, claiming that she owed no duty to mention the risks inherent in her advice to a client[8]. She had thought that a payment into court in settlement of another clinical negligence claim was less than the case was likely to be worth, provided she succeeded in an application to admit a new medical report, and so she advised Mr Moy that the offer be rejected. She failed to trouble her client with the knowledge that she thought there was a 50% chance of the court rejecting her application to admit the new medical report, because she believed he would have a claim against his solicitor for having failed to serve the report in time. In doing so, she ignored the fact that her client might lack the enthusiasm for further litigation, or that the solicitor might have a defence she had overlooked. The application to admit the report failed, and the payment into court was not beaten. When Mr Moy sued the solicitor, Miss Perry was sued as a co-defendant for failing to warn of the 50% risk that the application might fail. Truly one might suppose, a case of the biter bit.

The majority of the House of Lords found that barristers do not have a duty to spell out the reasons for their advice, that in Lady Hale's words '*there is still a respectable body of professional opinion that the client pays for the advocate's opinion not her doubts*'. Lord Carswell said that the court should be slow to hold advocates to blame '*if they concentrated on giving clear and readily understood advice to their clients about the course of action they recommended*' and that it would not be in the best interests of clients to adopt the practice of defensive advocacy in advising litigants about the course to be taken. The duty of an advocate does not require him to give full reasons for that advice, or the risks inherent in following it. This must seem odd to Mr Moy, who can hardly have intended to assign to his counsel the right to decide whether to take the risk. Most clients are advised by most counsel and solicitors that the law is a hazardous area and that half the cases argued are lost by one side or the other, so that the risks of disaster are much higher than they are in medicine. Outside the leafy groves of academe, lawyers level with their clients to the best of their ability and put the client in as good a position as possible to choose between unattractive options. The model for counsel as approved by the House of Lords still seems to be Sir Lancelot Spratt: *'Don't trouble, my man – this is doctors' business, nothing to do with you'* as he described a generous laparotomy with a crayon on a patient's abdomen.

We have since learned that *Afshar* does not apply to solicitors or independent financial advisers. One of the many problems with this situation is that we do not know how far it goes for doctors.

A host of surgical operations are now being replaced by less invasive interventions. Anaesthetists and radiologists now routinely undertake procedures which do not involve surgery in the traditional sense, but which are not without risk. There is no reason to suppose that different rules will apply to such procedures than to operations.

The risks of conservative advice?

It seems clear that the law Lords were influenced by the peculiar sensitivity of the law to any interference with a person's body. Yet, suppose that Mr Afshar had advised Miss Chester to persist with conservative management knowing, as he did, that there was a risk of her suffering an acute prolapse with permanent damage, and had failed to mention the risk involved, even though in the view of Professor Crockard it was greater than the risk of surgery. Would he become the insurer of that risk? The patient's right to self-determination surely involves her in being informed of the risks of following a doctor's advice whether that advice is to undergo surgery or not. If the answer is no, why? The choice he was helping her to make involved balancing two sets of risks, and it seems counter-intuitive that the obligation to explain should vary according to the nature of the advice. It seems even odder that the law's conception of causation of a complication should vary according to whether a doctor who advised one to take a risk ended up advising the patient to risk surgical rather than conservative treatment. The answer, according to Professor Honoré's argument, is that the surgeon has caused the damage by his operation, but in fact that is hardly the point because the surgeon was not negligent in the performance of the procedure. The patient who was properly counselled in the direction of conservative management and who did not wish to take the risk could easily obtain a second opinion. If an unmentioned risk eventuates, such a patient has suffered the damage as a result of accepting the doctor's advice.

What about medical therapy?

Many medical therapies involve risks as serious as those attached to surgery. For example, treatment with steroids commonly involves a high probability of significant side-effects in pursuit of desirable ends. Will a doctor be held to have caused the side-effects if the patient persuades the court that they were not mentioned, even if it is conceded that the patient would still have elected to take the medication once the reasons for the advice had been spelled out? Professor Honoré's policy considerations appear to be equally cogent. The implications of this proposition for anaesthetists are profound. You would be put in the position of insuring your patients against the side-effects of every drug you administer unless you explain those risks in detail, and it does not seem to matter whether the damage is a predictable side-effect or an unusual hazard, provided that there is a duty to warn. It is arguable that different considerations would apply to drugs you prescribe rather than administer, on the basis of the proposition that it is the administration of the drug that causes the damage, and the person who administers does something more tactile to the body of the patient than the prescriber. However this seems to be an unsatisfactory distinction.

And negative medical therapy? Is the doctor to be the patient's insurer in respect of all the risks that he should have mentioned as a result of not taking a pill?

One cannot advise that the position is clear: in reality, we do not know the answers to any of these questions and the law has shown a commendable agility in avoiding the consequences of apparently illogical previous decisions.

It is also worth pointing out that *Chester* does not displace *Sidaway* in setting the duty. An anaesthetist who fails to mention the risk of a drug he prescribes will still escape liability if he acts in accordance with a respectable body of opinion. However, the policy considerations which appear to upend logic when defining causation will find a ready ally in the *Bolitho*[9] exemption: a school of thought, however numerous or eminent its adherents may be, will not be respectable if it does not 'stand up to analysis.' Does this mean that the harassed anaesthetist must take pages from the Datasheet Compendium into every anaesthetic clinic and counsel patients about the risks inherent in each of the agents he may use? I do not think so, this year at least, but as we can see from the change between *Sidaway* and *Afshar*, the standard is shifting, and I think that doctors need to be much more aware of the model for their consultations which has been fashioned for them by the Judiciary. The present state of advice that I give still reflects that described in the Report of the Association of Anaesthetists of Great Britain and Ireland Working Party on Consent for Anaesthesia[10], which is available on the Association website.

The most obvious implication of *Afshar* is to bring home to doctors that, in the eyes of the law, the process of advising patients is now as important as taking their history, examining their bodies, forming a diagnosis or indeed delivering the treatment. The fact that patients do not agree, as Lemaire's review demonstrated, is irrelevant. If this proposition is indeed the basis of *Afshar* then it ought to apply equally to any risk, whether of surgical or medical treatment, or passive watchfulness.

It is fair to say that the decision of the majority in *Afshar* has been roundly criticized in many quarters. However, it may be decades before the House of Lords returns to the subject, and doctors will be well advised to act defensively in this situation.

What should doctors do about it?

It is easier to advise doctors what they should do about it than it will be for doctors to follow that advice. You should make detailed records of the advice you give and the risks you mention. You cannot rely on your memory or that of your patients. It was common ground that Mr Afshar spent 30 min discussing the implications of her surgery with Miss Chester. But as Lemaire's review demonstrates, it is not surprising that she did not remember any risks being mentioned. If it is not written down, the court is likely to find that it did not happen. The doctor's duty is to explain the risks in a fashion that the patient can understand, and this means that the record must demonstrate that that duty was discharged. The advice must be given in a comprehensive fashion. 'Nerve damage' or 'neurological damage' will not convey to many patients that their sexual, bowel, bladder, and lower limb functions are all at risk, or what may happen in practice if things go wrong.

Much use can be made of printed material, but the counsellor has a duty to ensure that it has been understood. This means that it must be in a language appropriate to the patient and his or her level of education.

I regularly see notes in which the history and the record of the examination run to many pages. The investigations are voluminous. However, it is unusual to see notes that list all of the options that were discussed with the patient, including the risks and benefits both of the options that were chosen and those which were not. When risks are recorded, it is usually in a summary form, which does not tell us explicitly what was said. The words:

risks - CNS, bleeding, infection

may provide an admirable aide memoire that the doctor could expand, but they do not make clear to a sceptical Judge, who is sympathetic to an unfortunate patient, quite what was said. Most doctors now realize that their role is to advise rather than dictate. They are there to put their knowledge at the disposal of the patient so that the patient can make a decision, which may not be that which the doctor would have taken. For some reason, they do not realize that, in this area as much as any other, although their skills are for their patients, their notes are for themselves. The modern doctor accepts an obligation to make a meticulous note of what the patient says, following Osler's advice that you should '*listen to the patient, he is telling you the diagnosis.*' Information of negative import is recorded in detail. If the modern doctor spends as long advising the patients and answering their questions, it is hard to understand why the clinical note is not as long. As a rough rule of thumb, I suggest that the wise doctor should not be surprised if the note of the advice given turns out to be as lengthy as the note of the history taken: the relationship should probably reflect the way in which time in the consultation was allocated. Obviously, a lot can be short-circuited by means of printed material supplementing the verbal explanation, but the precise text needs to be clearly identifiable years later, and the notes should record the steps taken to ensure that the patient had received and understood the material received.

References

1. *Schloendorff v Society of New York Hospital* (1914); 211 NY 125 cited with approval by House of Lords in Re F (1992) AC1 and in Airedale NHS Trust v Bland 1993 AC 789.
2. *Bolam v Friern Hospital Management Committee* (1957) [1WLR] 582.
3. *Chatterton v Gerson* (1981)1 ALL ER 257.
4. UKHL 41 (2004) http://www.publications.parliament.the-stationery-office.co.uk/pa/ld200304/ldjudgmt/jd041014/cheste-1.htm (last accessed 17th December 2008).
5. *Sidaway v Board of Governors of the Bethlem Royal Hospital and Maudsley Hospital* (1985) AC 76 1.
6. *Chappell v Hart* (1998) 72 ALJR 1344.
7. Lemaire R. (2006). Informed consent – a contemporary myth? *Journal of Bone and Joint Surgery. British Volume*, **88-B**, 2–7.
8. *Moy v Pettman Smith and Perry Lloyds* (2005) *Rep Med 205.*
9. *Bolitho v City & Hackney Health Authority* (1997) 4 All ER 771.
10. Consent for Anaesthesia. (2006). Association of Anaesthetists of Great Britain and Ireland, London.

Chapter 23

The patient's perspective

Ozzie Newell

In the 'dedicated upheaval,' which is the NHS, every day produces political spin and sound-bites, presented as Department of Health (DoH) policy. These are concerned mainly with reforms of the NHS and with targets of one kind or another, but are rarely about outcomes for patients. They do, however, offer myriad headings designed, it is said, to put patients at the centre of health care, the place where they should always have been. So, NHS policies present us with the *Patient and Public Involvement (PPI) Agenda*, *Partnership Working*, *Patient-centred Care*, a *Choice Agenda* for patients, and now, a *Patient-led NHS*. These reforms, we are told, are necessary to improve the delivery of health care and to ensure patient involvement.

In his letter to the Chairs and Chief Executives of Health and Social Care, dated 13 December 2005, which outlined the updated 'framework for Health Reforms', Sir Nigel Crisp, the chief executive of the NHS, stated that there will be '*More Choice and a much stronger voice for patients*'.

Unfortunately, as yet, it seems that such cultural reforms have no real commitment or support from front-line healthcare professionals. This is most probably due to the lack of financial resources required for committed support to become a reality. In the majority of cases, patient involvement is still a 'tick box' exercise, tokenistic, and patronizing in approach. However, I am pleased to say that this is not so for the hospital with which I am closely aligned, and I am encouraged and delighted to have been asked to contribute by providing a chapter written from a patient's viewpoint.

My own experiences over the past five years, in the varying roles I have occupied as a patient representative, have shown me that whenever patients are surveyed, by whatever means, there are constant themes which remain the same each time a survey is completed, namely:

- Access to services
- Environment
- Information and communication
- Manner and attitude
- Care and treatment
- Patient pathways

And within 'Care and treatment', the management of pain is always an issue. Rooted within these headings are patients' desires for

- Centres of excellence
- Shorter waiting lists
- More choice

But above all else, patients seek: well-being, reassurance, respect, dignity, and caring friendliness, and to be treated as partners in the provision of their own care.

Some patients can be extremely difficult; some have the most unrealistic ideas and demands. Some take no responsibility for their own health or recovery from ill-health at all. It seems to be someone else's problem, not theirs. Some are very rational and reasonable, but have families that are not. Some are very constructive and want to be fully involved in their own care. Others do not wish to be involved at all. However, all are now considered to be clients, under DoH Policy, and some involvement is now secured by the PPI agenda and under the Law.

To add to this potentially volatile mix, the Government's 'Choice Agenda,'—Choice of Providers, Clause 2.1, item 15—lists the range of service providers as:

- NHS Trusts
- Foundation Trusts
- NHS and Independent Sector Treatment Centres
- Independent Sector Hospitals
- General Practitioners with a Special Interest, or other extended Primary Care Treatment Services

This will mean a cultural upheaval for acute care hospitals and community care alike, with much more competition, more patient power, and the inherent risk of loss of income stream. On the other hand, it will perhaps offer the potential to gain additional income for some Trusts which are able to capture services from other Trusts.

Where then does 'consent, risk, and the patient's perspective' fit into this evolving maelstrom?

Based upon my own business experiences, a number of thoughts that will apply to this brave new world of the NHS come to mind immediately. First, the term 'Hospital of Choice' ceases to be a sound bite and becomes a reality. The public will need, in many circumstances, to be attracted to their hospital of choice, and in spite of the propaganda related to shorter waiting lists, the majority I think will opt for a place of excellence familiar to them, offering good outcomes for treatment and a demonstrable safety record: a place where the 'humanity of care' is paramount in the service provided for its patients. This will require the employment of the best available staff at every level, commitment to education, learning and research, and the provision of first-rate professional leadership, in centres of excellence, within appropriate specialities and functions. The facilities, the environment, and the issues discussed earlier will also be important in ensuring 'good patient experience' and all of this will apply to directorates of anaesthesia.

Coming now to what may be considered to be the mundane, having experienced surgery myself on two separate occasions, I have no recollection whatsoever of any protocol or procedure involving the kind of paperwork being discussed, or being asked personally to sign any consent form. This does not mean that it was not done, it simply means that I was so relaxed and laid-back that I cannot remember what actually happened. After all, both were fairly minor and common procedures and could not be considered to be life-threatening in any way at all. I do remember, however, the anaesthetists taking me through what would happen. However, I suppose it does raise the question of how memorable and effective the approach to consent was for me at that time.

Due to my own ignorance, I have being doing what I guess most members of the public with access to a personal computer would do if they wished to have information about anaesthesia. I have logged onto the Internet and gleaned what I can from this kind of research. There is a great deal of information readily available to anyone on a global basis. In fact, the amount of available information is overwhelming! Some of it is interesting and informative and some is not. Obtaining information on any specialist subject in this manner can be at best misleading, and at worst dangerous, if there is no expert available to interpret what can be seen and read.

Nevertheless, I have found many policy documents and guidelines relative to 'consent for treatment' in general terms, and others directly related to care or treatment given by an anaesthetist.

There is a document on policy from my local acute care Trust—*Policy on Consent to Treatment*, guidance from the GMC—*Purpose & Nature of Consent*, four documents from the Royal College of Anaesthetists—*What is anaesthesia? Who are anaesthetists? Frequently asked questions*, and *Pain Management*. There are pages and pages of information from across the world, with Australia being the most prolific, closely followed by the United States, and contributions from New Zealand, Ireland, and Scotland.

The main headings gathered from these documents can be listed as follows:

- What is anaesthesia?—(3 pages)
- Who are anaesthetists?—(2 pages)
- Frequently asked questions—(2 pages)
- Pain management
- When is consent required?
- Who may give consent?
- Consent must be voluntary
- Information to be provided to the patient prior to consent being given
- How patients may give consent
- Who should obtain consent?
- Timing of consent
- Associate guidelines and protocols (10 in number)
- References and documentation control
- 10 additional documents on Guidelines

In addition I have obtained and read 24 articles from Australia and the United States covering the subject, and in no sense could this be considered to be exhaustive, as there was much, much more information available. What is interesting is that there should be so much information available from varying places across the world, which can readily be accessed by lay people. There was a core of common themes, but also some significant variations and it would seem that perhaps we in the United Kingdom may be a little behind in making this kind of information available to the public. There was little or no real evidence to show that whatever was produced anywhere in the world was produced in partnership with patients or patient groups.

The whole spectrum seemed to me to be health professional driven, with large elements of it concerned with the legal perspective of adopting defensive positions if legal action from the public followed. Having said that, what was apparent was a core of articles surrounding the subject, described as 'informed consent.' Most thought that this was good practice and several related it to a valuable information base should legal proceedings become an issue later. The majority seemed to think patients wanted much better communication and more information made available to them before consent was given. Nor was anxiety seen to be a problem when associated with risks when these were discussed fully with individual patients.

It was Abraham Lincoln in a speech given in Peoria in 1854, who said,

No man is good enough to govern another man without that other's consent.

Nor is it acceptable for the establishment to impose its will as a right, in the sense that

The voice of Rome is the consent of Heaven.

(Ben Johnson, 1611)

I suggest that, with both of these quotations in mind, this is an appropriate place to begin to consider the concept of patients' consent with regard to anaesthesia.

The concept of consent given for anything, or to anyone else, conjures up an air of mistrust or unease, in the sense that, if what was being asked for was completely benign and nothing hidden, then consent would not be necessary at all. To some people it is likely to suggest that there is something that is not quite straightforward.

A dictionary definition of the word 'consent' gives the meaning to be:

- To give assent or permission, agree.
- Acquiescence to, or acceptance of, something done or planned by another.
- Harmony in opinion, agreement.

(The New Collins Dictionary—1985)

The use of the words harmony and agreement within the last phrase of the definition suggests something positive, whereas the remaining two phrases are somewhat negative, and reflect my comments around something that might be considered to be furtive.

It is most probable that the vast majority of patients who present for surgery of any kind, major or minor, are in a stressed and frightened state, or even terrified, prior to anaesthesia.

This part of patient treatment and care is like no other as the patient is unconscious for the majority of time when being treated. It has been calculated that, individually, we are likely to attend an acute care hospital on average only once every nine years.

With such a time scale, it is not possible for individual patients to become familiar with protocols, processes, and the treatment for which it is necessary for consent to be given. To be effective and meaningful, the consent required for anaesthesia for any kind of surgery, or indeed treatment for pain relief, must be obtained within an open and positive atmosphere, acceptable to anaesthetists, surgeons, and patients alike. Otherwise, difficulties will almost certainly result and recrimination may follow.

When patients are admitted to hospital, most tend to be intimidated by the environment in which they find themselves and by the thought of being taken to an operating theatre for what they must consider to be, potentially, an awful experience. They can also find it difficult to deal with, or listen carefully to, clinicians and other health professionals who attend them. Even when they accept that whatever has to be done will involve an anaesthetic of some kind to enable the procedure to actually take place, many will be disturbed by the thought that they will lose all control over what might happen to them. Some will fear that they will be put to sleep and never awaken again, others that they may awaken during the operation, feel the pain of the surgery and be unable to communicate this to the to the theatre staff involved.

Although it might be argued, as Jean-Paul Sartre did in his essay *Existentialism and Humanism*:

> Man is nothing else but that which he makes himself.

...such interventions are at best disturbing and at worst terrifying. So there is more than a little onus on the doctor to accommodate a smooth and positive acceptance of the situation.

Two quotations come to mind, which might illustrate such a process. The first is from Shakespeare's *As You like It*:

> Come woo me, woo me, for now I am in a holiday humour, and like enough to consent.

The second is that of Byron, in his work *Don Juan*:

> A little still she strove, and much repented, and whispering, I will ne'er consent – consented.

First-rate communication must lie at the very centre of the consent process. Proper time must be given to allay patients' fears and concerns. The communication process should be carried out using lay terms and in basic language, in a user-friendly manner, and with dignity and privacy. Patients can have a tendency not to be able to take in what is actually being said when in a stressed condition.

Discussion should also include subjects such as:

- What will happen before, during, and after the procedure?
- Are there any risks involved?
- Will there be any side-effects, such as headaches, nausea and vomiting, loss of appetite, and the ability to take food and drink?
- What length of recovery time is involved?

It seems to me that as the process of consent is two-way, it is in reality a *contract* between the parties involved. On the one hand, anaesthetists and surgeons contract to provide care and treatment, within specific parameters and involving some risks. Patients contract to receive such care and treatment, fully understanding what will be done and the risks involved. Thus, consent to proceed can follow only from such a contractual arrangement, signed off by all involved in it. Furthermore, it must also follow that, before any agreement can be reached at all, the whole matter must be discussed in some detail and fully understood and agreed by the parties involved.

To arrive at a basis for such 'contractual consent', the process needs to be agreed by all parties involved. To me, this also suggests that patients and patient groups must be involved in drafting such a process and in the resulting agreement. It is unacceptable for this to be arrived at by health professionals alone, or in isolation.

It is so important an approach that it should satisfy the notion that:

> Society is indeed a contract...It becomes a partnership not only between those who are living, but between those who are dead and those who are to be born.

(Edmund Blake—Reflections on the Revolution in France—1790)

It needs to be universal in application and what it must not be is what is reflected in the following quotation:

> The Social Contract is nothing more or less than a vast conspiracy of human beings to lie and humbug themselves and one another for the general good. Lies are the mortar that binds the savage individual man into the social masonry.

(H.G. Wells—Love and Mrs Lewisham)

Although it is accepted that clinical knowledge, skills, and proper governance are provided within the treatment and care available to patients, which falls outside public knowledge and patient expertise, the relevance of my opening comments does not. Government reforms, choice, people power, the cultural changes necessary to deal with a health service governed by payment, and the many other reforms, result from patient and public comment and the political response to this.

Such factors inevitably mean that patients will have choice and a much greater involvement in the care packages they receive. The elements of mutual interface discussed earlier will be vital in making sure that patients choose hospitals that not only provide excellent treatment and care, but which also give the patients what they desire from the health service that they provide via the taxes which they pay. This will be as applicable to Departments of Anaesthesia as it is for any other speciality, and the issues of patient involvement and competition will become more important than ever before. In addition, referring to the six common complaints listed at the beginning of this chapter, attitudes of staff to patients will also need to change. The NHS can be said to be *good at caring for people, but not good at caring about people*. Problems tend to arise not from the expertise of treatment or care, but from the smaller things related to the humanity of care, or lack of it, as broadly defined by the relationships between staff and patients.

Good or bad relationships mark every aspect of how we live our lives. Relationships are built upon trust, mutual respect, and honesty, and these are the aspects surrounding the humanity of care, which should be delivered to patients and which define staff attitudes. An individual's impression of the care delivered relates usually to their last experience of staff attitudes. If a bad experience is involved, it stays imprinted upon the mind permanently, defines the totality of care which that patient received, and consequently fixes the reputation of the place in which the care was delivered. We frequently refer to treatment and care, but there should be a much greater focus given to the process of healing, encompassing mind, body, and spirit.

Finally, how should we look at consent and the elements of risk relating to anaesthesia? Here are a few personal pointers:

- Patients and patient groups should be involved in the generation of protocols and systems, as partners in developing such processes. 'Partners' means equal partners, not as people who have been spoken to after decisions have been made so that a tick may be placed in a box to show that this has been done.

- The patients and or patient groups should work in partnership, challenging and supporting their professional partners in equal measure. They must not be confrontational, or adopt an attitude based on criticism, and then walk away; they must be prepared to work alongside their professional colleagues in a committed and constructive manner.

- Excellent communication and inter personal skills are required from health professionals, and much more information must be passed on to patients about their treatment and its potential risks.

- Perhaps most importantly, I see consent as a contract between the anaesthetist, the surgeon, and the patient. The professional side contracts to provide treatment and care within defined parameters and within acceptable risks. The patient contracts to accept this offer, having had the treatment, care, and risks explained very clearly, carefully, and understandably. Some of the papers read from Internet sources referred to earlier suggested that videotaped examples of the procedures might be helpful in clearly communicating what is involved in the anaesthetic procedures for which patients' consent is required.

Generally speaking, there is no doubt at all in my mind that contemporary patients wish to be much more informed about their treatment and care, in a much more detailed and clearly communicated manner. They also wish to be provided with information concerning their treatment, as well as understanding, at a personal level, who will administer the treatment and what is the knowledge base and experience of the person(s) delivering it.

Pain management is an extremely important issue in patients' minds, as illustrated by the vast majority of surveys undertaken. The subject of pain is ever present. Whilst accepting that tolerance of pain varies from individual to individual, and in part is a question of perception, it is an area which is often neglected in clinical terms, as it has no real priority attached in the overall scheme of things, perhaps because it has no financial reward. However, this is an issue which is high on the patient agenda and should not be underestimated or neglected in service development.

Government policies relating to those matters referred to earlier have informed, influenced, and generated public expectations to a level where a significant cultural change is necessary in all aspects of the NHS. The competitive and financial nature of the health service also demands a significant shift in the delivery of clinical services to the public at large. We have now entered a truly market-driven health service for the first time in the history of the NHS, with patients now thought of as clients. Clients will be a significant driver in the way that health services develop in the future and anaesthesia will be no different to any other discipline.

Maybe Thomas Carlyle was right when he wrote:

> Seldom can the unhappy be persuaded that the evil of the day is sufficient for it; and the ambitious will not be content with the present splendour, but paints yet more glorious triumphs, on the cloud curtain of the future.

(Signs of the Times—1829)

Index